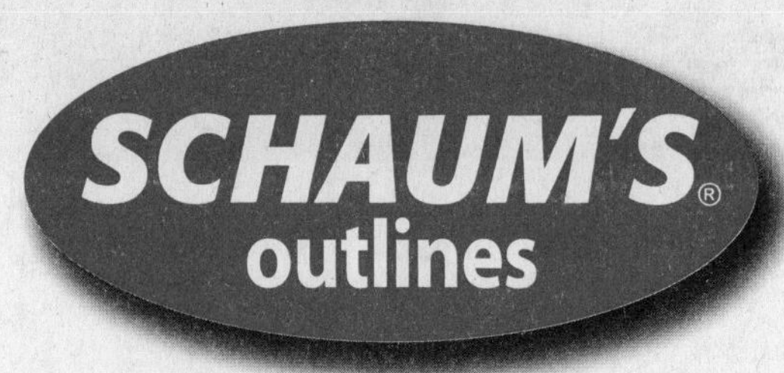

Maternal-Newborn Nursing

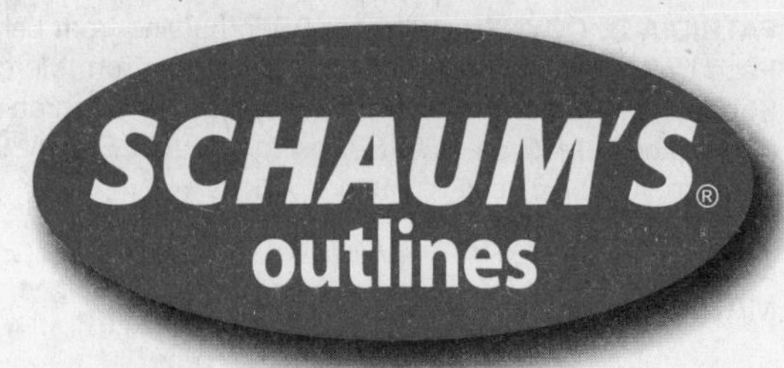

Maternal-Newborn Nursing

Patricia D. Coyne, RNC-MNN, MS, MPA
Instructor, Cochran School of Nursing and Rockland Community College

Schaum's Outline Series

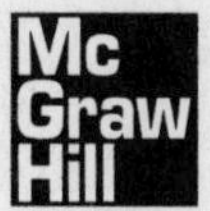

New York Chicago San Francisco Lisbon London Madrid
Mexico City Milan New Delhi San Juan Seoul
Singapore Sydney Toronto

The McGraw-Hill Companies

PATRICIA D. COYNE earned her BS in nursing from Lehman College-(CUNY), her MPA in health care administration from Pace University, her MS in nursing education from Mercy College, and is a PhD student in nursing at Rutgers University. She teaches maternal-newborn nursing at the Cochran School of Nursing and at Rockland Community College. She is a contributor to *McGraw-Hill's Review for the NCLEX-RN Examination* and is a reviewer for the National League for Nursing, Pearson, and Lippincott Williams & Wilkins.

Schaum's Outline of
MATERNAL-NEWBORN NURSING

1 2 3 4 5 6 7 8 9 10 QDB/QDB 1 9 8 7 6 5 4 3 2

ISBN 978-0-07-162361-2
MHID 0-07-162361-2

e-ISBN 978-0-07-162360-5
e-MHID 0-07-162360-4

This book is printed on acid-free paper.

Contents

Acknowledgments

I would like to dedicate this book to my family, my dear husband, Mike Coyne Sr., and my two beautiful daughters, Dawn Marie Aiello and Allison Ann Aiello. It was because of their love and support that I was able to complete this project. I am truly blessed!

Introduction to Contemporary Maternity Nursing

Objective A: To Understand the History of Maternity Care

1.1 History of Maternity Care

Prior to the late 19th century, childbirth in America occurred in the home setting with the assistance of a "granny midwife." This granny midwife obtained her training through attending births with a more experienced granny, or lay midwife.The wealthy patient was delivered by a trained midwife who attended the home birth and continued to care for the mother and newborn after birth.

In the late 19th century, technological developments available to physicians led to the increase in physician-assisted hospital births. These advances included the discovery of hygienic practices, the development of forceps, the discovery of chloroform used to control pain, the use of drugs to induce and strengthen labor, and advances in surgical procedures, such as cesarean birth. Many women were attracted to hospitals because this was a sign of affluence and hospitals provided pain management, which was not available for home births.

Maternity care became highly regimented with the shift to hospital care; however, despite the change to physician-assisted hospital births and technological advances, maternal and infant mortality rates declined slowly. The federal government, through the Sheppard-Towner Act of 1921, became involved in bettering maternity care. This act was the first to provide federal funding for maternal and infant health care by giving matching federal funds to states to establish women's health care clinics. Today the federal government supports several programs to improve the health of mothers, infants, and young children. These programs include Medicaid and WIC (Women, Infants, and Children), which provide funds for prenatal care and nutrition for pregnant women, breastfeeding women, and children up to age 6 who are economically disadvantaged or who are in a high-risk population.

1.2 Birth of Modern Maternity Care

The rise in ***consumerism*** in the 1950s led to couples wanting to be more involved in their health care decision making, and from that movement, the development of family-centered maternity care became the norm. Family-centered maternity care is a philosophy in which the family is the unit of care. It provides safe, quality physical and psychosocial care to the whole family. In family-centered care, support and respect for the uniqueness and diversity of the family are essential, along with encouragement and enhancement of their strengths. Family-centered care promotes greater family self-efficacy, decision-making abilities, control, and resulting sense of empowerment.

Objective B: Developing Frameworks for Maternal-Newborn Nursing Care

1.3 Framework for Maternal-Newborn Nursing Care

Ever since Florence Nightingale's pioneering work in the 1860s, helping patients and families gain an understanding of their health practices has been integral to the profession of nursing. Nightingale's model of nursing encouraged a focus on spiritual, environmental, physical, emotional, mental, and social needs of the patient—what has become known as the ***holistic model***. Nightingale believed that all people were equal in their abilities to attain health. She described nursing care as observation, experience, knowledge of sanitation and nutrition, and compassion, with the emphasis on the patient, not the illness (in contrast to the medical model, which focuses on illness).

Two modern-day theorists describe caring as the core of nursing. Jean Watson, who developed the *theory of human caring* (1979), contends that nursing care demands that attention be given not only to the body, but also to the soul and spiritual dimension of the patient, family, "and caregiver." Madeleine Leininger also believes that caring is the core of nursing. Her *theory of transcultural care diversity and universality* (1995) encourages understanding of the patient's cultural beliefs, values, methods of providing or demonstrating caring, causes of illness and how it is viewed, and how wellness is achieved, with the goal of providing culturally congruent holistic care.

Contemporary family health nursing has shifted to a framework that emphasizes health promotion, protection, prevention, maintenance, and caring for many reasons—well-educated consumers of care, the high cost of health care, managed care, and so on—all of which play roles in the delivery and quality of health care. Nurses use theoretical frameworks to guide their practice and help families achieve optimum health goals.

Objective C: Understanding Standards that Guide Delivery of Maternal-Newborn Nursing Care

1.4 Standards of Maternal-Newborn Nursing Care

While theory may give nurses a framework by which to define nursing and the care they give, nurses are governed legally by standards of nursing care and within a scope of practice for professional registered nurses.

Standards of care establish minimum criteria for competent, proficient delivery of nursing care. Such standards are designed to protect the public and are used to judge the quality of care provided. Legal interpretation of actions within standards of care is based upon what a reasonably prudent nurse with similar education and experience would do in a similar situation.

A number of different sources publish standards of care. The American Nurses Association (ANA) (2010) has published standards of professional practice. The ANA Divisions on Practice (2010) have also published standards for specific areas of nursing, including maternal-newborn nursing. Organizations such as the Association of Women's Health, Obstetric, and Neonatal Nurses (AWHONN) (2009) and the National Association of Neonatal Nurses (NANN) (2010) have developed standards for specialty practice.

Agency policies, procedures, and protocols also provide appropriate standards for care. It is important for the professional nurse to become familiar with the policies and procedures that are followed on the unit to which the nurse is assigned. Depending on the focus of the unit, health conditions may be treated differently than in other units. It is the responsibility of nurses to make sure they are properly following unit protocol.

Some standards carry the force of law, and even those without force of law carry important legal significance. Nurses who fail to meet appropriate standards of care may be subject to allegations of negligence or malpractice.

Negligence is omitting or committing an act that a reasonably prudent person would not omit or commit under the same or similar circumstances. Negligence consists of four elements: there was a duty to provide care, the duty was breached, injury occurred, and the breach of duty caused the injury. The injury that results may be physical and/or mental (pain and suffering).

Scope of practice acts protect the public by broadly defining the legal scope of practice within which every nurse must function. Although some state practice acts limit nurses to traditional nursing roles of providing nursing care related to health promotion and disease prevention, other states provide for expanded nursing roles, such as providing prescriptive privileges, diagnosing and managing uncomplicated pregnancies, and assisting in deliveries as certified nurse midwives.

Correctly interpreting and understanding state practice acts enable the nurse to provide safe care within the limits of nursing practice. Because practice acts change over time, it is the nurse's responsibility to remain up-to-date regarding scope of practice.

Objective D: Understanding Changes Affecting Maternal-Newborn Nursing

1.5 Family Structures and Relationships

The nurse working with the childbearing family is likely to encounter a variety of family types in the culturally diverse United States. There are a number of definitions of families in the literature. The United States Census Bureau (2007) defines ***family*** as a group of two or more persons related by birth, marriage, adoption, or residence in the same household. The broadest definition of family is one that consists of two or more members who "self-identify" as a family and interact and depend on one another socially, emotionally, and financially.

Within families, members are guided by a common set of values that bind them together. These family values are greatly influenced by external forces that may include cultural background, social norms, education, environmental influences, socioeconomic status, and influences of peers, coworkers, religious or political leaders, and other influences outside the family unit. Because of the influence of these external forces and domains, a family's values may change over time, as well as the family unit.

Nurses need to be respectful of their patients' identification of "family" and need to ask specific questions when patients are admitted to the maternity unit. Patients may choose to identify or not with biologic relatives, so it is important to ask upon admission to prevent any misunderstandings later on.

In contemporary society, the traditional ***nuclear family*** consists of a male and female married couple and their children. In the U.S. this makes up 50% of all households (CDC, National Center for Health Statistics, 2010).

Parents may be biologic or adoptive. Other family members may also be living in one household, often contributing financially and in taking care of the children. These are referred to as ***extended families.***

The ***single-parent family*** consists of an unmarried biologic or adoptive parent who lives with children. They may be unmarried due to several factors, including divorce, death, or desire to raise a child on their own. The single-parent family is becoming increasingly common in contemporary society.

The ***stepfamily*** consists of a biologic parent with children and a new spouse who may or may not have children of his or her own. This family structure is becoming increasingly common due to divorce and remarriage.

The ***binuclear family*** is a postdivorce family in which the children are part of two nuclear households, both that of the mother and the father. The children alternate between two homes. The binuclear family allows both parents to be involved in the children's upbringing and decisions regarding the children's well-being. It offers much support to the children through extended family members.

A ***nonmarital heterosexual cohabitating family*** describes a heterosexual family who may or may not have children and who live outside of marriage. Couples choose this option for many personal reasons, often citing financial reasons or for companionship.

Gay and lesbian families include those in which two or more people who share a same-sex orientation live together, with or without children. This family structure may also consist of a gay or lesbian single parent or multiple parenting figures raising a child.

Although the birth rate for teenagers in the United States has decreased over the last 15 years, ***adolescent parent families*** still represent a social and health care concern. Women in this age group most often have not completed their education, are at an increased likelihood of needing public assistance, have fewer employment opportunities, and are more likely to have unstable relationships. Children born to these mothers are at increased risk for low birth weight, infant mortality, and infant morbidity.

The ***no-parent family*** is one in which children live independently in foster or kinshipcare, such as living with a grandparent or aunt.

The nurse's understanding of the childbearing family's structure helps provide insight into the family's needs and support systems and helps guide nursing care.

Changes in Socioeconomic and Cultural Influences

The ***economic*** function of the family has changed in this century. In today's society, many women work outside the home. Two-income families are common and often necessary for economic stability. Low socioeconomic status typically has an adverse influence on an individual's health. Health care costs continue to rise with resultant increases in health care insurance rates. The family may not be able to afford food, health care, and housing; meals may be erratic, unbalanced, or insufficient. Housing may be over crowded or have poor sanitation.

A family's ***culture*** may influence its beliefs about and practices surrounding many aspects of childbearing and child rearing. Culture can be defined as the beliefs, values, attitudes, and practices that are accepted by an individual, group, or community. Nurses must be culturally sensitive and competent as they provide care to women and their families. Cultural attitudes and beliefs that are related to health can greatly affect how a patient will respond to and comply with health advice. ***Cultural competence*** includes attaining cultural knowledge, having an open attitude, and implementing appropriate, safe clinical nursing care. The professional registered nurse should be able to provide holistic care to diverse populations.

Families with Special Needs

Sometimes families are in special need of nursing intervention due to situational or developmental crises that go beyond the family's internal resources. The loss of a home, job, or family member, a fire, and hospitalization are all unexpected events that may force the family into chaos. They may need outside intervention to help reorganize.

Other situations, such as a member of the family with chronic mental illness, substance abuse, posttraumatic stress disorder, sexual, physical, or mental abuse, chronic physical illness, or death of a family member can negatively impact the childbearing family. Because the nurse is often the first to encounter the family during these times of stress, it is important for the nurse to identify and coordinate the resources and support to facilitate family empowerment.

Impact of Religion and Spirituality

A childbearing family's religious beliefs, affiliation, and practices may influence their experience and attitudes toward childbearing and childrearing. A religious history should be completed when a woman is admitted to the hospital. The assessment should include questions about current spiritual beliefs and practices that will affect the mother and baby during the hospital stay and preference for religious rituals during labor and birth. When possible, the nurse should attempt to accommodate religious rituals and practices requested by the childbearing family. Often the nurse will encounter families whose religious beliefs and practices conflict with her own. It is important for the nurse to provide nonjudgmental care to all families.

Complementary and Alternative Therapies

Today nurses are more likely to care for childbearing families who incorporate any number of nonconventional practices into their health practices. Some of these practices may be deeply rooted in their cultural or spiritual beliefs. It is important for the nurse to include this aspect in the health history when admitting a patient for labor and birth. It is important for the nurse to attempt to accommodate the childbearing families' needs for complementary and/or alternative therapies, providing it is safe and reasonable on the maternity unit.

A ***complementary therapy*** may be defined as any procedure or product that is used together with conventional medical treatment. In contrast, an ***alternative therapy*** is used in place of conventional medicine. Although there are many benefits to using complementary and alternative therapies, there are also many risks. The risks associated with some of these therapies include the lack of standardization of drugs, lack of research and regulation of remedies, inadequate training and certification of providers, and financial and health risks of unproven methods.

Objective E: To Understand Statistics Associated with Maternal-Newborn Nursing

1.6 Maternal-Newborn Health Statistics

Of women who become pregnant, 83.4% begin prenatal care within the first trimester of pregnancy. Prenatal care during the first trimester of pregnancy optimizes the chances for successful maternal and neonatal outcomes. This statistic is far more meaningful when considered in relation to subgroups of women. When viewed by ethnic and cultural subgroups, the percentage of women who started prenatal care during the first trimester varies considerably. These reasons may include poverty, lack of health insurance, cultures that do not feel the need for prenatal care as long as they "feel the baby moving," and situations in which the pregnancy is being hidden.

Some common statistics:

- ***Fertility rate*** compares births to the number of women in their childbearing years within a specific group.
- ***Birth rate*** refers to the number of live births per 1000 people.
- ***Maternal morbidity*** is defined as a condition outside of normal pregnancy, labor, and childbirth that negatively affects a woman's health during those times. It is reported in terms of 1000 live births.
- ***Maternal mortality*** is defined as pregnancy-related deaths that occurred during or within 1 year after pregnancy and resulted from (1) complications of pregnancy itself, (2) a chain of events initiated by pregnancy, or (3) aggravation of an unrelated condition by the physiologic effects of pregnancy-related deaths (Centers for Disease Control and Prevention, 2001).

Pregnancy-related mortality ratios are defined as the number of pregnancy-related deaths per 1000 live births. The risk for maternal mortality varies according to ethnic and racial groups and age, with mortality rates lower overall for younger women in all groups. ***Perinatal loss*** is death of a fetus or infant from the time of conception through the end of the newborn period (28 days after birth). Intrauterine fetal death after 20 weeks' gestation, often referred to as stillbirth, is termed ***fetal demise***. The ***perinatal mortality rate*** is defined by the National Center for Health Statistics (2006) as late fetal death (over 28 weeks' gestation) plus the first 6 days of life.

Objective F: To Understand Evidence-Based Nursing Care

1.7 Evidence-Based Practice

Evidence-based care is emerging as a driving force in health care today.

Evidence-based nursing care is care in which all interventions are supported by current, valid research evidence. It provides a useful approach to problem solving and decision making and to self-directed, client-centered, lifelong learning.

Research is vital to expanding the science of nursing, fostering evidence-based practice, and improving patient care. Through gathering of data and interpretation of statistics, guidelines can be established to enable the nurse to determine whether the patient's responses meet expected norms at any given time. Health-related statistics provide an objective basis for projecting client needs, planning the use of resources, and determining the effectiveness of specific treatments.

Objective G: To Identify Critical Thinking and the Nursing Process

1.8 Critical Thinking and the Nursing Process

Nurses must be concerned with refining the critical thinking skills needed to function in the rapidly changing clinical arena. ***Critical thinking*** is a higher-level, complex thought process through which competent, comprehensive decision making and problem solving can result in informed, intelligent decisions. Critical thinking is controlled and directed toward finding solutions and helps the nurse to make the best clinical judgments.

The ***nursing process*** forms the basis for maternal-newborn nursing, as for all nursing.The nursing process consists of five distinct steps:

1. Assessment
2. Analysis
3. Planning
4. Implementation
5. Evaluation

In maternal-newborn nursing, the process applies to a generally healthy population who is experiencing a life event that holds the potential for growth. Nursing activity in the maternal-newborn setting will most often focus on the assessment and diagnosis of client strengths and healthy functioning to achieve a higher or more satisfying level of wellness. This focus often is a stark contrast to providing care for patients who are ill, and the nurse must refocus her thought process when caring for healthy patients.

Objective H: To Understand Ethically Based Practice

1.9 Ethically Based Practice

Nurses must often deal with ethical and social dilemmas that affect individuals and families for whom they provide care. Nurses must know the best way to approach these issues in a knowledgeable and systematic way. Some issues are guided by law and others by nursing standards. The nurse must understand the legal basis for his or her scope of practice to reduce vulnerability and malpractice claims. Ethical behavior is discussed in such codes as the ANA's Code for Nurses (2010).

An ***ethical dilemma*** is a situation in which no solution appears completely satisfactory. Ethical dilemmas are among the most difficult situations in nursing practice. They are solved by applying ethical theories and principles and the steps of the nursing process.

The two major theories that guide ethical decision making are deontologic and utilitarian. Few people use one theory but examine both theories and determine which is more appropriate for the situation at hand. The ***deontologic approach*** determines what is right by applying ethical principles and moral rules. It does not vary the solution according to individual situations. Under this approach, life should be maintained at all costs and in all circumstances. The ***utilitarian theory*** approaches ethical dilemmas by analyzing the benefits and burdens of any course of action to find one that will result in the greatest amount of good. With this theory, appropriate actions may vary according to the situation. This approach is more concerned with the consequences of actions than the actions themselves.

Ethical principles are also important for solving ethical dilemmas. The four major principles are beneficence, nonmaleficence, respect for autonomy, and justice. They are defined below:

1. **Beneficence:** people are required to do or promote good for others.
2. **Nonmaleficence:** people must avoid risking or causing harm to others.
3. **Autonomy:** people have the right to self-determination. This includes the right to respect, privacy, and information necessary to make decisions.
4. **Justice:** all people should be treated equally and fairly regardless of disease or social or economic status.

Some of the ethical issues seen in reproductive health are abortion, mandated contraception, fetal injury, infertility treatment, privacy issues, poverty, homelessness, access to health care, allocation of health care resources, early discharge, and delegation to unlicensed assistive personnel.

Objective I: To Identify Roles for Professional Nurses in Maternal-Newborn Nursing

1.10 Roles for Professional Nurses in Maternal-Newborn Nursing

Greater complexity of care and the need to contain costs have increased the need for nurses with advanced preparation. Advanced practice nurses may practice as certified nurse midwives, nurse practitioners, nurse educators, nurse administrators, nurse anesthetists, and nurse educators. Preparation for advanced practice involves obtaining a master's or doctoral degree, depending on the specialty.

Certified nurse midwives(CNMs) are registered nurses who have completed an extensive program of study and clinical experience. They must pass a certification exam administered by the American College of Nurse-Midwives. CNMs are qualified to take complete health histories and perform physical examinations. They can provide complete care during pregnancy, childbirth, and the postpartum period as long as the mother's progress is normal. They spend a great deal of time counseling and supporting the childbearing family. The practice approach of the CNM is noninterventionist and supportive, as pregnancy and childbirth are a normal process.

Nurse practitioners(NPs) are registered nurses with advanced preparation that allows them to provide primary care for specific groups of clients. The women's health nurse practitioner (WHNP) provides wellness-focused, primary, reproductive, and gynecologic care over the lifespan. Hospitals may employ NPs for clinics or to screen patients in emergency rooms. Unlike CNMs, NPs do not assist with childbirth.

Pediatric nurse practitioners (PNPs) provide health maintenance care for infants and children who do not require the care of physicians. They may see infants at well-baby visits and for common illnesses.

Review Exercises

Completion

1. ____________________ in the 1950s led to couples wanting to take a more active role in their health care decision making.

2. The first federally funded program to provide funds for state-managed programs for mothers and children was established by the ____________________ Act.

3. ____________________ advocates birth without medication and focuses on relaxation techniques.

4. The ____________________approach recognizes that the health and functioning of the family affects the health of the client and other members of the family.

True/False

1. ______The theory of human caring contends that nursing care demands that attention be given to the body, soul, and spiritual dimensions of the patient, family, and caregiver.

2. ______The theory of transcultural care diversity and universality only encourages health care practices of the patient's cultural origin.

3. ______Standards of care establish minimum criteria for competent, proficient delivery ofnursing care.

4. ______Children of adolescent mothers are at an increased risk for low birth weight, infant mortality, and infant morbidity.

5. ______ Family is whatever the client "self-identifies" as his or her family.

6. ______ Scope of practice acts protect the public by broadly defining the legal scope of practice within which every nurse must practice.

7. ______ Negligence is defined as omitting or committing an act that a reasonably prudent person would not omit or commit under the same or similar circumstances.

8. ______ Cultural competence includes attaining cultural knowledge, having an open attitude, and implementing appropriate, safe clinical nursing care.

9. ______ Spirituality is mostly concerned with an institutionalized religion.

10. ______ Perinatal loss is the death of a fetus or infant from the time of conception through the end of the newborn period (28 days after birth).

11. ______ Evidence-based nursing care is care that is supported by current, valid research evidence.

12. ______ Critical thinking is not controlled but in-time decision making.

13. ______ Maternal morbidity is the normal pregnancy state.

14. ______ Maternal mortality is the term for pregnancy-related deaths that occur during or within 1 year after pregnancy and result from complications of the pregnancy itself.

15. ______ In the utilitarian approach to ethical dilemmas, life should be maintained at all costs.

Answers

Completion

1. Consumerism
2. Sheppard–Towner (Act of 1921)
3. Natural childbirth
4. Family-centered

True/False

1. True
2. False. The theory of transcultural care diversity and universality encourages understanding of the patient's cultural beliefs, values, methods of providing or demonstrating caring, causes of illness and how it is viewed, and how wellness is achieved.
3. True
4. True
5. True
6. True
7. True
8. True
9. False. Spirituality refers to a person's concern with the spirit or soul.
10. True
11. True
12. False. Critical thinking is controlled and involves a complex thought process.
13. False. Maternal morbidity refers to conditions outside of normal pregnancy, labor, or childbirth that negatively affect the woman during those times.
14. True
15. False. The deontologic view maintains that life must be maintained at all costs.

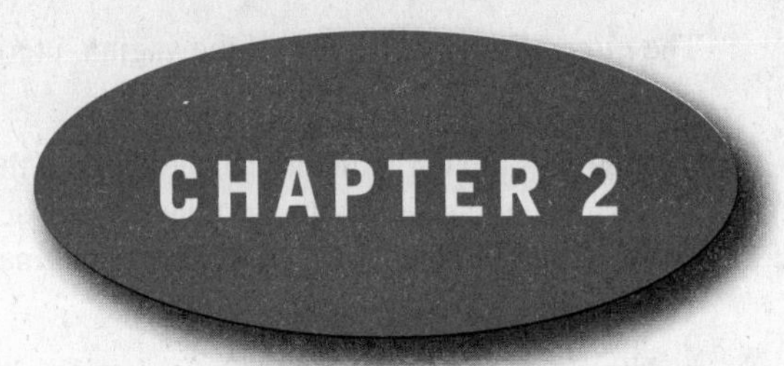

Anatomy and Physiology of the Reproductive System

Objective A: To Describe the Parts of the Female Reproductive System

2.1 The Female Reproductive System

The female reproductive system consists of external genitals, internal genitals, supportive structures, accessory organs of the breasts, and the bony pelvis. The ***external genitals*** consist of the mons pubis, labia majora, labia minora, prepuce, clitoris, vestibule, Bartholin glands, fourchette, and perineum.

- **Mons pubis**—a rounded pad of fatty tissue over the symphysis pubis covered with pubic hair; protects symphysis during intercourse
- **Labia majora**—two round folds of fatty and connective tissues covered with pubic hair; extend from the mons pubis to the perineum; function is the protection of the vaginal introitus
- **Labia minora**—narrow folds of hairless skin located within the labia majora; begin beneath the clitoris and extend to the fourchette; highly vascular and rich in nerves; glans lubricate the vagina; respond to stimulation by becoming engorged with blood
- **Prepuce**—hoodlike covering of the clitoris; function is the protection of the clitoris
- **Clitoris**—a small projection at the anterior junction of the labia minora; highly sensitive erectile organ located beneath the pubic arch that consists of shaft and glans; secretes smegma (pheromone); function is sexual stimulation
- **Vestibule**—an oval-shaped area whose boundaries are the clitoris, fourchette, and labia minora; contains (1) the urethral meatus, (2) Skene glands (which produce mucus for lubrication), (3) hymen (tough, elastic mucosa-covered tissue across the vaginal introitus), and (4) Bartholin glands (located at the base of each labia minora; produce mucus during coitus favorable to sperm)
- **Fourchette**—point located below the vaginal opening where the labia majora and labia minora merge
- **Perineum**—skin-covered muscular tissue located between the vaginal opening and the anus; the most posterior part of the female reproductive organs

The ***internal organs*** consist of the vagina, uterus, fallopian tubes (oviducts), and ovaries (female gonads).

- **Vagina**—tubular structure located behind the bladder and in front of the rectum extending from the introitus to the cervix; thin-walled, composed of smooth muscle; highly vascular; functions as the out flow track for menstrual flow and for vaginal and cervical secretions, the birth canal, and the organ for coitus
- **Uterus**—located behind the symphysis pubis between the bladder and the rectum; muscular, pear-shaped cavity; smooth, nontender, firm, and symmetric; composed of four parts: fundus (the upper, rounded portion above the insertion of the fallopian tubes; corpus (body), the main portion of the uterus, located between the cervix and the fundus; isthmus, the lower uterine segment that connects the corpus to the cervix; and the cervix (also called the neck), composed of fibrous connective tissue; produces mucus in response to cyclic hormones; thickened mucus prevents the passage of bacteria and sperm
- **Uterine wall**—composed of three layers: (1) the endometrium, a highly vascular mucous membrane that responds to hormone stimulation first by hypertrophy and then by secretion to prepare to receive the developing ovum; sloughs if pregnancy does not occur, resulting in menstruation; (2) the myometrium, composed of smooth muscle in layers, predominantly in the fundus; provides power to expel the fetus; a middle layer is composed of fibers interlaced with blood vessels, contraction after childbirth helps to control blood loss; an inner layer is composed of circular fibers concentrated around the internal cervical os; provides sphincter action to help keep the cervix closed during pregnancy; and (3) the peritoneum, which covers most of the uterus, except for the cervix and a portion of the anterior corpus
- **Fallopian tubes**—attached to the uterine fundus, curve around each ovary, and connect to the uterus; functions include capture of the ovum, transportation of the ovum into the uterus by peristaltic activity and wavelike movements of the cilia, and secretion of nutrients to support the ovum during transport
- **Ovaries**—located on either side of the uterus; almond-sized, smooth, tender, mobile, firm; functions include ovulation and production of hormones (estrogen, progesterone,and androgens); comparable to the testes in the male
- **Supportive structures**—consist of the circulation, pelvic floor and perineum, ligaments, bony pelvis, and nervous innervation; the bony pelvis supports and protects the lower abdominal and internal reproductive organs; muscles and ligaments provide added support for the internal organs of the pelvis against the downward force of gravity
- **Circulation**—the uterine blood supply is carried by the uterine arteries, which are branches of the internal iliac artery; major pelvic arteries are the uterine, vaginal pudendal, and perineal; ovarian arteries branch directly from the aorta; lymphatic drainage is accomplished from the uterus, ovaries, and fallopian tubes to nodes around the aorta, with some use of the femoral, iliac, and hypogastric nodes
- **Bony pelvis**—a basin-shaped structure at the lower end of the spine; the posterior wall is formed by the sacrum; functions include support and protection of the pelvic structures and internal reproductive organs; provides support for a growing fetus during gestation
- **Muscles**—paired muscles enclose the lower pelvis and provide support for internal reproductive, urinary, and bowel structures; the muscles supporting the internal pelvic structures include the pubovaginal, puborectal, and iliococcygeus
- **Ligaments**—seven pairs of ligaments support the internal reproductive organs
- **Nerve supply**—most functions of the reproductive system are under involuntary or unconscious control; nerves of the autonomic nervous system, sensory and motor nerves that innervate the reproductive organs, enter the spinal cord at the T12 through L2 levels

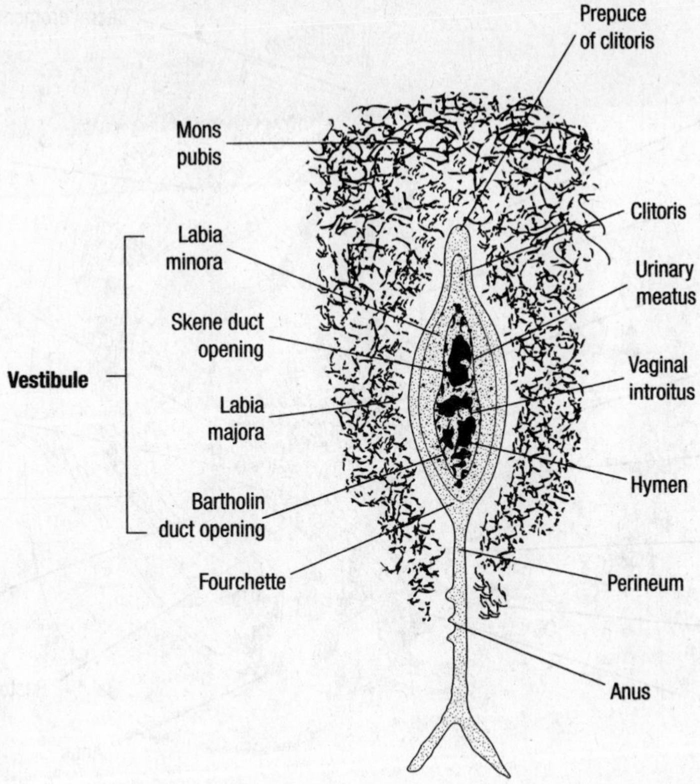

Figure 2.1 External female reproductive structures.

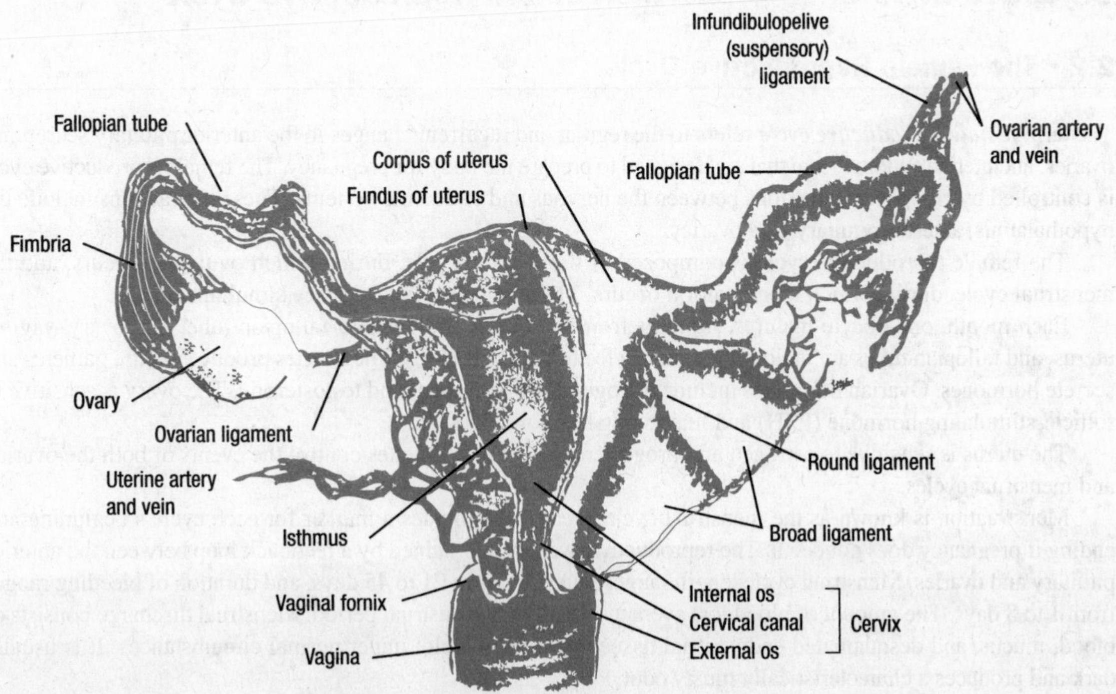

Figure 2.2 Internal female reproductive structures, anterior veiw.

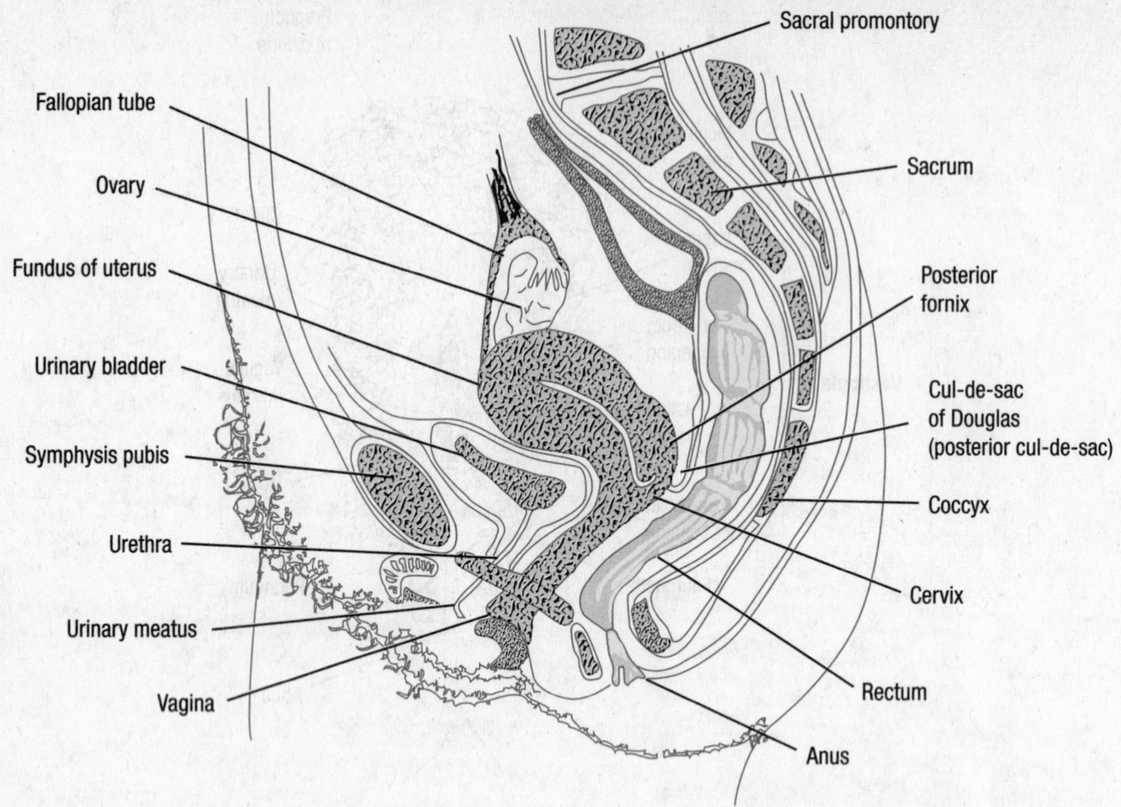

Figure 2.3 Internal female reproductive structures, midsagittal veiw.

Objective B: To Understand the Female Reproductive Cycle

2.2 The Female Reproductive Cycle

The term ***female reproductive cycle*** refers to the regular and recurrent changes in the anterior pituitary secretions, ovaries, and uterine endometrium that are designed to prepare the body for pregnancy. The female reproductive cycle is controlled by complex interactions between the nervous and endocrine systems. These interactions include the hypothalamus, anterior pituitary, and ovaries.

The female reproductive cycle is composed of the ovarian cycle, during which ovulation occurs, and the menstrual cycle, during which menstruation occurs. These two cycles take place simultaneously.

Each month, one oocyte matures, ruptures from the ovary, and enters a fallopian tube. The ovary, vagina, uterus, and fallopian tubes are major target organs for female hormones. The ovaries produce mature gametes and secrete hormones. Ovarian hormones include estrogens, progesterone, and testosterone. The ovary is sensitive to follicle-stimulating hormone (FSH) and luteinizing hormone (LH).

The uterus is sensitive to estrogen and progesterone. These hormones control the events of both the ovarian and menstrual cycles.

Menstruation is known as the menstrual cycle because it provides a marker for each cycle's beginning and ending if pregnancy does not occur. The reproductive cycle is maintained by a feedback loop between the anterior pituitary and ovaries. Menstrual cycle length ranges normally from 21 to 45 days, and duration of bleeding ranges from 1 to 8 days. The amount of blood lost averages 30 mL per menstrual period. Menstrual discharge consists of blood, mucus, and desquamated endometrial tissue and does not clot under normal circumstances. It is usually dark and produces a characteristically musty odor.

Menarche (the first menstrual period) normally occurs between the ages of 9 and 17 (mean 12.5 years) in girls in the United States. Menstrual cycles in the first two years are known as ***postmenarche,*** which tend to be irregular and are associated with irregular ovulation. During adulthood, menstruation continues to recur in a recognizable and characteristic pattern, predictable by the third decade of life. The length of the menstrual cycle varies considerably among women. Cessation of menses (***menopause***) occurs between the ages of 35 and 60 (average 51 years) in women in the United States.

Menstrual cycles are timed from the first day of menstrual bleeding and are considered the first day of the cycle. The menstrual cycle consists of three phases of one event, ovulation. During ovulation, an ovum from a mature ovarian follicle is released. The three phases of the menstrual cycle are the

1. Follicular/proliferative phase
2. Luteal/secretory phase
3. Ischemic/menstrual phase

During menstruation, the functional layer of the endometrium disintegrates and is discharged through the vagina. Menstruation is followed by the follicular/proliferative phase. During the follicular/proliferative phase, the anterior pituitary gland secretes FSH, which causes an ovarian follicle to develop. While the follicle develops, estrogen causes cells of the endometrium to proliferate. By the time the ovarian follicle matures, the endometrial lining is restored, and ovulation occurs.

Ovulation marks the beginning of the luteal/secretory phase of the menstrual cycle. The ovarian follicle begins its transformation into a corpus luteum. LH from the anterior pituitary stimulates the corpus luteum to secrete progesterone, which then stimulates the secretory phase of endometrial development. Glands and blood-vessels in the endometrium begin to secrete a thin, glycogen-containing fluid.

If conception occurs, the nutrient-laden endometrium is ready for implantation. If conception and implantation do not occur, the corpus luteum degenerates and ceases its production of progesterone and estrogen. Without progesterone or estrogen to maintain it, the endometrium enters the ischemic/menstrual phase and disintegrates. Menstruation then occurs, marking the beginning of another cycle.

Objective C: To Understand Breasts and Their Function

2.3 Breasts

Breasts, also called mammary glands, are considered accessories of the reproductive system and are specialized sebaceous glands. They are specialized to produce milk after pregnancy. They overlie the pectoralis major muscles and extend from the second to the sixth ribs and from the sternum to the axilla. Each breast has a nipple located near the tip, surrounded by a pigmented area called the areola. Each breast is composed of lobes that contain glands and lactiferous ducts, which lead to the nipple and open to the outside of the breast. The breast also consists of adipose tissue and connective tissue,which helps to support the weight of the breasts.

During pregnancy, placental estrogen and progesterone stimulate the development of the mammary glands. The breasts often double in size during pregnancy. Glandular tissue replaces adipose tissue during pregnancy.

With the expulsion of the placenta, there is a sharp decrease in the placental hormones, progesterone and lactogen, and the action of prolactin is stimulated. Prolactin stimulates the production of milk within a few days after childbirth. In the meantime, a thick yellowish fluid called colostrum is secreted. Colostrum contains more minerals and protein, but less sugar and fat, than mature breast milk does. Colostrum is also rich in maternal antibodies, especially immunoglobulin A (IgA), which offers protection for the newborn against enteric pathogens.

Nursing stimulates the nipple and areola, sending sensory input via the spinal cord to the hypothalamus, which releases oxytocin. Oxytocin stimulates contraction of the myoepithelial cells, which causes ejection, or let-down, of milk.

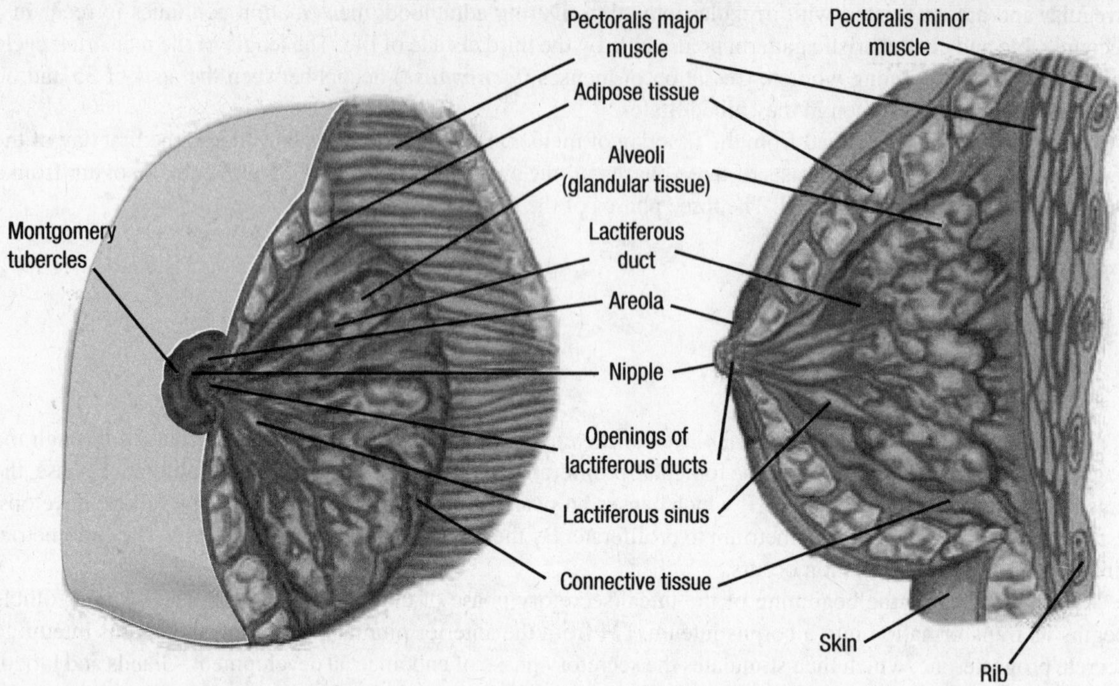

Figure 2.4 Structures of the female breast.

Objective D: To Understand the Male Reproductive System

2.4 The Male Reproductive System

The male reproductive system consists of the external and internal genitals. The primary reproductive functions of the male genitals are to produce and transport the male sex cells (sperm) through and out of the genital tract into the female reproductive tract.

Sperm are produced in the male gonads, the testes, and delivered to the female vagina by the penis. The internal male genitalia have a more accessory function. They consist of conducting tubes and fluid-producing glands, all of which aid in the transport of sperm from the testes to the urethral opening of the penis. ***External genitals*** consist of the penis and the scrotum.

- **Penis**—elongated, cylindrical structure consisting of a body, termed the shaft, and a cone-shaped end called the glans. The primary reproductive function of the penis is to deposit sperm in the female vagina during sexual intercourse so that fertilization of the ovum can occur.

  The shaft of the penis is made up of three longitudinal columns of erectile tissue that are innervated by the pudendal nerve. These columns are covered by fibrous connective tissue and enclosed by elastic tissue. The penis is covered with a thin layer of skin. At the distal end of the penis, the urethral meatus is located. A circular fold of skin called the prepuce, or foreskin, arises just behind the glans and covers it.

  Sexual stimulation causes the penis to become erect, elongate, and harden in a process called erection. The penis becomes erect when its blood vessels become engorged from parasympathetic nerve stimulation. With intense sexual stimulation, forceful expulsion of semen occurs through the rhythmic contractions of the penile muscles. This phenomenon is called ejaculation. The penis serves as the reproductive organ of intercourse. The penis lies in front of the scrotum.
- **Scrotum**—a pouchlike structure that hangs in front of the anus and behind the penis. The function of the scrotum is to protect the testes and the sperm by maintaining a temperature lower than that of the body. The skin of the scrotum is thin and has rugae (wrinkles), which enable it to enlarge or relax

away from the body. At puberty the scrotal skin darkens and develops sebaceous glands, and becomes sparsely covered with hair.

Under the skin lies a layer of connective tissue (fascia) and smooth muscle, the tunica dartos. The tunica dartos forms a septum that separates the two testes. Exposure to cold temperatures causes the tunica dartos to contract and pull the testes close to the warm body. In warm temperatures the tunica dartos relaxes, causing the testes to move away from the body.

The ***internal organs*** consist of the gonads (testes), a system of ducts (epididymis, vans deferens, ejaculatory duct, and urethra), and accessory glands (seminal vesicles, bulbourethral glands, prostate gland, and urethral glands).

- **Testes**—pair of oval compound glandular organs contained in the scrotum. The testes have two functions: the production of gametes (sperm) and the production of sex hormones (androgens and testosterone).

  Each testis is covered by a serous membrane and an inner capsule that is tough, white, and fibrous. Inward extensions form septa that separate the testis into compartments, or lobules, each of which contains ducts called seminiferous tubules, which are the site of sperm production. The tubules also contain Sertoli cells, which nourish and protect the spermatocytes. The tissue surrounding seminiferous tubules contain blood and lymphatic vessels, fibroblastic support cells, macrophages, mast cells, and Leydig cells. Leydig cells produce androgens, mainly testosterone. Sperm travel from the seminiferous tubules to the epididymis, where they mature.

  The process of spermatogenesis and other functions of the testes are the result of complex neural and hormonal controls. The hypothalamus secretes releasing factors that stimulate the anterior pituitary to release FSH and LH. The hormones cause the testes to produce testosterone, which maintains spermatogenesis.
- **Epididymis**—a duct that arises from the top of the testis, runs downward, and then rises upward, where it becomes the vans deferens. An epididymis lies behind each testis. The epididymis provides a reservoir for maturing spermatozoa. When discharged from the seminiferous tubules into the epididymis, the sperm are immobile and incapable of fertilizing an ovum. The spermatozoa usually remain in the epididymis for 2 to 10 days.
- **Vans deferens**—connects the epididymis with the prostate gland. The main function of the vans deferens is to rapidly squeeze the sperm from their storage sites into the urethra. One vans deferens arises from the posterior border of each test is and joins the spermatic cord; it weaves over pelvic structures until it meets the vans deferens from the other side. It then unites with the seminal vesicle duct to form the ejaculatory duct, which enters the prostate gland and ends in the prostate urethra. The ejaculatory ducts serve as a passageway for semen and fluids secreted by the seminal vesicles and pass through the prostate gland.
- **Accessory glands**—consist of the seminal vesicles, prostate gland, bulbourethral glands, and urethral glands.
- **Seminal vesicles**—two glands composed of many lobes. They are situated between the bladder and the rectum, immediately above the base of the prostate. The epithelium lining the seminal vesicles secretes an alkaline, viscous, clear fluid rich in fructose, prostaglandins, fibrinogen, and amino acids. During ejaculation, this fluid mixes with sperm in the ejaculatory ducts. This fluid provides an environment favorable to sperm metabolism and motility.
- **Prostate gland**—encircles the upper part of the urethra and lies below the neck of the bladder. It is made up of several lobes and composed of glandular and muscular tissue. Prostatic fluid is a thin, milky substance with an alkaline pH that helps sperm survive in the acidic environment of the female reproductive tract.
- **Bulbourethral glands**—a pair of small, round structures whose ducts secrete mucus into the urethra near the base of the penis. The glands secrete a thick, clear, alkaline fluid rich in mucoproteins that become part of the semen. This secretion also lubricates the penile urethra during sexual excitement.
- **Urethral glands**—tiny mucus-secreting glands found throughout the membranes lining the penile urethra. Their secretions add to those of the bulbourethral glands.

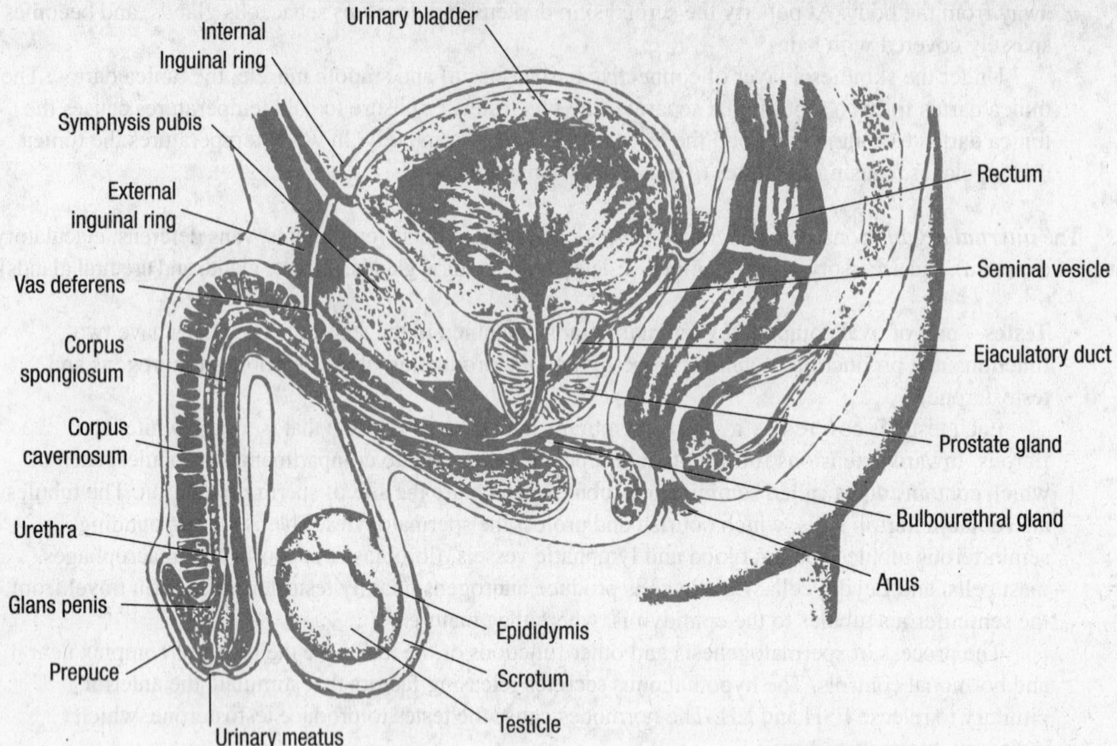

Figure 2.5 Structures of the male reproductive system, midsagittal view.

Objective E: To Understand Reproductive Development

2.5 Reproductive Development

The primary functions of both the female and male reproductive systems are to produce sex cells and transport them to locations where their union can occur. The female and male reproductive systems are considered homologous; they are similar in terms of function and structure.

The ***primary sex organs***, or ***gonads***, are the ***testes*** in the male and the ***ovaries*** in the female. The gonads function as mixed glands in that they produce both hormones and gametes. The secondary, or accessory, sex organs are those structures that mature at puberty. The fallopian tubes of the female and the epididymides of the male transport ova and spermatozoa. The female reproduction system produces the female reproductive cells (ova, or eggs) and an organ (the uterus) where the fetus develops. The male reproductive system produces the male reproductive cells (sperm) and contains an organ (penis) that deposits the sperm into the female reproductive system.

Reproductive and sexual development begins at conception when the genetic sex is determined by the union of an ovum and a sperm. The male and female reproductive systems are undifferentiated for the first 8 weeks of gestation. By the ninth week of gestation, the external structures begin to change. Differentiation of the external sexual organs is complete by the 12th week of gestation.

Every egg available for maturation during a woman's reproductive life is present at her birth. Production of sperm continues throughout the male's lifetime, although a decrease in sperm production and sexual functioning starts to occur in the late 40s and 50s. During childhood the sex organs are inactive. They become active during puberty as the person begins sexual maturation.

Objective F: To Understand Sexuality and Sexual Identity

2.6 Sexuality and Sexual Identity

Development of sexuality is an important part of each person's identity. Although sexuality is different from reproduction, they are often spoken about interchangeably. They are separate in that not all sexual activity results in reproduction; engagement in sexual activity may be for pleasure only.

The reproductive organs are inactive during childhood. The physiological and psychological tasks of childhood are the growth and development of other body organs and systems, cognition, language, and socialization to the gender role.

Children proceed through predictable stages in which they are likely to identify with a certain sex. By the time a toddler is 24 months old, he or she is able to identify differences in sex organs and genders of other children; by 6 or 7 years old, the child has been socialized to assume and accept the gender identity and roles that match his or her biologic gender. Those stages include comfort with a certain sex (gender role development), affirmation of gender identity, adoption of the stereotypical roles or behaviors associated with that gender, and expression of gender superiority. Some children, regardless of their biologic sex determination, identify with the opposite sex and adopt its associated sexual behaviors (gay [male] and lesbian [female])).

Objective G: To Understand Puberty

2.7 Puberty

Puberty, also called ***adolescence,*** is the developmental period between childhood and the attainment of adult sexual characteristics and functioning. After an accelerated growth spurt (adolescent growth spurt), puberty lasts between 1.5 and 5 years and involves profound physical, psychological, and emotional changes. These changes include an altered body image, changing roles, and changing societal expectations and responses as the child matures into an adult. Most people have reached their adult height and are physically mature by age 20.

During puberty, girls experience a broadening of hips, budding of the breasts, the appearance of pubic and axillary hair, and then the onset of menstruation called ***menarche*** ("first period"). The average time between breast development and menarche is 2.3 years. Boys experience an increase in the size of the external genitalia, the appearance of pubic, axillary, and facial hair, deepening of the voice, and nocturnal emissions ("wet dreams") without sexual stimulation. These early emissions do not usually contain mature sperm.

Puberty is initiated by the maturation of the hypothalamic-pituitary-gonad complex and input from the central nervous system. The central nervous system releases a neurotransmitter that stimulates the hypothalamus to synthesize and release gonadotropin-releasing hormone (GnRH). GnRH is then transmitted to the anterior pituitary, where it causes the synthesis and secretion of gonadotropins FSH and LH.

Although the gonads do produce small amounts of androgens (male sex hormones) and estrogens (female sex hormones) before the onset of puberty, FSH and LH stimulate increased secretion of these hormones. Androgens and estrogens influence the development of secondary sex characteristics. FSH and LH stimulate the processes of maturation of ova and spermatogenesis. The external and internal female reproductive organs develop and mature in response to estrogen and progesterone.

Objective H: To Understand Human Sexual Response

2.8 Human Sexual Response

The physiology of the male sexual response consists of penile erection, lubrication, ejaculation of semen through the internal urethra, and resolution. With sexual stimulation, the arteries leading to the penis dilate and increase blood flow into erectile tissues. At the same time, the erectile tissue compresses the veins of the penis, reducing blood flow away from the penis. Blood accumulates, causing the penis to swell and elongate, producing an erection. Through continued stimulation of the penis through intercourse or other mechanisms, the internal urethra ejects a fluid that lubricates the receptacle and further heightens sexual arousal.

Orgasm is accompanied by emission of sperm from the testes and fluids from the accessory glands into the urethra, where it is mixed to form semen. As the urethra fills with sperm, the base of the erect penis contracts, which increases pressure and forces it through the urethra, where the sperm, seminal fluid, and prostatic fluid mix, and is discharged through the urethra to the outside (ejaculation). Resolution occurs after ejaculation as the penis returns to normal size and sexual excitement disappears.

In women, stimulation of the external genitalia (labia majora, labia minora, and clitoris) and breasts causes sexual arousal. Once aroused, genital vasocongestion results, the labia minora and majora darken and swell, and the vestibular glands secrete mucus to moisten and lubricate the tissues to allow for insertion of the penis.

Lubricating fluid allows vigorous penetration of the vagina with the male penis without pain. At the same time, the vagina begins to expand and elongate to accommodate the penis. Rapid firing of nerve impulses exceeds the threshold, resulting in orgasm, the spasmodic and involuntary contractions of the muscles in the region of the vulva, the uterus, and the vagina that produce a pleasurable sensation to the woman. Typically, the woman feels warm and relaxed after an orgasm. During resolution, sexual excitement decreases, and the neurons return to the normal state. Women have a longer resolution phase, thus enabling them to experience more than one orgasm if stimulation continues.

Coitus, also known as ***copulation***, is ***sexual intercourse***. Coitus produces ejaculation of sperm through the copulatory organ (the penis) into the vagina, where spermatozoa can remain alive for up to 5 days. If exposed to the air, ejaculated sperm will dry out and die within minutes. Generally, between 1.5 and 5 mL of semen is released during an ejaculation, and normally, 200 million to 500 million sperm are ejected.

Objective I: To Identify Disorders of Sexual Functioning

2.9 Disorders of Sexual Functioning

During menopause there is a decrease in estrogen resulting in thinning of the vaginal wall, increased vaginal dryness, and atrophy of the vaginal canal. These changes often make sexual intercourse painful or difficult. Both FSH and LH also decrease, and the ova are used up or fail to mature.

In ***andropause*** (male "menopause") there is a decreased production of androgens, occurring as early as 40 years of age, resulting from decreased testosterone, which accompanies aging. Because of the decreased testosterone, men experience a delay in erections. With less testosterone there is also decreased sperm, the testes become firm, and ejaculations are less forceful. Unlike women who can no longer reproduce, men continue to produce sperm and can reproduce over their lifetime.

A thorough health and sexual history needs to be done in the older patient. Many older couples who desire to have children together have problems with infertility. Sexual dysfunction needs to be ruled out before the couple goes through invasive procedures to identify the cause of infertility. Many couples remain sexually active well past menopause and andropause. A thorough sexual health history helps to identify problems in sexual relationships. As people age, sexual expression needs to be adapted to reflect physical limitations and capabilities.

Some medications the older client may be taking may cause sexual dysfunction problems. Often men will not take medications fearing resultant sexual dysfunction. Other methods are available to couples, such as lubricating gels, medications to enhance sexual pleasure, and medications that may improve erectile dysfunction.

The nurse needs to communicate openly, provide accurate information, and listen actively to be effective in assisting the couple with disorders of sexual functioning.

Review Exercises

Multiple Choice

1. Which of the following is not part of the female external genitalia?
   - A. Labia majora
   - B. Labia minora
   - C. Ovaries
   - D. Vaginal orifice

2. The primary female sex organ(s) is/are
   - A. uterus
   - B. fallopian tubes
   - C. ovaries
   - D. breasts

3. The penis is
   A. the male primary sex organ
   B. a copulatory organ
   C. composed of three layers of tissue
   D. homologous to the female vagina

4. Which of the following is not an accessory male reproductive organ?
   A. Penis
   B. Bulbourethral gland
   C. Prostate
   D. Seminal vesicle

5. Fertilization normally occurs in
   A. the uterine tube
   B. the ovary
   C. the uterus
   D. the vagina

6. Menstruation is initiated by
   A. a sudden drop in luteinizing hormone (LH)
   B. a sudden release of follicle-stimulating hormone (FSH) from the anterior pituitary
   C. a lack of estrogens and progesterone due to degeneration of the corpus luteum
   D. an increase in the release of estrogen and progesterone from the corpus luteum

7. The ovarian hormones include all of the following except
   A. testosterone
   B. estrogen
   C. progesterone
   D. oxytocin

8. A toddler is able to identify differences in the sex organs and genders of other children by the age of
   A. 12 months
   B. 36 months
   C. 24 months
   D. 48 months

9. The uterus is a(n)
   A. almond-shaped organ
   B. pear-shaped, hollow organ
   C. tubular ligament
   D. fluid-filled sac

10. Mammary glands are also known as
    A. testicles
    B. breasts
    C. vestibular glands
    D. internal female genitalia

True/False

1. ______ The primary functions of both the female and male reproductive systems are to produce sex cells and transport them to locations where their union can occur.

2. ______ Reproductive and sexual development begins at conception.

3. ______ Differentiation of the external sexual organs is completed by the 16th week of gestation.

4. ______ The reproductive organs are inactive during childhood.

5. ______ Puberty is the developmental period between childhood and the attainment of adult sexual characteristics and functioning.

6. ______ Bartholin glands produce mucus during coitus favorable to sperm.

7. ______ The perineum is located between the vaginal opening and the anus.

8. ______ The cervix is considered the neck of the uterus.

9. ______ The uterine wall is composed of five layers.

10. ______ The function of the ovaries includes ovulation and production of hormones.

11. ______ The female reproduction cycle is composed of the ovarian cycle and the menstrual cycle.

12. ______ The length of the menstrual cycle does not vary among women.

13. ______ The male external genitalia comprise the penis and the scrotum.

14. ______ The testes are the male equivalent of the ovaries in females.

15. ______ During menstruation, the functional layer of the myometrium disintegrates and is discharged through the vagina.

16. ______ Sexual development is an important aspect of an individual's identity.

17. ______ The prostate gland secretes a thin, milky substance with an alkaline pH that helps sperm survive in the acidic environment of the female reproductive tract.

18. ______ The menstrual cycle is timed from the last day of menstrual bleeding which is considered the first day of the cycle.

19. ______ The female reproductive cycle is controlled by interactions among the hypothalamus, anterior pituitary, and ovaries.

20. ______ Approximately 200,000 to 500,000 sperm are released during an ejaculation.

Completion

1. The first menstrual period is called ______________________.

2. ______________________ stimulates milk production.

3. ______________________ is a baby's first food and provides important maternal immunity to the infant.

4. ______________________ is the mixture of fluids that is ejaculated from the erect penis.

5. Menopause is the cessation of ______________________________.

6. Puberty is initiated by the maturation of the hypothalamic-pituitary-gonad complex and input from the ______________________________.

7. Experts have categorized phases of sexual arousal and orgasm as the ______________________________.

8. Every egg available for maturation during a woman's reproductive life is present______________________.

9. The hormones that cause the testes to produce testosterone, which maintains spermatogenesis, are ______________________ and ______________________.

10. Each month ______________________oocyte matures, ruptures from the ovary, and enters a fallopian tube, where fertilization can take place.

11. The ______________________ acts as support and protection of the pelvic structures and internal reproductive organs and provides support for a growing fetus during gestation.

12. Sensory nerves that innervate the reproductive organs enter the spinal cord at the____________ through ____________ level.

13. Coitus is another term for ______________________________.

14. Once ejaculated into the vagina, spermatozoa have a life expectancy of______________________.

15. ______________________ is responsible for let-down of milk during nursing.

Answers

Multiple Choice

1. C
2. C
3. B
4. A
5. A
6. C
7. D
8. C
9. B
10. B

True/False

1. True
2. True
3. False. Differentiation of the external sexual organs is completed by the 12th week of gestation.
4. True
5. True
6. True
7. True
8. True
9. False. The uterine wall is composed of three layers.
10. True
11. True
12. False. The length of the menstrual cycle does vary from woman to woman.
13. True

14. True

15. False. During menstruation, the endometrium is shed.

16. True

17. True

18. False. The first day of menstrual bleeding is considered the first day of the cycle.

19. True

20. False. Approximately 200 million to 500 million sperm are ejected.

Completion

1. Menarche

2. Prolactin

3. Colostrum

4. Semen

5. Menstruation

6. Central nervous system

7. Human sexual response

8. At birth

9. FSH and LH

10. One

11. Bony pelvis

12. T12–L2

13. Sexual intercourse

14. 5 days

15. Oxytocin

Health Promotion in Reproductive and Sexual Health

Objective A: To Understand Health Promotion and Disease Prevention

3.1 Health Promotion and Disease Prevention

The World Health Organization (WHO) (1948) defines health as a state of complete physical, mental, and social well-being and not merely the absence of disease or infirmity. In helping to achieve this state, the WHO (1986) defines health promotion as the process of enabling people to increase control over and to improve their health.

Health promotion is behavior motivated by the desire to increase well-being and actualize human health potential. ***Disease prevention,*** also called health protection, is behavior motivated by a desire to actively avoid illness, detect illness early, or maintain functioning within the constraints of illness.

For the past 3 decades, the Department of Health and Human Services (HHS) has issued a national agenda aimed at improving the health of all Americans over each 10-year span. Although the mission of Healthy People 2020 is broad in scope, the overarching goals include enabling the nation to achieve health equity and eliminate disparities; create social and physical environments that promote good health; and promote quality of life, healthy development, and healthy behaviors across life stages.

Healthy People 2020 lists 42 topics and nearly 600 objectives. There are 33 maternal, infant, and child health objectives (see **Table 3.1**). Also, HHS asked the Institute of Medicine (IOM) to identify leading health indicators, or measurements of health-related concepts that reflect major public health concerns. The IOM determined that increasing the proportion of healthy births was a leading health indicator for maternal-infant health.

As a result, the health care system has moved from reactive treatment strategies in hospitals to a proactive approach in the community. This has resulted in an increasing emphasis on health promotion and illness prevention within the community.

Primary prevention encompasses health promotion as well as activities specifically meant to prevent disease from occurring. ***Secondary prevention*** refers to early identification and prompt treatment of a health problem before it has an opportunity to spread or become more serious. In ***tertiary prevention,*** the goal is to restore health to the highest level of functioning possible.

Of particular concern are vulnerable populations who often have inadequate health care, low-paying jobs without health insurance coverage, and chronic exposure to hazardous environments. Health promotion and illness prevention programs for these populations also need to be culturally appropriate, as some people may be new immigrants to the United States.

TABLE 3.1 Healthy People 2020 Maternal, Infant, and Child Health Objectives

1. Reduce the number of fetal and infant deaths
2. Reduce the 1-year mortality rate for infants with Down syndrome
3. Reduce the rate of child deaths
4. Reduce the rate of adolescent and young adult deaths
5. Reduce the rate of maternal mortality
6. Reduce maternal illness and complications due to pregnancy
7. Reduce cesarean births among low-risk women
8. Reduce the rate of low birth weight (LBW) and very low birth weight (VLBW)
9. Reduce preterm births
10. Increase the proportion of pregnant women who receive early and adequate prenatal care
11. Increase abstinence from alcohol, cigarettes, and illicit drugs among pregnant women
12. Increase the proportion of women who attend a series of prepared childbirth classes
13. Increase the proportion of mothers who achieve a recommended weight gain during their pregnancies
14. Increase the proportion of women of childbearing potential with intake of at least 400 mg of folic acid from fortified foods or dietary supplements
15. Reduce the proportion of women of childbearing potential who have low red blood cell folate concentrations
16. Increase the proportion of women delivering a live birth who received preconception care services and practiced key recommended preconception health behaviors
17. Reduce the proportion of persons ages 18 to 44 years who have impaired fecundity (ie, a physical barrier preventing pregnancy or carrying a pregnancy to term)
18. Reduce postpartum relapse of smoking among women who quit smoking during pregnancy
19. Increase the proportion of women giving birth who attend a postpartum care visit with a health worker
20. Increase the proportion of infants who are put to sleep on their backs
21. Increase the proportion of infants who are breastfed
22. Increase the proportion of employers that have worksite lactation support programs
23. Reduce the proportion of breastfed newborns who receive formula supplementation in the first 2 days of life
24. Increase the proportion of live births that occur in facilities that provide recommended care for lactating mothers and their babies
25. Reduce the occurrence of fetal alcohol syndrome (FAS)
26. Reduce the number of children diagnosed with a disorder through newborn blood-spot screening who experience developmental delays
27. Reduce the proportion of children with cerebral palsy born as LBW infants
28. Reduce the number of neural tube defects
29. Increase the proportion of young children with an autism spectrum disorder (ASD) and other developmental delays who are screened, evaluated, and enrolled in early intervention services in a timely manner
30. Increase the proportion of children, including those with special health care needs, who have access to a medical home
31. Increase the proportion of children with special health care needs who receive their care in family-centered, comprehensive, coordinated systems
32. Increase appropriate newborn blood-spot screening and follow-up testing
33. Increase the proportion of VLBW infants born at level III hospitals or subspecialty perinatal centers

Services provided by health professionals in the United States are increasingly directed toward the goal of assisting individuals, families, and populations to achieve their full health potential through the adoption of healthy behaviors. Health promotion and primary prevention of disease have been shown to have substantial benefits in improving quality of life and longevity. Individuals have the potential for change. ***Self-change*** is defined as new behaviors that clients willingly undertake to achieve self-selected goals or desired outcomes.

Objective B: To Understand Health Promotion Theories and Models

3.2 Health Promotion Theories and Models

Theories and conceptual models are the primary mechanisms by which researchers organize findings into a broader conceptual context. Scientists have used theory to refer to an abstract generalization that presents a systematic explanation about how phenomena are interrelated. A conceptual model deals with abstractions (concepts) that are assembled because of their relevance to a common theme. A conceptual model broadly presents an understanding of the phenomenon of interest and generates assumptions about the phenomenon of interest. Conceptual models and theories also serve as important starting points for the generation of hypotheses to be tested. A number of theories and models have been developed to understand human behavior and to use in formulating plans for supporting health promotion behavior in individuals, families, and communities.

The ***health belief model (HBM)*** (1988), the most commonly used theory in health education and promotion, was proposed as a framework for exploring why some people who are illness-free take actions to avoid illness, whereas others fail to take preventive actions. The model was viewed as potentially useful to predict individuals who would or would not use preventive measures and to suggest interventions that might increase the predisposition of resistant individuals to engage in preventive behaviors. The HBM suggests that behavior is influenced by cues to action, which are events, people, or things that move people to change their behavior. Examples include watching a family member breastfeed, advice from others (health education), and reminder cards from health professionals. The HBM is derived from cognitive theory.

Social cognitive theory (1985) is a broad theoretical approach to explaining human behavior, based on the work of Bandura. In social cognitive theory, environmental events, personal factors, and behavior act as reciprocal determinants of each other. The theory places major emphasis on self-direction, self-regulation, and perceptions of self-efficacy.

Social cognitive theory proposes that human beings possess the following basic capabilities: symbolization, forethought, vicarious learning, self-regulation, and self-reflection. Given these basic capabilities, behavior is neither solely driven by inner forces nor automatically shaped by external stimuli. Instead, cognitions and other personal factors, as well as behavior and environmental events, are interactive.

Pender's ***health promotion model*** (1996) describes the multidimensional nature of persons as they interact within their environment to pursue health. The health promotion model integrates a number of constructs from both social cognitive theory and expectancy-value theory. According to the ***expectancy-value model,*** behavior is rational and economical. A person engages in a given action and persists in it to the extent that the outcome of taking action is of positive personal value and to the degree that based on available information, taking the course of action is likely to bring about the desired outcome. The subjective value of change is based on prior knowledge of personal successes or the successes of others in attaining the change and one's own personal confidence that he or she can achieve the same or superior results. The ***revised health promotion model*** (1996) added three new variables to the model: activity-related affect, commitment to a plan of action, and immediate competing demands and preference.

Knowledge of individual theories of health behavior makes it possible for the nurse to select the best model for the client and the anticipated health maintenance activities or behavior changes. These theories, models, and strategies proposed with each will enable the nurse to give informed, evidenced-based counseling and behavioral intervention for health promotion in diverse populations.

Objective C: To Understand Cultural Beliefs Regarding Health Promotion Issues

3.3 Cultural Beliefs Regarding Health Promotion Issues

Cultural beliefs of women affect their use of the health care system, confidence in their practitioners, recommended prevention guidelines, and general health beliefs.

Women are frequently the primary caregivers for their families, extended families, as well as for community members. Because they are busy caring for their families, women may not take time to care for themselves adequately.

The maternity patient often presents with unique issues related to her cultural beliefs such as superstitions, rituals, or thoughts that prenatal care is not important as long as she can feel the fetus moving. Nurses must educate women on health care practices within a cultural framework that communicates respect for their value systems. The nurse and patient should explore ways to promote seeking preventive care and medical treatment consistent with the patient's value system.

Review Exercises

Completion

1. ________________ prevention encompasses health promotion as well as activities specifically meant to prevent disease from occurring.
2. The ________________ model is a framework used to explain why some people who are illness-free take actions to avoid illness, whereas others do not.
3. ________________ is the current blueprint for health services in the United States.
4. The World Health Organization defines health as a state of complete physical, mental, and social well-being, and not merely the absence of ____________ or ________.
5. ________________ is defined as behaviors that patients willingly undertake to achieve self-selected goals or desired outcomes.
6. In ____________ prevention, the goal is to restore health to the highest level of functioning.
7. ________________ theory is a broad theoretical approach to explaining human behavior.
8. According to the ________________ model, the value of change is based on prior knowledge of personal success and one's own confidence in achieving the desired outcome.

True/False

1. _______ Social cognitive theory is based on the work of Bandura.
2. _______ The Health Belief Model is derived from cognitive theory.
3. _______ Cultural beliefs of women affect their use of the health care system, confidence in their practitioners, recommended prevention guidelines, and general health beliefs.
4. _______ Regular prenatal care is important to the health of the pregnant woman as well as her fetus.

5. _______ Health promotion must be geared to families and communities, not just to individuals.

6. _______ Health promotion is behavior motivated to increase well-being and actualize human potential.

7. _______ Health promotion and primary prevention of disease have been shown to have substantial benefits in improving quality of life and longevity.

Answers

Completion

1. Primary
2. Health belief
3. Healthy People 2020
4. Disease or infirmity
5. Disease prevention (or health protection)
6. Tertiary
7. Social cognitive
8. Health promotion

True/False

1. True
2. True
3. True
4. True
5. True
6. True
7. True

Common Reproductive Issues

Objective A: To Understand Menstrual Disorders

4.1 Menstrual Disorders

Monthly menstruation normally involves some minor discomfort, including breast tenderness, a feeling of congestion in the pelvic area, uterine cramping, and lower backache. Some women experience more serious effects, both physiologic and psychological.

4.2 Premenstrual Syndrome

Premenstrual syndrome (PMS) is a complex syndrome manifested by mood swings, breast tenderness, fatigue, irritability, food cravings, and depression. Although the pathophysiology of PMS is not clearly understood, it is believed to be due to hormonal changes, such as altered estrogen-progesterone ratios, increased prolactin levels, and rise in aldosterone levels during the luteal phase of the menstrual cycle (7 to 10 days prior to the onset of menstruation). Increased production of aldosterone results in sodium retention and edema. Decreased levels of monoamine oxidase in the brain are associated with depression, and reduced levels of serotonin can lead to mood swings.

It is estimated that three out of four women experience mild to moderate symptoms (Mayo Clinic, 2011), and up to 5% have severe symptoms. For some women, PMS is so disabling that it is referred to by the psychiatric label ***premenstrual dysphoric disorder (PMDD).***

PMS can be a factor in absenteeism from work or school, decreased productivity, interpersonal relationship difficulties, and lifestyle disruption.

The syndrome is seen less frequently in the teens and 20s, reaching a peak in women in their mid-30s. Major life stressors, age greater than 30 years, and depression are risk factors associated with PMS.

The intensity of symptoms is individualized for each woman and may manifest differently in a woman from month to month. There are no definitive diagnostic tests for PMS. The regular recurrence of symptoms preceding the onset of menses for at least 3 months leads to a diagnosis of PMS.

Interdisciplinary care often is focused on relieving symptoms. If no organic cause can be identified, the goals are to relieve symptoms and to develop self-care patterns that will help the woman anticipate and cope more effectively with future episodes of PMS. Treatment of PMS integrates self-monitoring of symptoms, regular exercise, avoidance of caffeine, and a diet low in sugars and high in lean protein. Although many different medications, vitamins, and herbal supplements have been used to treat PMS, the most promising medication appears to be selective serotonin reuptake inhibitors (SSRIs).

If the symptoms are severe or incapacitating, ovulation may be suppressed by the use of gonadotropin-releasing hormone (GnRH) agonists, oral contraceptives, or danazol. Nonsteroidal anti inflammatory drugs (NSAIDs) may help relieve cramping. Diuretics may be prescribed to relieve bloating. SSRIs such as Prozac, Zoloft, and Paxil may be used to manage mood symptoms.

Nursing care for the woman with PMS focuses on relieving symptoms. Most women require interventions to manage pain and enhance coping.

- Teach effective pharmacologic and nonpharmacologic self-care measures to relieve pain, including relaxation techniques, application of heat, and exercise.
- Review daily activities and suggest ways to balance rest periods with activity.
- Encourage the woman to keep a diary of symptoms; try to correlate symptoms with dietary patterns and activity levels.
- Encourage the woman to keep a record of mood changes in the 7 to 10 days prior to menstruation; explore what self-care measures have helped in coping with PMS in the past.

4.3 Dysmenorrhea

Dysmenorrhea is pain or discomfort associated with menstruation. It is experienced by a significant number of women. ***Primary dysmenorrhea*** occurs without specific pelvic pathology and is most often seen in teenagers who are having their first period, becoming less severe in their 20s or after giving birth.

In primary dysmenorrhea, excessive production of prostaglandins stimulates muscle fibers to contract. As the muscle fibers contract, uterine circulation is compromised, resulting in uterine ischemia and pain. ***Secondary dysmenorrhea*** is related to underlying conditions that involve scarring or injury to the reproductive tract (endometriosis, fibroid tumors, pelvic inflammatory disease, or ovarian cancer).

A careful history and physical assessment are performed to rule out any underlying organic cause of dysmenorrhea. If no underlying cause is found, the diagnosis of primary dysmenorrhea is given. Counseling regarding expectations about menstruation and lifestyle disruption is helpful.

Various diagnostic tests are performed to identify structural abnormalities, hormonal imbalances, and pathologic conditions that may cause menstrual pain. Diagnosis is made based on findings from a pelvic exam and diagnostic procedures (Pap smear, cervical and vaginal cultures, ultrasound of the pelvis and vagina, and computed tomography [CT] scans or magnetic resonance imaging [MRI] to detect structural abnormalities, malignancy, or infection). Lab tests include follicle-stimulating hormone (FSH) and luteinizing hormone (LH) levels, progesterone and estradiol levels, and thyroid function tests. A laparoscopy may be used to diagnose structural defects and blockage caused by scarring, endometriosis, tumors, and cysts.

Treatment may include analgesics, prostaglandin inhibitors such as NSAIDs, oral contraceptives, or a dilatation and curettage (D&C) to relieve heavy menstrual bleeding. Interdisciplinary care of the woman with menstrual pain focuses on identifying the underlying cause, reestablishing functional capacity, and managing pain.

Nursing care for the woman with dysmenorrhea focuses on controlling symptoms and providing education about the normal physiology of the menstrual cycle and self-care measures. Nursing interventions previously described for the woman with PMS are also appropriate for the woman with dysmenorrhea.

4.4 Other Menstrual Disorders

Dysfunctional uterine bleeding refers to vaginal bleeding that is usually painless but abnormal in amount, duration, or time of occurrence.

Amenorrhea is the absence of menses. It can either indicate normal physiologic processes or pathology in the reproductive system. Amenorrhea before menarche, during pregnancy, during postpartum and lactation, and after menopause is normal.

Amenorrhea at other times is abnormal and is termed primary or secondary amenorrhea, according to when it occurs. ***Primary amenorrhea*** is when onset of menstrual periods has not occurred; causes may be genetic or systemic or may involve abnormalities of the reproductive tract. If secondary sex characteristics are present, incomplete development of internal reproductive organs may be the cause; other causes include hormonal imbalances, cancer with its associated therapy, abnormalities of the hypothalamic-pituitary axis, chronic stress, hypothyroidism, abnormal steroid secretion, central nervous system diseases, and drug use. ***Secondary amenorrhea*** is the absence of menses for at least 6 months in a previously menstruating female. It may be caused by anorexia nervosa, excessive athletic activity or training, a large weight loss, hormonal imbalance, or ovarian tumors.

Oligomenorrhea is scant menses and is usually related to hormonal imbalances.

Menorrhagia is excessive or prolonged menstruation. This condition may be caused by thyroid disorders, endometriosis, pelvic inflammatory disease, functional ovarian cysts, uterine polyps or fibroids, clotting disorders, or anticoagulant medications.

Metrorrhagia is bleeding between menstrual periods. It may be caused by hormonal imbalances, pelvic inflammatory disease, cervical or uterine polyps, uterine fibroids, or cervical or uterine cancer. Midcycle bleeding associated with ovulation, or ***mittelschmerz***, is not considered metrorrhagia.

Postmenopausal bleeding may be caused by endometrial polyps, endometrial hyperplasia, or uterine cancer.

Interdisciplinary care of the woman with dysfunctional uterine bleeding focuses on identifying and treating the underlying disease. A careful history and physical exam are performed. Abdominal and pelvic exams are performed to rule out abdominal masses. The woman may need to keep a menstrual history and basal body temperature chart for several months to determine whether or not ovulation is occurring.

A variety of diagnostic tests are used to diagnose the cause of dysfunctional uterine bleeding, including a Pap smear, pelvic ultrasound, hysteroscopy, and an endometrial biopsy to obtain tissue for histologic examination. Laboratory tests may include a complete blood count (CBC), thyroid function studies, endocrine studies to evaluate pituitary and adrenal function, and serum progesterone.

For many women, hormonal agents can correct menstrual irregularities. For anovulatory dysfunctional bleeding, oral contraceptives may be prescribed. Progesterone may be prescribed to regulate uterine bleeding. Ovulatory dysfunctional uterine bleeding may be treated with progestins during the luteal phase. Oral iron supplements may be prescribed to replace iron lost through menstrual bleeding. Surgical intervention is sometimes needed, and the least invasive method that proves effective relief is performed. The first surgical intervention would be a D&C. In a therapeutic D&C, the cervical canal is dilated, and the uterine wall is scraped. It is used to correct excessive or prolonged bleeding.

If a woman is not responsive to pharmacologic management or a D&C, an endometrial ablation is performed. In an endometrial ablation, the endometrial layer of the uterus is permanently destroyed using laser surgery or electrosurgical resection. The woman needs to understand that this procedure ends menstruation and reproduction.

Hysterectomy, or removal of the uterus, may be performed when medical management of bleeding disorders is unsuccessful or malignancy is present, particularly if the woman no longer wishes to bear children. In premenopausal women, the ovaries are usually left in place. In postmenopausal women, a total hysterectomy may be done (removal of the uterus, fallopian tubes, and ovaries).

Nursing care and interventions for the woman with dysfunctional uterine bleeding commonly address the problems with anxiety and sexual functioning.

4.5 Endometriosis

Endometriosis is a benign disorder of the reproductive tract characterized by the presence and growth of endometrial tissue outside the uterus. Women ages 30 to 40 are most likely to develop endometriosis.

Endometrial tissue may implant on the fallopian tubes, ovaries, and tissues surrounding and lining the pelvis. The endometrial tissue responds to hormonal influences during the secretory and proliferative stages of the menstrual cycle, where it grows and thickens, in a similar fashion to the endometrial tissue lining the uterus.

However, during the ischemic and menstrual phases of the cycle, the misplaced endometrial tissue breaks down and bleeds into the surrounding tissue, causing inflammation. The blood becomes trapped in the surrounding tissues, resulting in the development of blood-containing cysts.

Recurring inflammation in the area outside the uterus eventually results in scarring, fibrosis, and the development of adhesions (scar tissue) that bind the organs together, causing increased abdominal pain and a risk of infertility.

Although the etiology of endometriosis is unknown, the most commonly held theory is retrograde menstruation. During menstruation, endometrial tissue is refluxed through the fallopian tubes and out into the peritoneal cavity, where it implants on the ovaries and surrounding organs. Although 90% of all women experience retrograde menstruation, only 5% to 10% of women develop endometriosis, indicating a possible difference in immune function, genetic predisposition, or environmental influence.

Abdominal pain of varying intensity is the most common symptom associated with endometriosis. However, the degree of pain associated with endometriosis is not a reliable indicator of the extent of the disorder, as women may experience pain during ovulation, may have dyspareunia, or have pain during defecation.

The diagnosis of endometriosis may be made by pelvic examination, although it is often impossible to palpate small areas of localized endometrial tissue. A vaginal ultrasound may be performed to provide imaging of the displaced endometrial tissue or cyst. A laparoscopy may also be performed to visualize the abdominal organs and locate signs of abnormally located endometrial tissue.

Medical management includes pain control, the use of hormonal therapy to shrink the abnormal tissue, and surgery to remove the abnormal tissue. The pain associated with tissue inflammation may be managed with NSAIDs (eg, ibuprofen) to reduce inflammation and inhibit prostaglandin production.

When pregnancy is not an immediate goal, oral contraceptives with a low estrogen-progesterone ratio may be used to inhibit the production of hormones and suppress ovulation.

When pharmacologic approaches are not successful or when pregnancy is desired, the endometrial tissue growths, scar tissue, and adhesions can be removed laparoscopically. When endometriosis is severe, salpingo-oophorectomy (removal of the ovaries, fallopian tubes, and uterus) may be indicated. Nursing care of the woman with endometriosis involves providing support and comfort, as well as accurate information concerning treatment.

Objective B: To Understand Infertility

4.6 Infertility

Infertility is the inability to conceive within 12 months of actively attempting a pregnancy. It is estimated that 10% to 15% of heterosexual couples are infertile in the United States. Approximately 40% of cases can be attributed to female problems, 40% can be attributed to male causes, and the remaining cases of infertility are attributed to a combination of female and male factors or are undeterminable. In ***primary infertility,*** the couple has never been able to achieve a pregnancy. In ***secondary infertility,*** the couple has had a child previously but cannot successfully become pregnant again.

Fertility requires that the sperm and the ovum can meet; that the sperm is viable, normal, and able to penetrate a normal, viable egg; and that the uterus is able to support the implanted embryo. A variety of structural and functional abnormalities may contribute to a couple's infertility. The man may have abnormalities of the sperm or the seminal fluid or with ejaculation. The woman may have ovulation disorders, anatomical problems, such as fallopian tube occlusion, or physiologic disorders, such as hormone imbalances.

Delays in childbearing and increased consumer awareness of reproductive technology have prompted more couples, single women, and same-sex couples to seek fertility assistance than ever before.

Nurses may encounter couples having infertility problems in a variety of settings other than a fertility clinic, such as maternity or gynecologic services, urology services, the perioperative area, and in the emergency department. The nurse's role in infertility care begins with education and counseling during the initial assessment. Couples need to be made aware that because many factors in reproduction exist, identification and correction of problems in one or both partners may not necessarily resolve their infertility.

Before starting extensive workups for infertility, it is important to establish that the timing of intercourse and length of coital exposure are adequate. The nurse evaluates the couple's understanding of the most fertile times to have intercourse during the menstrual cycle. Educating couples about the signs and timing of ovulation, the most effective times for intercourse (every 48 hours around ovulation), and positions to enhance sperm retention is an important nursing intervention during the initial evaluation.

A systematic evaluation of both partners, proceeding from simple to complex, identifies therapy that is most likely to be successful and cost effective. The couple may decide to stop evaluation or therapy at any point. Infertility represents a crisis for the couple and often for the extended family. Either or both partners may feel that the inability to conceive represents a personal failure. Infertile couples must make choices at many points during evaluation and treatment. Some major decisions include personal, social, cultural, and religious values; difficulty of treatment; cost of treatment; probability of success; and age, especially the woman's.

The partners' general health history is reviewed to determine problems that affect general health and fertility. A reproductive history is done and includes the woman's menstrual pattern; any pregnancies and outcomes; contraceptive methods used; previous history of infertility of both partners with other partners; pattern of intercourse; length of time the couple has had intercourse without contraception; exposure to potential toxins, such as prescribed medicine, over-the-counter medicine, and herbal therapies; family history of multiple pregnancy loss, birth defects, or mental retardation; home tests the couple may have used, such as ovulation kits or basal body temperature kits; past surgeries, pelvic inflammatory disease, abnormal Pap tests and treatment; and past medical history, including childhood illnesses and surgeries. The couple's past and present occupations may identify exposure to stress, toxins, and other adverse influences on reproduction.

Common diagnostic tests for early infertility evaluation include the following:

- Basal body temperature
- Hormone evaluations, such as estrogen, progesterone, LH, FSH, and thyroid function
- Ultrasound
- Hysterosalpingogram
- Endometrial biopsy
- Semen analysis

Therapies to facilitate pregnancy include medications, ovulation induction, surgical procedures, therapeutic insemination, egg donation, surrogate parenting, and assisted reproductive technology. Hormones and other medications may be given to either the man or the woman. A medication may be given to improve semen quality, induce ovulation (Clomid or Serophene), prepare the uterine endometrium, or support the pregnancy once it is established. Medications may also be given to correct infections.

Medication (Viagra) can be given to men when erectile dysfunction is the primary problem.

Surgical procedures may be used to correct obstructions with minimal invasiveness in either the man or the woman. The woman may need a laparotomy to correct obstructions caused by endometriosis, infection, or previous surgical procedures if these cannot be corrected via laparoscopy. Laser surgery may be done to reduce adhesions. Correction of a varicocele by ligating or embolizing the dilated vein may improve sperm quality and quantity. Microsurgical techniques may be attempted for obstructions in the fallopian tubes or male tubal structures. Transcervical balloon tuboplasty is a minimally invasive method to unblock the fallopian tubes.

Therapeutic insemination may use either the partner's semen or that of a donor to overcome a low sperm count. Donor insemination may also be used if the partner carries a genetic defect or if a woman wants a biologic child without having a relationship with a male partner.

Egg donation is the use of donor oocytes and may be an option for some women who do not produce ova because of premature ovarian failure, who do not respond to ovarian stimulation, or whose ova are not successfully fertilized despite apparently normal sperm.

Surrogate parenting is when a surrogate mother may be used if the woman is infertile or cannot carry a fetus to live birth. The surrogate mother may supply her uterus only (gestational surrogate), with the infertile couple supplying the sperm and the ovum, or she may be inseminated with the male partner's sperm and carry the fetus to birth, thus supplying the genetic component and the gestational component.

Assisted reproductive technology (ART) uses advanced techniques that bypass many natural obstacles to conception by placing intact gametes together to allow fertilization. These techniques include in vitro fertilization (IVF), gamete intrafallopian transfer (GIFT), and zygote intrafallopian transfer (ZIFT). Each procedure begins with ovulation induction to permit retrieval of several ova, thus improving the likelihood of a successful pregnancy. Sperm are prepared and concentrated. The success rate for ART therapy in carefully selected couples is ~35%, according to the Centers for Disease Control and Prevention (2004).

In vitro insemination (IVF) involves bypassing blocked or absent fallopian tubes. The physician removes the ova by laparoscope or ultrasound-guided transvaginal retrieval and mixes them with prepared sperm from the woman's partner or a donor. Fertilized ova are returned to the uterus 1 or 2 days after conception. The number of fertilized ova returned is individualized but is usually three or four. Supplemental progesterone is given to the woman to promote implantation and support the early pregnancy. Four weeks after implantation, transvaginal ultrasound is used to determine whether one or more gestational sacs are present and to identify if an ectopic pregnancy occurred.

GIFT begins in a similar manner as that of IVF, with retrieval of multiple ova and washed sperm. Ova may be retrieved either laparoscopically or transvaginally with ultrasound guidance. The retrieved ova are drawn into a catheter that also carries prepared sperm. Sperm and up to two ova per tube are injected into each fallopian tube through a laparoscope, in which fertilization may occur. Additional prepared sperm may be injected into the uterus through the cervix to improve the chance of successful fertilization. Progesterone is often given to enhance implantation, as in IVF.

ZIFT is a combination of IVF and GIFT. The woman's ova are fertilized outside her body, and the resulting fertilized ova are placed in the fallopian tubes and enter the uterus naturally for implantation. The possible outcomes after infertility therapy may present new challenges for infertile couples. Many nursing care needs may be identified as the couple evaluates their choices.

Objective C: To Understand Contraception

4.7 Contraception

Contraception, often called ***family planning,*** is the prevention of pregnancy. In the broadest sense, family planning involves choosing if and when to have children. It includes the prevention of pregnancy as well as methods to achieve pregnancy.

If both partners are fertile, ~90% of women will conceive within 1 year if they do not use contraception. Approximately half of the pregnancies that occur in the United States are unintended. A Healthy People 2020 goal is to increase the number of intended pregnancies to 56%.

Unintended pregnancies may cause major disruptions in a woman's life. They may result in economic hardship, interference with educational or career plans, health problems, relationship problems, and other disruptions in the woman's and her family's lives.

In the United States, ~98% of women have used contraception. Because most contraceptive measures must be practiced by women, some method of contraception is used by women who are sexually active and who do not wish a pregnancy. During a woman's reproductive life, her needs change, and many women will use various methods of contraception before they reach menopause.

The role of the nurse in assisting couples with family planning is that of counselor and educator. The nurse must provide current, accurate information about contraception and assist them in finding a method that best meets their needs.

The perfect contraceptive method does not exist. The only 100% effective method for preventing a pregnancy is through abstinence, or the avoidance of sexual intercourse and any activity that may allow sperm to enter the vagina. It must be practiced perfectly to avoid pregnancy or sexually transmitted infections (STIs), however. The least perfect methods of contraception are breastfeeding and coitus interruptus (removal of the penis before ejaculation).

No contraceptive method is 100% effective against STIs, other than abstinence practiced perfectly. The risk for STIs should be considered in counseling women about contraceptive choices. The male condom offers the best protection available. It should be used whenever there is a risk that one partner may have an STI, even when another form of contraception is practiced.

The methods of contraception are

- Sterilization
- Hormonal contraceptives
- Intrauterine devices
- Barrier methods
- Natural family planning
- Abstinence

Sterilization is a permanent method of contraception. Couples considering this method need counseling to ensure they understand all aspects of the procedure.

Female sterilization (also called ***tubal ligation***) is the second leading method of contraception in the United States. The surgery includes cutting or mechanically occluding the fallopian tubes and can be performed at any time. The procedure is usually performed in one of three ways. (1) In the first method, a mini-laparotomy incision is made near the umbilicus in the postpartum period or just above the symphysis pubis for interval sterilization. (2) In the second method, surgery is performed through a laparoscope inserted through a small incision. (3) The third method is performed generally along with a cesarean section. The fallopian tubes can be occluded by removing a section and tying the ends, by using clips, bands, or rings, or by destroying a portion of the tubes with electrocoagulation.

General, regional, or local anesthesia may be used. A nonsurgical method of female sterilization involves vaginal insertion of a tiny coil through the cervix and into each fallopian tube. The tubes become permanently blocked over the following 3 months as tissue grows into the inserts. This procedure can be done in the physician's office.

After sterilization the woman should rest for 24 hours and should not lift heavy objects for 1 week. Intercourse should be avoided for 1 week. Mild analgesics may be needed. The woman should be counseled to contact her health care provider if bleeding, fever, fainting, or severe pain should occur.

Complications of sterilization are rare but are the same as that for any surgical procedure, including hemorrhage, infection, and anesthesia complications. Although pregnancy is rare, the possibility of failure should be discussed. Pregnancies occurring after sterilization are more likely to be ectopic in nature.

Vasectomy, the ***male sterilization*** procedure, involves making a small incision or puncture in the scrotum to lift out the vans deferens, which carries sperm from the testes to the penis. Ligation and removal of a section of the vas or cautery may be used. After vasectomy, semen no longer contain sperm. Although performed less frequently than female sterilization, it involves lower morbidity rates than tubal ligation and can be performed in the physician's office under local anesthesia.

After surgery the man needs to rest for 48 hours, applies ice to the area, uses a scrotal support for 2 days, and takes a mild analgesic, if necessary. Strenuous activity should be avoided for 1 week to prevent bleeding. Intercourse may be resumed in 2 or 3 days, but the man is not yet sterile at that time, so contraception must be used to avoid a pregnancy. The male is not completely sterile until sperm are no longer present in the semen, which can take 3 months or longer. The man needs to give semen samples for analysis for 3 months or more until specimens show no sperm present.

Hormonal contraceptives alter the normal hormone fluctuations of the menstrual cycle. Hormones may be delivered by implant, injection, patch, or vaginal ring or may be taken orally.

The progestin ***hormonal implant*** Implanon consists of a single rod implanted subcutaneously into the upper inner arm. The implant releases progestin continuously and acts to inhibit ovulation and thicken cervical mucus. Side effects include irregular menstrual bleeding and bleeding between periods. When the implant is removed, fertility returns immediately.

Depo-Provera is an ***injectable progestin*** that prevents ovulation for 12 weeks. It is convenient, contains no estrogen, and has a failure rate of only 3%. Action and side effects are similar to those of other progestin contraceptives. Menstrual irregularities are often the major reason for discontinuation. Other side effects include weight gain, headaches, nervousness, breast discomfort, decreased libido, and depression.

Depo-Provera is given by deep intramuscular injection. The site should be massaged for maximum absorption. It should be given within 5 days of the menstrual period. In breastfeeding women, it is started 6 weeks postpartum, when lactation is well established. Fertility returns in approximately 10 to 18 months after discontinuing.

Oral hormonal contraceptives are the leading contraceptive methods used in the United States. They are available as combination pills, which contain both estrogen and progestin, and as "mini-pills," which contain only progestin. The failure rate is ~8%.

Estrogen and progestin combinations are the most common oral contraceptives. The major action of combination oral contraceptives is to cause thickening of the cervical mucus, which prevents sperm from entering the upper genital tract. Oral contraceptives also block the LH surge from the pituitary, which inhibits maturation of the follicle and ovulation. In addition, capacitation of sperm is impaired, tubal motility is slowed, and the endometrium becomes less favorable for implantation.

Mini-pills, or progestin-only pills, are less effective at inhibiting ovulation but cause thickening of the cervical mucus to prevent penetration by sperm. They also make the endometrium unfavorable for implantation.

When oral contraceptives are being considered, benefits, risks, and cautions must be considered for each woman on an individual basis. Benefits include the reduction of heavy bleeding, dysmenorrhea, PMS, and anemia. Other benefits are cycle control and improved bone density.

Women who smoke should not use estrogen-containing contraceptives. Other risk factors are hypertension, high cholesterol levels, obesity, and diabetes with vascular involvement. Oral contraceptives provide no protection against STIs, and women should be encouraged to use condoms and spermicide if their partners may be infected.

Most side effects are minor, often decrease after a few months of use, and are less frequent in lower-dose oral contraceptives. Some side effects mimic those during pregnancy. Side effects include weight gain or loss, nausea, breast tenderness, fluid retention, amenorrhea, and melasma.

Maintaining a constant blood level is important for effectiveness, so women need to take the pill at the same time every day. Instructions should be given if the woman misses a dose. Women who frequently miss taking pills should be counseled on other methods of contraception.

Combination oral contraceptives reduce milk production in lactating women, and most experts recommend that combination oral contraceptives should not be used during lactation. Progestin-only pills are a better choice for women who are lactating. They are usually started at 6 weeks' postpartum. Because of their increased risk for thrombus formation, postpartum women who are not breastfeeding should wait at least 3 to 4 weeks to begin oral contraceptives.

Oral contraceptives may interact with other drugs, and the effectiveness of the contraceptives may be changed, especially with antibiotics and anticonvulsants. The health care provider needs to instruct the patient that additional contraceptive methods may need to be used when on certain medications.

The woman who takes oral contraceptives needs yearly follow-up visits. A breast examination and blood pressure measurement need to be done. The woman's ability to remember to take a pill every day should be evaluated. Return of fertility usually occurs within 2 to 3 months after the pills are discontinued.

The ***contraceptive patch*** releases small amounts of estrogen and progestin to suppress ovulation and make the cervical mucus thick. It also regulates menstrual cycles. The contraceptive patch is as effective as oral contraceptives and may be more effective because it is used once a week instead of daily. It is a more effective method for those who forget to take their pill daily. A new patch is applied to a different site weekly on the same day of the week for 3 weeks and worn continuously for 7 days. The woman then goes without a patch for 1 week and during that week will have her period.

The patch is applied to the skin on the abdomen, upper torso excluding the breasts, buttock, or upper outer arm. Adherence to skin is good even in the shower or when exercising or swimming. The patch should not be cut or altered in any way. Side effects include breakthrough bleeding, breast tenderness, headaches, and skin reactions. The patch has been shown to be less effective in women who weigh over 90 kg (198 lb).

The ***contraceptive vaginal ring*** releases small amounts of estrogen and progestin continuously to prevent ovulation. The soft, flexible ring is inserted high into the vagina. The woman removes the ring after the third week, and she has her period. Women need to be comfortable touching their body in order to use this method. The most common side effect is headache. Other side effects are nausea, breast tenderness, vaginitis, expulsion, and vaginal discharge or discomfort. Some women or their partners may feel the ring during intercourse, but it is generally not a problem.

Emergency contraception is often called the ***"morning after" pill***, or ***Plan B***. This method is used to prevent pregnancy after unprotected intercourse. It involves taking two tablets that contain a high dose of progestin. The first tablet should be taken as soon as possible after unprotected intercourse and the second within the first 12 hours after. Both may be taken together with no increase in side effects. This method can also be used after contraceptive failure, rape, or incorrect contraceptive use.

The effectiveness is greatest if the contraception is used within 72 hours after unprotected intercourse, although it may be used up to 120 hours after. This method reduces the risk of pregnancy by 89%. It does not work, however, if implantation has already taken place, and it will not harm a developing fetus.

Intrauterine devices (IUDs) are inserted to provide continuous pregnancy prevention. The mechanism of action for IUDs is a sterile inflammatory response resulting in a hostile environment for sperm. Very few sperm reach the fallopian tubes. A T-shaped device is implanted into the uterine wall and is effective for up to 10 years. IUDs are appropriate for women who cannot use hormonal contraception. They are often inserted at the 6-week postpartum checkup and are safe for use during lactation.

Side effects include cramping and bleeding with insertion, menorrhagia, irregular periods with light bleeding, and spotting between periods. Complications include perforation of the uterus with insertion, expulsion of the device, and risk of infection. Fertility returns promptly when the device is removed.

Barrier methods of contraception involve chemicals or devices that prevent sperm from entering the uterus. The method may kill sperm or place a barrier between the penis and the cervix. All methods are coitus related and may interfere with spontaneity.

Chemical barriers, or spermicides, kill sperm and come in many forms. Foams, foaming tablets, suppositories, and vaginal film may be used alone or with another contraceptive measure. Gels and creams are generally used with mechanical barriers, such as the diaphragm or the cervical cap. They are inserted deep into the vagina before intercourse.

Spermicides are available without prescriptions and are inexpensive and easy to use. When spermicides are used alone, the failure rate is 29%. Effectiveness is increased when used with a mechanical barrier. Sensitivity to the product may cause genital irritation.

Mechanical barriers are devices placed over the penis or cervix to prevent passage of sperm into the uterus. They include the condom, sponge, diaphragm, and cervical cap.

The ***male condom*** is the only male contraceptive device currently available. It covers the penis to prevent sperm from entering the vagina. Condoms are most often made of latex and may be lubricated. Couples allergic to latex may use condoms made from other substances, such as polyurethane, other synthetic materials, or natural membranes (sheep). Latex condoms provide the best protection available against STIs.

Condoms are readily available and are inexpensive. The failure rate is 15% and can be reduced when using another method, such as spermicide. Because condoms must be applied before intercourse, some couples feel it interferes with spontaneity. Some men feel that it interferes with sensation.

The ***female condom,*** also called the ***"vaginal pouch,"*** is a polyurethane sheath inserted into the vagina. A flexible ring fits over the cervix like a diaphragm, and another ring extends outside the vagina to partially cover the perineum. The female condom is less effective than the male condom, with a failure rate of 21%. Many women object to its use based on esthetics. It does give some protection against STIs. The male and female condoms should not be used together, as they may adhere to each other.

The ***contraceptive sponge*** is made of soft polyurethane that contains spermicide. It traps and absorbs semen, and the spermicide kills the sperm. The sponge provides contraception for 24 hours without the need for added spermicide for repeated intercourse. The sponge does not require a prescription and is inexpensive. It can be inserted right before intercourse or can be inserted hours before intercourse is expected. It needs to remain in place for 6 hours after intercourse.

Side effects are rare. Sensitivity to the product may cause irritation. Prolonged use or use during menstruation increases the risk of toxic shock syndrome. The sponge should not be left in for more than 30 hours. It may be difficult to remove for some women.

The ***diaphragm*** is a latex dome surrounded by a spring or a coil. The woman places spermicidal gel around the rim, then inserts the diaphragm over the cervix. Because it covers the cervix, it prevents passage of sperm. The spermicidal gel adds protection. The typical failure rate is 16%. Women must be fitted for a diaphragm by their health care provider and need to be refitted after a weight gain or loss of 20% and after an abortion or pregnancy. The diaphragm may be inserted in advance of intercourse. It needs to remain in place for 6 to 8 hours after intercourse. If intercourse is repeated, the woman should leave the diaphragm in place and insert additional spermicide into the vagina.

Side effects include urinary tract infections and irritation from the spermicidal gels. The diaphragm should be replaced every 2 years.

The ***cervical cap*** is a firm cap that differs from the diaphragm in that a seal forms between the cervical surface or vaginal wall, with the rim of the cap holding the mechanism in place. The typical failure rates are 20% for nulliparous women and up to 40% for multiparous women. The reason for the high failure rate in multiparous patients is because pregnancy and childbirth cause the cervix to become softer and more pliable, making the cervical cap less capable of remaining in place. The cervical cap must be fitted by a health care provider and requires a prescription.

Before inserting the cap, the dome is filled with spermicidal jelly, and a thin coating is placed on the brim and outside the dome. For repeated intercourse, no additional spermicide is needed. The cap should be left in for 6 hours after intercourse but no longer than 48 hours. It should not be used during menstruation.

Latex allergies, sensitivities to spermicides, and an uneven-shaped cervix are all contraindicated for cervical cap use. The U.S. Food and Drug Administration (FDA) recommends that the woman have a follow-up Pap smear after 3 months of use, then return to normal yearly screening.

The cervical cap should be replaced after 2 years or a pregnancy.

Fertility awareness methods of contraception focus on determining a woman's time of ovulation. Natural family planning relies on sex only during nonfertile periods and abstinence during the determined period of fertility. The couple may choose to follow the rhythm (calendar) method, the cervical mucus ovulation detection method, or the symptothermal method. All have a typical failure rate of 25%.

Couples who choose ***natural family planning*** must be highly motivated to abstain from intercourse during the fertile days. They also must be capable of understanding the concept of fertile days and of tracking daily temperature. If using the cervical mucus ovulation detection or symptothermal method, the woman must be comfortable with checking her cervical mucus. Breastfeeding, recent childbirth, and pregnancy loss may affect signs of fertility and thus make these methods unreliable. There are no side effects to natural family planning methods. These methods are often endorsed by religious groups.

The ***rhythm method,*** or ***calendar method,*** calls on the woman to track the length of her menstrual cycles. Ovulation takes place 12 to 16 days before the start of the next menstrual period. The first day of the fertile time cannot be predicted with perfect accuracy but may be estimated by tracking six menstrual cycles and subtracting 18 from the shortest cycle (day 1 of menses to day 1 of next menses). The last day of the fertile period would be the longest cycle length minus 11. To prevent conception, the patient needs to abstain from intercourse on the first day of fertility through the last day of the fertile period. Women with irregular cycles cannot accurately predict ovulation and therefore would not be good candidates for this method.

In the ***cervical mucus ovulation detection method,*** the woman's cervical mucus is clear and stretchy when she is ovulating. To prevent pregnancy, women should use a barrier method or abstain from intercourse at the first appearance of fertile mucus through the third day after the last appearance of fertile mucus.

The ***basal body temperature (BBT) method*** is based on the woman's temperature changes around the time of ovulation, with an ~0.5°F decrease before ovulation and a 0.4° to 0.8°F increase with ovulation. The woman needs to take her temperature every day at approximately the same time, usually when she first awakens, and definitely before getting out of bed or eating, which may alter the temperature.

As temperature may not always drop, the ***symptothermal method,*** which combines BBT with cervical mucus changes, provides more accuracy in predicting the fertile period. Women using the symptothermal method mark the beginning of the fertile period with the appearance of fertile mucus and the end of the fertile period with the fourth day after an elevated temperature.

The ***lactational amenorrhea method (LAM)*** is appropriate for breastfeeding mothers in the first 6 months after childbirth, provided that these women have no periods and they breastfeed exclusively. LAM suppresses ovulation because breastfeeding continually releases prolactin, which inhibits the FSH and LH cycle. The typical use failure rate is 2%. The nurse needs to emphasize to the patient that this method is only effective if she breastfeeds exclusively. She must also wake the baby during the night to feed, which maintains prolactin stimulation and prevents ovulation.

Abortion may be defined as the termination of pregnancy before the fetus reaches the age of viability, or the point at which vital organs are able to support life independently outside the uterus. In most cases, viability is considered to be the end of the second trimester, or 24 weeks' gestation. Although it is preferable to control conception, some women with an unintended pregnancy may elect to terminate a pregnancy for a variety of reasons. Religion, culture, and legal access to safe abortion services all affect a woman's utilization of abortion services.

The landmark 1973 decision by the U.S. Supreme Court in *Roe v. Wade* affirmed that a woman has a basic right to privacy and autonomy that permits first-trimester abortion on demand. The court left decisions about second-trimester abortions to the discretion of the states and strongly discouraged third-trimester abortions. This decision has been argued ever since; most arguments against abortion assert that the fetus, as well as the mother, has certain rights. Approximately 50% of all pregnancies are unintended, and ~50% of those unintended pregnancies end in abortion.

The nurse's role should be to evaluate the patient's condition; to provide factual, nondirective teaching about the types of abortion available and other possible alternatives such as adoption; and to ensure the patient feels comfortable and confident that the choice is the best possible alternative, given the circumstances surrounding the pregnancy.

The method of pregnancy termination available to the woman depends largely on the length of the gestation. Most first-trimester abortions are performed by vacuum extraction in the physician's office or clinic. The patient may visit the office or clinic the day before the procedure for insertion of laminaria tents. Laminaria tents are small dried cones of seaweed that, when exposed to moisture, expand and painlessly dilate the cervix.

The patient wears a tampon to hold the laminaria in place. An alternative is the placement of prostaglandin gel to the cervix to soften it.

A mild sedative may be given to the patient prior to the procedure. Local anesthesia in the form of a lidocaine paracervical block is common. The physician will do a bimanual exam to document the size of the uterus and threads a small catheter through the cervix, which is connected to a vacuum aspirator or syringe. The aspirator or syringe then evacuates the contents of the uterus.

The patient needs to be monitored for 1 to 2 hours following the procedure to ensure that her vital signs are stable and that she is not experiencing excessive blood loss. She should be instructed that her bleeding will be like a heavy menstrual period in duration and intensity. Also, she should avoid using tampons and avoid sexual intercourse while she is actively bleeding. The patient should be instructed to call the physician if she has an elevated temperature, excessive cramping or tenderness, or excessive bleeding and to expect resumption of menses 4 to 6 weeks after the procedure.

Some health care providers require a follow-up visit, at which time they perform a pelvic exam and do a pregnancy test to ensure that the pregnancy has been terminated successfully. Instructions on contraceptives and a prescription may be given at this time.

The drugs methotrexate and misoprostol are lethal to proliferating trophoblastic tissues and lead to abortion by blocking folic acid in fetal cells, preventing them from dividing. Used together, there is a 95% success rate in early pregnancy termination.

Treatment regimens vary, but they usually require at least two visits to the health care provider. Typically, the patient is given an injection of methotrexate and a misoprostol suppository to insert 3 to 7 days later. Bleeding will ensue. The patient then returns to the office or clinic 3 to 7 days after the misoprostol insertion to ensure that the abortion is complete. Some cases require a second dose of misoprostol or a vacuum extraction if the medical procedure is not effective in terminating the pregnancy.

Mifepristone, or RU-486, acts as a progesterone antagonist. It is used as emergency contraception in many countries throughout the world. Supplementing it with misoprostol enhances its efficacy. Patients who use mifepristone report abortion experiences similar to those who experience spontaneous abortions, with cramping and bleeding. Two weeks later, the patient returns to the clinic for an examination to ensure the abortion is complete.

Contraindications to using these medications include suspected ectopic pregnancy, renal failure, and concurrent use of steroids or anticoagulant therapy.

Infusions of hypertonic solutions such as saline and urea are used to terminate second-trimester pregnancies. Typically, the clinician will insert laminaria tents before the procedure, have the patient urinate, and do an amniocentesis, removing amniotic fluid and infusing the same amount of saline. The goal is to stimulate uterine contractions, resulting in expulsion of the uterine contents.

A second-trimester D&C may be performed. The procedure is similar to a first-trimester vacuum aspiration but requires greater cervical dilation because of the increased volume of uterine contents. It is also more uncomfortable for the patient.

Aftercare for the patient who has an abortion includes ensuring the woman receives RhoGAM if she is Rh negative, as well as instructions that include reporting warning signs, such as fever, chills, abdominal pain or tenderness, excessive or prolonged bleeding, foul-smelling vaginal discharge, and/or lack of menses by 6 weeks after the procedure. The client may be fertile immediately after undergoing an abortion. The nurse should offer information about contraceptives as appropriate.

Objective D: To Understand Reproductive Needs of Couples with Mental or Physical Challenges

4.8 Reproduction and Mental and Physical Challenges

Couples who present with mental and/or physical challenges regarding reproductive issues need counseling and may need extra services depending on their individual situations. It is important for the nurse to spend extra time when counseling couples with mental and physical challenges and make the appropriate referrals as necessary. Follow-up should be done to ensure that these couples are getting the appropriate assistance and care related to their needs.

Review Exercises

Completion

1. ____________________ is pain or discomfort associated with menstruation.

2. Nursing care for women with premenstrual syndrome (PMS) focuses on relieving ________________.

3. Hysterectomy refers to removal of the ________________________.

4. In treating endometriosis, when pregnancy is not an immediate goal, oral contraceptives with a low estrogen-progesterone ratio may be used to inhibit the production of hormones and suppress ________________________.

5. Midcycle bleeding associated with ovulation is called ______________.

6. ________________________ is a benign disorder of the reproductive tract characterized by the presence of growth of endometrial tissue outside the uterus.

7. ______________________ is the most common symptom associated with endometriosis.

8. ______________________ is the inability to conceive within 12 months of actively attempting a pregnancy.

9. A Healthy People 2020 goal is to increase the number of intended pregnancies to ________________.

10. ______________ contraceptive method is 100% effective against sexually transmitted infections (STIs).

11. ____________________________________ uses advanced techniques that bypass many natural obstacles to conception by placing intact gametes together to allow fertilization.

12. The ____________________ is the contraceptive method that offers the best protection available against STIs.

13. Pregnancies occurring after female sterilization are ______________ in nature.

14. After male sterilization, the male is not fully sterile until ______________ are no longer present in his ______________.

15. The regular recurrence of symptoms preceding the onset of menses for at least______________ leads to a diagnosis of PMS.

True/False

1. _______ PMS is a complex syndrome manifested by mood swings, breast tenderness, fatigue, irritability, food cravings, and depression.

2. _______ PMS is seen more frequently in teenagers than any other age group.

3. _______ Secondary amenorrhea is related to underlying conditions that involve scarring or injury to the reproductive tract.

4. _______ Dysfunctional uterine bleeding refers to vaginal bleeding that is usually painless but abnormal in amount, duration, or time of occurrence.

5. _______ For many women, hormonal agents can correct menstrual irregularities.

6. _______ A therapeutic dilatation and curettage (D&C) can be used to correct excessive or prolonged bleeding.

7. _______ Infertility is defined as the inability to conceive within 6 months of actively attempting a pregnancy.

8. _______ Before starting extensive fertility workups, it is important to establish that the timing of intercourse and length of coital exposure are adequate.

9. _______ Common diagnostic tests for early infertility evaluation include basal body temperature; hormone evaluations, such as estrogen, progesterone, luteinizing hormone, follicle-stimulating hormone, and thyroid function; ultrasound; hysterosalpingogram; and zygote intrafallopian transfer (ZIFT).

10. _______ In vitro insemination involves bypassing blocked or absent fallopian tubes.

11. _______ The only contraceptive method that is 100% effective against STIs is abstinence.

12. _______ The least effective methods of contraception are breastfeeding and coitus interruptus.

13. _______ Female sterilization can be reversed at a later time in the woman's life.

14. _______ After a vasectomy, semen no longer carries sperm.

15. _______ Depo-Provera is an injectable hormonal contraceptive that lasts for 6 months.

16. _______ Progestin-only pills are the most commonly taken oral contraceptives.

17. _______ Benefits of taking oral contraceptives include cycle control and improved bone density.

18. _______ Barrier methods of contraception involve chemicals or devices that prevent sperm from entering the uterus.

19. _______ The mechanism of action of an intrauterine device is a sterile inflammatory response resulting in a hostile environment for sperm.

20. _______ The "morning after" pill is only effective if taken within the first 24 hours after unprotected sexual intercourse.

21. _______ The male condom is the only male contraceptive device currently available.

22. _______ The diaphragm needs to be refitted after a pregnancy or weight gain or loss of 20%.

23. _______ The diaphragm must be left in place for 24 hours in order to be effective.

24. _______ The cervical cap can be used during menstruation.

25. _______ Couples who choose fertility awareness methods of contraception must be highly motivated.

26. _______ Fertility awareness methods of contraception have a typical failure rate of 50%.

27. _______ Breastfeeding is a reliable method of contraception until breastfeeding ends.

28. _______ When using the basal body temperature method, the woman's temperature increases before ovulation and decreases with ovulation.

29. _______ When using the cervical mucus ovulation detection method, the woman needs to know that her mucus will be clear and stretchy when she is ovulating.

30. _______ Primary infertility refers to a couple who have never conceived together.

Answers

Completion

1. Dysmenorrhea
2. Symptoms
3. Uterus
4. Ovulation
5. Mittelschmerz
6. Endometriosis
7. Pelvic pain
8. Infertility
9. 56%
10. No
11. Assisted reproductive technology (ART)
12. Male condom
13. Ectopic
14. Sperm, semen
15. 3 months

True/False

1. True
2. False. Women in their 30s are more likely to have PMS.
3. True
4. True
5. True
6. True
7. False. Infertility is defined as the inability to conceive after 12 months of actively trying.
8. True
9. False. ZIFT is a procedure that can be done after diagnosis.
10. True
11. True
12. True
13. False. Sterilization is irreversible.
14. True
15. False. Depo-Provera injections are effective for up to 12 weeks.
16. False. The most commonly taken oral contraceptives are the combination estrogen and progesterone pills.
17. True
18. True
19. True

20. **False. The "morning after" pill can be taken up to 72 hours after unprotected intercourse.**

21. **True**

22. **True**

23. **True**

24. **False. The cervical cap cannot be used during menstruation.**

25. **True**

26. **False. Fertility awareness methods typically have a 25% failure rate.**

27. **False. If breastfeeding exclusively, breastfeeding can be used as a form of contraception for up to 6 months only.**

28. **False. Temperature decreases before ovulation and increases with ovulation.**

29. **True**

30. **True**

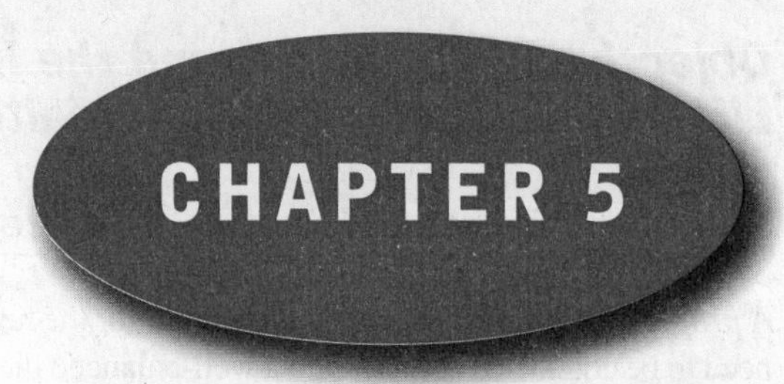

Preconception Health Promotion

Objective A: To Understand the Importance of Preconception Health Promotion

5.1 Importance of Preconception Health Promotion

Evidence is accumulating that preconception health promotion can positively affect pregnancy outcomes. The goal of preconception health promotion is to provide women with information to make timely, informed decisions about their reproductive futures. This goal is accomplished by helping them prevent unintended pregnancies, identifying risk factors that could affect reproductive outcomes, and initiating education and prevention interventions before pregnancy.

Health care providers need to offer information about the effects of lifestyle choices, health status, and medical treatments on embryonic and placental development before becoming pregnant so that patients have the information necessary to maximize their chance of having a healthy pregnancy. For most women, preconception recommendations mimic those for general good health: guidance regarding nutritional health and supplements; prescription, nonprescription, and herbal remedies; alcohol, tobacco, and illicit drug use; safety at home and in the workplace; routine exercise patterns; disease screening; and appropriate immunizations.

Approximately half of the pregnancies each year in the United States are unintended or unplanned. Even with planned pregnancies, most women start their traditional prenatal care after the critical period of organogenesis and many obstetric outcomes have already been determined. The period of greatest environmental sensitivity for the developing fetus is between 17 and 56 days after conception. During this period of embryogenesis, cells multiply and divide faster than at any other time and form organ systems. Any insult that interrupts normal cell organization and differentiation can result in abnormal development. It is therefore imperative that preconception care begin before a woman contemplates pregnancy.

Nurses are in a unique position to educate women on preconception health promotion, as many are now working in the community, and people look to nurses for information about health measures. Nurses see patients in different settings where education can be done. Every nurse who works with women of reproductive age should be aware of opportunities to help their patients consider if and when they want to conceive and how to actively prepare for a pregnancy and promote healthy outcomes for themselves and their infants.

Objective B: To Understand the Importance of Diet, Exercise, and Lifestyle on Preconception Health

5.2 Diet, Exercise, Lifestyle, and Preconception Health

A proper diet and body weight are essential for the health of a woman and when pregnant, that of her fetus. Women need to be counseled about eating a well-balanced diet of three meals a day. They need to be encouraged to achieve height-to-weight goals set by standard guidelines. A woman who is underweight may have delayed conception or infertility. A woman who is pregnant and underweight is at a greater risk for having a premature or low-weight infant. Overweight or obese women also may be at risk for delayed conception, as well as an increased risk of hypertension, thromboembolytic disease, preeclampsia, diabetes mellitus, gestational diabetes, macrosomic infant, dysfunctional labors, birth trauma, and operative deliveries. Additionally, preconception obesity has been linked to babies born with neural tube defects.

The Institute of Medicine (IOM) and the U.S. Public Health Service recommend that women of childbearing age take a multivitamin daily and eat foods containing at least of 0.4 mg of folic acid to prevent neural tube defects in the developing fetus. The neural tube closes during the fourth week of gestation before women may know they are pregnant. Foods containing folate include whole grain breads and cereals and green, leafy vegetables, such as spinach and broccoli. A multivitamin is ideal, as some women are deficient in other vitamins as well. Infants born to vitamin-deficient mothers are at a risk for malnutrition, fetal death, or mental retardation. Caution should be maintained in taking a supplement, as oversupplementation can have negative effects, some associated with birth defects or mental retardation.

Women who consume a vegetarian diet may have nutrient deficiencies that may affect the normal growth and development of the embryo/fetus. Deficiencies in folic acid, vitamin B_{12}, zinc, and calcium are common for vegetarians. Carefully planned vegetarian diets can be safe in pregnancy.

Special or restricted diets and unusual food habits, such as pica, fad dieting, anorexia, and bulimia, may result in insufficient absorption of vitamins and minerals needed by the pregnant woman and her unborn child; patients therefore need to be counseled about potential risks. They should be referred to a nutritionist for a thorough nutritional assessment if they have a medical condition or habits that could interfere with their nutritional health.

A potentially overlooked nutritional risk exists for the women of reproductive age in the United States who have ***phenylketonuria (PKU)***. PKU is an autosomal recessive disorder of phenylalanine that, if untreated, causes severe mental retardation. Through routine newborn screening, individuals affected by this disorder are identified and placed on treatment that involves restricting nutritional intake to phenylalanine-free foods and supplements. Many young men and women have benefited from this screening and therapy program and as a result have IQs in the normal range. Many individuals abandon this regimen during late adolescence, and it does not appear to affect the health of young women negatively; however, should a woman with PKU become pregnant, the fetus is likely to be affected by her high circulating phenylalanine levels, even when the fetus does not have PKU. Outcomes for these infants include a high risk for mental retardation, microcephaly, and heart defects.

Caffeine acts as a central nervous system (CNS) stimulant, causing tachycardia and hypertension. Because caffeine readily crosses the placenta to the fetus, the effects of caffeine affect fetal heart rate and movement. High caffeine intake during pregnancy has been associated with preterm labor and birth, as well as intrauterine growth restriction. Pregnant women are encouraged to limit their consumption of caffeine to < 300 mg/day, which is equivalent to two caffeinated drinks per day.

Exercise is an important component in promoting a healthy lifestyle. Not only is it important in achieving or maintaining a healthy weight, but it has many other benefits, including promotion of cardiovascular health; stress reduction; improved mood, balance, and flexibility; and increased bone mass. Nurses should emphasize the relationship between diet and exercise in health promotion teaching plans for clients. Well-woman care should include emphasis on social and lifestyle circumstances and choices, because these are areas where education, counseling, and strategies for behavioral health modification can make a difference in preventing future health problems and adverse pregnancy outcomes.

Routine assessment of hobbies, habits, and home and employment environments may reveal exposures associated with adverse reproductive consequences that can be minimized in the periconceptual period. Some examples are exposures to solvents, pesticides, vinyl polymers, and heavy metals, such as lead and mercury, which can lead to spontaneous abortions, infertility, low birth weight, and malformations. In general, it is best to avoid the avoidable and to take precautions, such as wearing a mask and gloves and making sure there is adequate ventilation when encountering toxic environments.

Although ***environmental exposures*** are a frequent concern of couples considering a pregnancy, use of alcohol and tobacco and other mood-altering drugs is far more hazardous for women and their unborn children than are most other lifestyle choices.

Alcohol is a leading cause of preventable mental retardation in the United States. ***Fetal alcohol syndrome***, the most severe consequence of in utero alcohol exposure, occurs if alcohol is consumed between the second and eighth weeks of pregnancy. First described in 1973, fetal alcohol syndrome is based on three criteria: prenatal and/or postnatal growth retardation, characteristic facial anomalies, and CNS dysfunctions.

Beyond the syndrome, alcohol exposure in pregnancy is associated with spontaneous abortion, placental abruption, fetal death, low birth weight, behavioral problems, and CNS dysfunctions.

The goal of preconception education is to provide women with timely prevention messages. It is important for women to understand when fetal alcohol syndrome occurs before getting pregnant. The safest choice is to avoid all alcohol if pregnancy is a possibility.

Smoking during pregnancy nearly doubles the risk for a low birth weight baby. It also increases the risk for premature delivery, other pregnancy complications, and sudden infant death syndrome (SIDS). Smoking may also make it more difficult to conceive. One advantage of addressing cessation of smoking prior to pregnancy is that all first-line pharmacotherapies approved by the Food and Drug Administration (FDA) are safe and effective for tobacco dependence treatment.

Taking ***illegal drugs*** and prescription drugs not prescribed for a woman poses many risks, including premature deliveries, low birth weight, birth defects, learning or behavioral problems, and withdrawal symptoms. Identification of addictions in nonpregnant women should be addressed, irrespective of the likelihood of future pregnancy. In those contemplating a pregnancy, treatment for addiction can be started before the most vulnerable weeks of gestation.

Objective C: To Understand the Importance of Psychosocial Health Promotion

5.3 Psychosocial Health Promotion

Mental health is an important component of overall health and should be included as part of a health promotion assessment. A person's mental state can help promote general health or can prevent health promotion behavior. Nurses should assess women for indicators that problems exist or put them at risk should a pregnancy occur. Self-esteem issues, history of depression, intimate partner violence, sexually transmitted infections, difficulties in partner relationships, limited financial resources, substance use, poor social support systems, low educational level, unintended pregnancies, and other mental conditions may interfere with normal daily living as well as pose risks that could interfere with the patient's ability to bond with and take care of an infant.

Intimate partner violence, formerly known as domestic violence, is the most common form of violence experienced by women worldwide. Approximately one out of every six women has been a victim of domestic violence, according to the World Health Organization (WHO, 2005). Up to 45% of victims of intimate partner abuse before pregnancy continue to be abused during pregnancy.

Because partner violence affects reproductive outcomes, the well-woman visit should investigate its occurrence not only as it relates to the woman's health and safety, but also as an opportunity to educate women about how violence can escalate during a pregnancy and jeopardize the likelihood of having a healthy pregnancy and a healthy baby. Women need to know that they do not deserve to be abused and that help is available to them.

Objective D: To Understand Cardiovascular Health as a Means of Health Promotion

5.4 Cardiovascular Health

Some forms of ***heart disease*** pose a life-threatening risk for both the pregnant woman and her fetus. Chronic high blood pressure can increase the risk of pregnancy complications, such as placental problems, preeclampsia, and poor fetal growth.

Primary pulmonary hypertension has a maternal mortality rate that approaches 50% and an infant mortality rate that exceeds 40%. (National Institutes of Health, 2005). Nurses must identify and offer preconception counseling to all women whose life expectancy could be altered by a pregnancy or whose infants are at risk of associated complications, so that they can make informed decisions about the level of risk they are willing to accept.

Objective E: To Understand the Need for Controlling Diabetes Preconceptually

5.5 Diabetes

Women with poorly controlled ***diabetes*** that started before pregnancy are 2–4 times more likely to have a baby born with serious birth defects than nondiabetic mothers (March of Dimes, 2009). They are also at an increased risk for miscarriage and stillbirth and for having a baby that is very large.

Controlling blood sugar before pregnancy and during the first few months of pregnancy can help prevent birth defects. Most oral hypoglycemic agents have not been proven to be safe in pregnancy. It is appropriate to switch to insulin for glucose control in the preconception period to prepare for use in pregnancy. Insulin does not cross the placenta, thereby making it safer for use during pregnancy. Nurses need to provide education and support in assuming a new aspect of self-care.

Objective F: To Understand the Importance of Sexual and Reproductive Health Preconceptually

5.6 Sexual and Reproductive Health

Reproductive history is an important tool in identifying health risks for women and future pregnancies. Awareness of these risks is important in determining appropriate screening for the woman at her routine visits; early detection of disease and appropriate pre-pregnancy management are important to future pregnancy outcomes.

The ***occurrence of sexually transmitted infections (STIs)*** has increased over the past 3 decades. The nurse caring for a woman with infection can be most helpful by providing accurate, sensitive, and supportive health care and health information. Nurses need to be nonjudgmental and respectful and draw on their counseling skills in sharing information.

STIs are an epidemic today, with the highest incidence among adolescents and young adults. For many reasons, these diseases remain a major health problem despite advancements in the development of antibiotics. Multiple sex partners, inadequate knowledge of transmission and prevention, and feelings of invincibility are common in this age group.

Because the vagina may have microscopic tears after intercourse that provide favorable conditions for an infection, women are twice as likely to have an STI.

Bacterial vaginosis is the most prevalent form of vaginal infection in the United States and worldwide. It is more prevalent in sexually active females. Bacterial vaginosis, formerly known as nonspecific vaginosis or *Gardnerella* vaginitis, is an alteration of normal vaginal bacterial flora, resulting in the loss of hydrogen-producing lactobacilli and an overgrowth of predominantly anaerobic bacteria. The process is poorly understood, and the causes leading to overgrowth are not clear. Frequent sexual intercourse without condom use, trauma from douching, and an upset in normal vaginal flora are all predisposing factors. Research also suggests that increased psychosocial stress is associated with an increased incidence and greater prevalence of bacterial vaginosis.

The infected woman often notices an excessive amount of thin, watery, white or gray discharge, with a foul odor often described as "fishy." The characteristic cells are seen on a wet-mount preparation, and leukocytes are conspicuously absent.

Women with bacterial vaginosis have an increased risk of pelvic inflammatory disease (PID), abnormal cervical cytology, postoperative cuff infections after hysterectomy, and postabortion PID. The pregnant woman with bacterial vaginosis is at risk for premature rupture of the membranes (PROM), preterm labor, chorioamnionitis, and postcesarean endometritis.

Therapeutic treatment is with metronidazole (Flagyl) 500 mg orally twice daily for 7 days or one full applicator of metronidazole gel 0.75% intravaginally once daily for 5 days. The currently recommended treatment during pregnancy is metronidazole 500 mg orally twice daily, metronidazole 250 mg orally three times daily, or clindamycin 300 mg orally twice daily.

Vulvovaginal candidiasis (VVC), also known as a ***candidiasis*** or ***fungal yeast infection,*** is a very common vaginal infection. *Candida albicans* is responsible for the vast majority of vaginal yeast infections. Predisposing factors include the use of oral contraceptives, glycosuria, antibiotic use, pregnancy, diabetes mellitus, and the use of immunosuppressant drugs.

The woman with vulvovaginal candidiasis often complains of a white, thick vaginal discharge, severe itching, dysuria, and dyspareunia. A male sexual partner may experience a rash or excoriation of the skin of the penis and possibly pruritis. The male may be symptomatic and the female asymptomatic.

On physical examination, the female's labia may be swollen and excoriated if pruritis has been severe. A speculum exam will reveal thick, white, tenacious, curdy patches adhering to the vaginal mucosa. A Gram stain or culture positive for fungus is an accurate way of diagnosing the causative organism.

Local vaginal treatment with intravaginal butoconazole, clotrimazole, miconazole, nystatin, terconazole, or tioconazole cream, tablets, or suppositories is recommended. Women with severe symptoms are treated with oral fluconazole and may need a repeat dose in 4 days. Treatment of the male partner is usually not necessary. For men who have candidal balanitis (inflammation of the glans penis), treatment with a topical antifungal medication is indicated. Recurrent VVC, defined as four episodes of symptomatic VVC in 1 year, should be tested for an elevated blood glucose level to determine whether a diabetic or prediabetic condition is present.

Pregnant women with VVC should be treated only with topical azole preparations applied for 7 days. Infection at the time of birth may cause ***thrush*** (a candidal infection of the mouth) in the newborn.

Trichomoniasis is a commonly occurring STI caused by *Trichomonas vaginalis*, a microscopic motile protozoan that thrives in an alkaline environment. The single-celled parasite, called a trichomonad, is an anaerobic microorganism that has the ability to generate hydrogen, which combines with oxygen to create an anaerobic environment. Most infections are acquired through sexual intimacy. Fomite transmission by shared bath facilities, wet towels, or wet swimsuits may also be possible.

Many women with trichomoniasis are asymptomatic or have only mild symptoms. More pronounced symptoms of trichomoniasis may include a yellow-green, frothy, odorous discharge and vulvar itching. The woman may also complain of dysuria and dyspareunia. Microscopic visualization of mobile trichomonads and increased leukocytes, a vaginal pH of 4.5 or higher, and a positive whiff test are diagnostic of *T.vaginalis*. Pregnant women with trichomoniasis may be at an increased risk for PROM, preterm birth, and low birth weight.

Recommended treatment for trichomoniasis is metronidazole administered in a single 2 g dose, tinidazole in a single 2 g dose, or metronidazole 500 mg twice daily for 7 days for both male and female sexual partners. Partners should not have intercourse until both are cured. Pregnant women who are symptomatic should be treated with a single 2 g dose of metronidazole orally to reduce their symptoms.

Chlamydial infection, caused by *Chlamydia trachomatis*, is the most common bacterial STI in the United States. It is found most often in sexually active adolescents and young adults. The organism is an intracellular bacterium with several different immunotypes.

In women, chlamydia can infect the fallopian tubes, cervix, urethra, and Bartholin glands. Severe sequelae can result from untreated chlamydial infection, including PID, infertility, and ectopic pregnancy. In men, chlamydia can result in epididymitis and infertility. Newborn exposure to chlamydia in the birth canal of the mother can result in blindness in the newborn. The newborn may also develop chlamydial pneumonia. This newborn eye infection responds to the erythromycin ophthalmic ointment given at birth.

Symptoms of chlamydial infection include a thin or mucopurulent discharge, cervical ectopia, friable cervix (bleeds easily), burning and frequency of urination, and lower abdominal pain. Chlamydia is a major cause of nongonococcal urethritis in men. Nucleic acid amplification is the most sensitive test for diagnosis. Other tests used for diagnosis are culture, direct immunofluorescence, enzyme immunoassay (EIA), and nucleic acid hybridization.

The recommended treatment is a single dose of azithromycin 1 g orally or doxycycline 100 mg by mouth twice daily for 7 days. Sexual partners should also be treated, and the couple should abstain from intercourse for 7 days after taking the single-dose treatment or for the entire 7 days of the doxycycline therapy. For pregnant women, the Centers for Disease Control and Prevention (CDC) recommends treatment with azithromycin or amoxicillin, as doxycycline is contraindicated during pregnancy. Repeat testing is recommended 3 weeks after the completion of the recommended treatment as a test of cure.

Because many females and males are asymptomatic, the CDC recommends annual screening for chlamydia as the primary method of decreasing the incidence of chlamydia.

Gonorrhea, an infection caused by the bacterium *Neisseria gonorrhoeae*, is the second most common reported STI in the United States. Most men seek treatment for gonorrhea early because of symptoms, but many women with the infection are asymptomatic until complications such as PID occur.

Transmission can occur through vaginal, anal, or oral sex. If a pregnant woman becomes infected after the third month of pregnancy, the mucus plug in the cervix prevents the infection from ascending, and it will remain localized until the membranes rupture, when it can then spread upward and infect the fetus. A newborn exposed to a gonococcal-infected birth canal is at risk for developing ophthalmia neonatorum. Eye prophylaxis (erythromycin) for all newborns is provided to prevent this complication.

The most common symptoms of gonorrheal infection are a purulent, greenish yellow vaginal discharge, dysuria, and urinary frequency. Some women also develop inflammation and swelling of the vulva. The cervix may appear swollen and eroded and may secrete a foul-smelling discharge. Bilateral lower abdominal or pelvic pain may also occur. Diagnosis is through culture. Reculture is needed to verify cure.

Treatment for nonpregnant women consists of antibiotic therapy with cefixime, ciproflaxin, ofloxacin, or levofloxacin orally plus doxycycline or azithromycin administered orally if chlamydia has not been ruled out. This combined approach provides dual treatment for gonorrhea and chlamydia because the two infections often occur together. Additional treatment may be needed if the cultures remain positive 7 to 14 days after completion of treatment. All sexual partners must be treated, or the woman may become reinfected.

Pregnant women should be treated with a recommended cephalosporin orally, combined with azithromycin or amoxicillin to address the risk of coinfection with chlamydia.

The herpes simplex virus (HSV) causes ***herpes infections,*** which are recurrent, lifelong infections. Two serotypes cause human infections: HSV1 and HSV2, with HSV2 causing most cases of genital herpes. Genital herpes is spread through vaginal, anal, or oral sex. It can also be spread through skin-to-skin contact with an infected site, such as a finger.

The primary episode (first outbreak) of herpes genitalis is characterized by the development of single or multiple blisterlike vesicles, which usually occur in the genital area and sometimes affect the vaginal walls, cervix, urethra, and anus. The vesicles may appear within a few hours or up to 20 days after exposure and rupture spontaneously to form very painful, open, ulcerated lesions. Inflammation and pain secondary to the presence of lesions can cause difficult urination. Enlargement of the inguinal lymph nodes may be present, as well as flu-like symptoms. Primary episodes are the most severe. Lesions heal in approximately 2 to 4 weeks, and the virus lays dormant, residing in the nerve ganglia of the affected area. Recurrences are usually less severe and brought on by stress, menstruation, ovulation, pregnancy, frequent or vigorous intercourse, poor health, tight clothing, or overheating. Diagnosis is made on the basis of the clinical appearance of the lesions, culture of the lesions, polymerase chain reaction (PCR) identification, and glycoprotein G-based type-specific assays.

No known cure for herpes exists, although medications are available to provide relief from pain. The recommended treatment of the first clinical episode is oral acyclovir, valacyclovir, or famciclovir. These same medications, in different dosages, are also recommended for recurrent herpes infection and for daily suppressive therapy.

Acyclovir may be administered orally to pregnant women. It is used in the third trimester of pregnancy to suppress outbreaks and reduce the number of cesarean births. If herpes is present in the genital tract of a pregnant woman during childbirth, it can prove fatal for the newborn, and delivery by cesarean section is recommended.

Syphilis is a chronic infection caused by the spirochete *Treponema pallidum*. Syphilis is acquired through vaginal, anal, or oral sex. Less commonly, it can be contracted from nonsexual exposure to exudates from an infected individual. Congenital transmission through transplacental inoculation may occur.

Syphilis is divided into early and late stages. During the early stage, a chancre, or painless ulcer, appears at the site where the organism entered the body. Symptoms include fever, loss of weight, and malaise. The chancre persists for approximately 4 weeks and disappears. In 6 weeks to 6 months, symptoms may reappear with secondary symptoms. Skin eruptions called condylomata, which resemble warts, may appear on the vulva. Other secondary symptoms are acute arthritis, enlargement of the liver and spleen, enlarged lymph nodes, iritis, and chronic sore throat with hoarseness.

Transplacental transmission of syphilis is as high as 95%, and congenital syphilis may cause intrauterine growth restriction, preterm birth, and stillbirth. Because of the impact of this disease on the fetus, most states require serologic prenatal testing at the first prenatal visit that is repeated during the last trimester of pregnancy.

Diagnosis is made in the early stage by microscopic examination of the chancre and in the later stage by serologic tests, such as the VDRL (Venereal Disease Research Laboratories) or the RPR (rapid plasma reagin), or the more specific FTA-ABS (fluorescent treponemal antibody absorption test).

For pregnant and nonpregnant women with syphilis of under 1 year's duration, the recommended treatment by the CDC is 2.4 million units of benzathine penicillin G given intramuscularly in one dose. If syphilis is of long duration (over 1 year) or of unknown origin, the recommended dosage is 2.4 million units of benzathine penicillin G intramuscularly once weekly for 3 weeks. Patients who are allergic to penicillin and nonpregnant should be given doxycycline or tetracycline. The pregnant woman who is allergic to penicillin should be desensitized to penicillin and then treated.

Because of the impact of the disease on a fetus, serologic testing is routinely done on every pregnant woman during her first trimester (as required by most states by law) and again in her third trimester. It is often repeated as part of admission blood work when the woman goes to the hospital to deliver her baby. It is important to remember that maternal serologic testing may remain positive for 8 months, and the newborn may have a positive test for 3 months.

Condylomata acuminata, also called genital or venereal warts, are a common STI caused by the ***human papilloma virus (HPV).*** Transmission can occur through vaginal, oral, or anal sex.

Most HPV infections are unrecognized, asymptomatic, or subclinical. There is increased evidence of a link between HPV and cervical and anorectal cancers.

Symptoms include single or multiple soft, grayish pink, cauliflower-like lesions in the genital area. Depending on their size and location, they may cause itching (pruritis), be friable (bleed easily), or be painful. Diagnosis is usually made by visual inspection and visual appearance. However, vaginal and cervical warts are more common than those on external genitalia. Most of these are flat lesions visible only by colposcopy. Subclinical diagnosis can be made if characteristic changes are present on a Pap smear.

The CDC does not specify a treatment of choice for genital warts but recommends that treatment be determined by client preference, available resources, and experience of the health care provider. Client-applied treatments include podofilox solution or gel or imiquimod cream. Provider-administered therapies include cryotherapy with liquid nitrogen or cryoprobe; topical podophyllin, trichloroacetic acid, bichloroacetic acid, and surgical removal by shave excision, curettage, or electrosurgery. Alternate therapies include intralesional interferon and laser surgery. Pregnant women should not be treated with imiquimod, podophyllin, or podofilox because they are thought to be teratogenic and in large doses have been associated with fetal death.

The use of condoms may reduce the risk of transmitting the virus to an uninfected partner. In 2006 the first vaccine was approved for use designed to protect against four types of HPV, which together account for 90% of all cases of HPV. The vaccine, Gardasil, is given in three doses and is recommended in young girls as early as 9 years of age. It is recommended in all women up to 26 years of age.

HIV/AIDS is one of today's major health issues worldwide. ***Acquired immunodeficiency syndrome (AIDS)*** is caused by the ***human immunodeficiency virus (HIV).*** Adult and adolescent males are the largest group of infected individuals (73%) (Center for Disease Control, 2011). Infection in this group occurs by homosexual contact, intravenous (IV) drug use, heterosexual contact, and homosexual IV drug use. Among female cases of HIV/AIDS, heterosexual contact and IV drug use are the major sources of infection.

HIV found in blood, semen, vaginal fluid, and breast milk has been implicated in disease transmission, although the virus has been isolated in urine, tears, cerebrospinal fluid, lymph nodes, brain tissue, and bone marrow. HIV shedding has also been detected in the genital tract of women. Of the known pediatric cases, the vast majority became infected perinatally, according to the CDC (2005).

Once infected with the virus, the individual develops antibodies that can be detected with enzyme-linked immunosorbent assay (ELISA) and is confirmed with a Western blot test. Antibodies can be detected in most individuals within 6 months of exposure; however, in rare circumstances the latent phase may be longer. A symptomatic period lasting from a few months to up to 17 years follows seroconversion. The majority of infected pregnant women fall into this category. The diagnosis of AIDS is usually made when a person with HIV is identified as having one of several specific opportunistic infections.

Many women who are HIV positive choose to avoid pregnancy because of the risk of infecting the fetus and the likelihood of dying before the child is raised. Many states now mandate prenatal serologic testing of pregnant women to detect HIV. The goal is to identify those women in order to start prophylactic treatment to prevent transmission to the fetus.

The use of zidovudine (ZDV, formerly called AZT) during pregnancy reduces the risk of transmitting HIV to the fetus, and most medications taken during pregnancy to treat HIV can be taken safely during pregnancy. A triple therapy approach is recommended during the perinatal period. It includes ZDV, a nucleoside analogue, plus a second nucleoside analogue, such as zalcitabine, didanosine, or lamivudine, combined with a protease inhibitor, such as indinavir, ritonavir, or saquinavir.

HIV transmission can occur during pregnancy and through breast milk, although it is believed that at least half of all infections occur during labor and birth. For HIV-infected pregnant women who do not receive treatment, the transmission rate to the newborn is 25% (Centers for Disease Control, 2011). For HIV-infected pregnant women who receive prophylactic treatment with ZDV, give birth by elective cesarean section at 38 weeks before the rupture of membranes, and avoid breastfeeding, the rate drops to $< 2\%$.

Following birth, infants will often have a positive antibody titer, which reflects the passive transfer of maternal antibodies and does not indicate HIV infection. Although infected infants are usually asymptomatic at birth, they are likely to be premature, low birth weight, and small for gestational age (SGA). The signs of AIDS in infants include failure to thrive, hepatosplenomegaly, pneumonia, recurrent cradle cap, encephalopathy, and delayed developmental milestones or the loss of acquired skills, including cognitive abilities. The prognosis for an infected child remains poor.

Objective G: To Understand the Need for Vaccinations Before Pregnancy

5.7 Vaccinations

At a preconception visit, the health care provider may do a blood test to see if a woman is immune to ***rubella (German measles)*** and ***chickenpox***. Both of these diseases can cause birth defects and other complications if a woman gets them during pregnancy. If a woman is not immune, she should be vaccinated before pregnancy. She should then wait 1 month before attempting to get pregnant.

Congenital rubella syndrome is associated with abnormalities of the heart, eyes, and ears. Congenital varicella syndrome is rare, but infants born to women with acute infection may suffer significant morbidity.

Women who are at high risk for ***hepatitis B,*** such as health care workers, and have not been vaccinated for it should consider getting vaccinated before or during pregnancy. The disease can be passed on to the baby during delivery. Children who are infected as fetuses have a 25% chance of dying from a liver-related disease unless treated within days of birth. The health care provider may also recommend other vaccines, such as a flu shot.

Objective H: To Understand the Need to Treat Other Maternal Illnesses Before Pregnancy

5.8 Other Maternal Illnesses

Chronic ***high blood pressure*** can increase the risk of pregnancy complications, including placental problems, poor fetal growth, and preeclampsia, and should be treated before a pregnancy occurs.

The autoimmune disorder ***systemic lupus erythematosus (SLE)*** can cause arthritis-like symptoms, kidney disease, skin rashes, and other problems. Affected pregnant women are at an increased risk for miscarriage, poor fetal growth, preterm labor, and stillbirth. If symptoms are well controlled before pregnancy, the risk of complications is reduced.

Some ***seizure*** control medications increase the risk of birth defects. During a preconception visit, a provider may adjust a woman's dosage or switch her to a drug that is safer for a fetus. A woman should not stop taking seizure medication without first talking with her provider.

Some women with ***kidney disease*** may suffer additional kidney damage during pregnancy, and their babies may be at an increased risk for premature delivery, poor growth, or death.

Although 30% of the population is immune to ***toxoplasmosis,*** toxoplasmosis can cause serious birth defects, including hydrocephaly, microcephaly, and hepatosplenomegaly, if infection occurs in the first trimester. Women who are planning a pregnancy who own cats should be counseled to have someone else change the litter box or to wear gloves and a mask when changing cat litter, and to avoid soil that is used by cats for defecation. All women should be encouraged to thoroughly cook meats (to 105°F, or 41°C).

Periodontal disease is associated with increased risk for low birth weight infants. Dental care should be encouraged and is safe during pregnancy.

Objective I: To Understand the Need for Preconception Genetic Risk Assessment

5.9 Genetic Risk Assessment

Preconception evaluation of genetic risk offers advantages over genetic evaluation at the first prenatal visit. Couples at risk for having a child with a genetic disorder have several reproductive options: choosing to remain childless, accepting the risk and having children, choosing to have prenatal diagnosis to determine if the child is affected, using artificial insemination or oocyte donation to avoid passing on the mutant gene, or undergoing preimplantation diagnosis.

Carrier screening is of special importance because it allows for relevant counseling before the first affected pregnancy. Each racial or ethnic group is at risk for one or more autosomal recessive diseases, and screening can be individualized to specific racial or ethnic groups.

Women identified as carriers of autosomal recessive genes should receive posttest counseling; partner status may then be explored. Because the likelihood of bearing a child with certain life-threatening autosomal recessive diseases can be determined before conception, women and their partners deserve the option of being tested before pregnancy occurs. Individuals should have the opportunity to know their reproductive risks so they can make informed and timely decisions about how they wish to handle those risks.

Objective J: To Understand Paternal Considerations in Preconception Health

5.10 Paternal Considerations

Beyond infertility, little is known about the effects of male environmental exposures and disease on human reproductive outcomes. The male's contribution to congenital anomalies could originate from a number of different affluences, including personal and family medical histories; his habits and environmental exposures to chemicals, drugs, and radiation; and his infectious disease history and risks.

Evidence is growing that alcohol or tobacco use by the father negatively affects birth weight. It is unclear how much of the effect is direct and how much is related to the female's use of the same drugs. In addition, male tobacco use has been associated with a 10% decrease in fertility. Advancing paternal age ($\geq$ 40 years) has been associated with an increased likelihood of autosomal dominant disease from new mutations in the offspring. Approximately 20% of Down syndrome appears to be caused by advanced paternal age, as well as 5% of congenital cardiac defects.

Counseling to promote preconception health should be approached as an occasion for both members of a couple to learn about opportunities to maximize their chances of having a healthy pregnancy and healthy baby.

Review Exercises

True/False

1. _______ The goal of preconception health promotion is to provide women with information to make timely, informed decisions about their reproductive futures.

2. _______ Half of all pregnancies each year in the United States are unplanned.

3. _______ The period of greatest environmental sensitivity for the developing fetus is between the 17th and 56th day after conception.

4. _______ Nurses are in a unique position to educate women on preconception health promotion.

5. _______ A woman who is underweight may have trouble conceiving.

6. _______ Infants born to mothers who are vitamin deficient are at risk for malnutrition, fetal death, or mental retardation.

7. _______ Preconception obesity has been linked to neural tube defects in infants.

8. _______ Women who have unusual food habits, such as pica, should be referred to a nutritionist.

9. _______ Phenylketonuria (PKU) is an autosomal dominant disorder of phenylalanine that if left untreated in the pregnant woman could cause severe mental retardation in her infant.

10. _______ Caffeine intake in the pregnant woman should be limited to five drinks per day.

11. _______ Exercise is contraindicated in the pregnant woman.

12. _______ Mental health is an important component of overall health and should be included as part of a health promotion assessment.

13. _______ Controlling blood sugar before pregnancy and during the first few months of pregnancy can help prevent birth defects.

14. _______ Newborn exposure to chlamydia during birth can result in blindness in the newborn.

15. _______ The vaccine Gardasil, used for the treatment of human papilloma virus (HPV), is given in one dose and recommended for all women of childbearing age.

Completion

1. ______________________ ingestion is recommended for the prevention of neural tube defects by women of childbearing age.

2. Foods containing high folate content include ______________, ______________, and ______________.

3. According to the World Health Organization, 1 in every ___________ women have been the target of intimate partner violence.

4. Women with poorly controlled diabetes that started before pregnancy are ____________ more likely to have a baby born with serious birth defects than nondiabetic mothers.

5. ____________ is the leading cause of preventable mental retardation in the United States.

6. Syphilis, a chronic sexually transmitted infection, can cause intrauterine ____________, ____________, or ____________ of the fetus.

7. Of the known pediatric cases of human immunodeficiency virus (HIV), the vast majority became infected ____________.

8. The Institute of Medicine and U.S. Public Health Service recommend that all women of childbearing age consume ____________ of folic acid a day and eat foods high in folate.

9. Women with untreated PKU disease are at risk for giving birth to infants with ____________, ____________, or ____________.

10. It is important for women to know when fetal alcohol syndrome occurs ____________ they become pregnant.

11. ____________ does not cross the placenta, making it safer for use in pregnant mothers over oral hypoglycemic medications.

12. The most sensitive test for diagnosing chlamydia is ____________.

13. Pregnant women with trichomoniasis are at risk for ____________, ____________, and ____________.

14. A newborn exposed to gonorrhea during birth is at risk for developing ____________.

15. Acyclovir is given during the third trimester of pregnancy to suppress outbreaks and reduce the number of ____________.

16. Breastfeeding is ____________ for HIV-positive women.

17. ____________ can be contracted from infected cat litter.

18. Women should be vaccinated against ____________ and ____________ before becoming pregnant, as the diseases can affect the fetus seriously.

19. The father's use of alcohol and tobacco has negative effects on the fetus's ____________.

20. Advanced paternal age is associated with ____________, ____________, and ____________ in the fetus.

21. If herpes is present in the genital tract of the woman during childbirth, delivery by ____________ is recommended.

22. The risk of an infant contracting HIV from his mother who did take prophylactic treatment is ____________.

23. The outcomes for pediatric cases of HIV are ____________.

Matching Columns

1. Treatment for HIV _______
2. Treatment for syphillis _______
3. Treatment for trichomoniasis _______
4. Vaccine for HPV _______
5. Treatment for yeast infection _______
6. Treatment for gonorrhea _______
7. Treatment for herpes _______
8. Treatment for chlamydia _______

A. Penicillin G
B. Acyclovir
C. Azithromycin
D. Flagyl
E. Ciproflaxin
F. Gardasil
G. ZDV
H. Clotrimazole

Answers

True/False

1. True
2. True
3. True
4. True
5. True
6. True
7. True
8. True
9. False. PKU is an autosomal recessive disease.
10. False. Caffeine intake should be limited to two drinks per day for the pregnant woman.
11. False. Exercise is encouraged for the pregnant woman.
12. True
13. True
14. True
15. False. Gardasil is given in three doses in women ages 9 to 26 years.

Completion

1. Folic acid
2. Cereal, whole grain bread, green, leafy vegetables (spinach, broccoli)
3. 6
4. Three times
5. Alcohol
6. Death, preterm birth, intrauterine growth restriction (IUGR)
7. Perinatally
8. 0.4 mg
9. Mental retardation, microcephaly, heart defects
10. Before
11. Insulin
12. Nucleic acid amplification
13. Premature rupture of the membranes (PROM), preterm birth, low birth weight
14. Ophthalmia neonatorum

15. Cesarean births
16. Contraindicated
17. Toxoplasmosis
18. Rubella, chicken pox
19. Birth weight
20. Autosomal dominant disease, Down syndrome, cardiac defects
21. Cesarean section
22. less than 2%
23. poor

Matching Columns

1. G
2. A
3. D
4. F
5. H
6. E
7. B
8. C

Antepartum Nursing Assessment

Objective A: To Understand What Is Involved in the Antepartum Nursing Assessment

6.1 Antepartum Nursing Assessment

Today nurses are assuming a more significant role in prenatal care, particularly in the area of assessment. The certified nurse midwife and nurse practitioner may share assessment responsibilities with the physician. The nurse needs to establish an environment of comfort and open communication with each prenatal office visit, conveying concern for the woman as an individual and being available to listen to the woman's concerns. The information gathered through the antepartum visits should enable the nurse to identify needed areas of education and counseling. Counseling and education of the pregnant woman and her partner are critical to ensure healthy outcomes for the mother and her infant.

The ultimate goal of any pregnancy is the birth of a healthy newborn. To address issues and foster the overall well-being of pregnant women and their fetuses, specific national health goals have been established. Healthy People 2020 lists 33 maternal, infant, and child health objectives with the goal of strengthening the health of families and communities, as well as the health of the nation (Chapter 3, **Table 3.1**).

Appropriate nursing management starting at conception and continuing throughout pregnancy has a positive impact on the health of pregnant women and their unborn children. Nurses not only see patients during the antepartum office visits, but also teach many classes in the community related to pregnancy, labor and birth, and breastfeeding, along with a variety of other classes of interest to childbearing families. The nurse acts as educator and patient advocate for women and their partners in the childbearing phases of their lives.

It is important for the nurse to enter into a collaborative partnership with the pregnant woman and her partner, enabling the couple to examine their own health and practices and their influence on the health of their future baby. Providing information to the couple allows them to make timely, informed decisions about childbearing.

Objective B: To Understand What Is Involved in the Initial Prenatal Assessment

6.2 The Initial Prenatal Assessment

Once a pregnancy is suspected, the woman usually will seek prenatal care for confirmation and information about pregnancy. The assessment process begins at this initial prenatal visit and continues throughout the pregnancy. The initial visit is an ideal time to screen for factors that may place the woman and her fetus at risk for problems. The initial visit is also an optimal time to begin educating the client about changes that will affect her life.

Pregnant women and their partners frequently have questions, misinformation, and misconceptions about pregnancy. The nurse needs to allow time to answer questions and provide anticipatory guidance during pregnancy and to make appropriate community agency referrals to meet the needs of patients.

6.3 Components of the Comprehensive Health History

During the initial visit, a comprehensive health history is obtained. The initial health history typically includes three major areas: the reason for seeking care; the patient's past medical, surgical, and personal history, including that of her family and her partner; and the patient's reproductive history.

6.4 Reason for Seeking Care

The woman commonly comes for prenatal care based on the suspicion that she is pregnant. She may have missed a period or had a positive result on a home pregnancy test. The nurse should ask the date of the woman's last menstrual period and about any presumptive or probable signs she might be experiencing.

Presumptive signs are mainly subjective changes that are experienced and reported by the woman. Presumptive changes are the least reliable indicators of pregnancy because any of them can be caused by conditions other than pregnancy. These typically include amenorrhea, nausea and vomiting, fatigue, breast and skin changes, vaginal and cervical color changes, and fetal movement.

Probable signs of pregnancy are objective findings that can be documented by an examiner. They are primarily related to physical changes in the reproductive organs. Although these signs are stronger indicators of pregnancy, a positive diagnosis cannot be made because they may have other causes. These include abdominal enlargement, cervical softening, changes in uterine consistency, ballottement, Braxton Hicks contractions, and home pregnancy tests.

Only three signs are accepted as positive confirmation of pregnancy:

1. Auscultation of ***fetal heart sounds***
2. ***Fetal movement*** felt by an examiner
3. ***Visualization of the fetus*** with sonography

Typically, a blood or urine test is done to detect human chorionic gonadotropin (hCG) to confirm the pregnancy.

6.5 Past History

The woman's past medical and surgical history should be obtained. This information is important because conditions the woman may have experienced in the past may recur or be exacerbated by pregnancy. Chronic conditions can increase the risk of complications. The woman's personal history is important. Her occupation, possible exposure to teratogens, exercise and activity level, use of substances including tobacco, illegal drugs, and homeopathic remedies, sleep patterns, nutritional habits, and general lifestyle issues can all have a significant impact on the outcome of the pregnancy. Mental health issues should be identified, and similar information on the woman's family and partner should be obtained.

6.6 Reproductive History

The woman's reproductive history should be obtained and includes a menstrual, gynecologic, and obstetrical history. The history begins with a description of the woman's menstrual cycle, including her age at menarche, number of days in her cycle, typical flow characteristics, and any discomfort experienced. The use of contraception and date last used are also important to ascertain.

A full-term pregnancy is one that finishes at 40 weeks' gestation or 9 full lunar months. Any pregnancy that delivers between 20 and 37 weeks is considered ***preterm***. To determine the estimated or expected date of birth (EDB) or delivery (EDD), the date of the woman's first day of her last menstrual period is obtained. ***Naegele's rule*** is used to determine the date of birth. Using this rule, take the first day of the last menstrual period (LMP) and subtract 3 months, then add 7 days. Depending on the month, you may have to correct the year by adding 1 year to it. For example, if the woman reports that her LMP was April 1, 2011, you would subtract 3 months (January), add 7 days (January 8), and add one year (2012). The EDD or EDB is January 8, 2012. This date has a margin of error of plus or minus 2 weeks, due to normal variations in a woman's cycle, conception while breastfeeding, ovulating while amenorrheic, discontinuance of oral contraception, and errors in dating.

An obstetric history provides information about the woman's past pregnancies. Such information can provide clues to problems that might develop in the current pregnancy. Some common terms used to describe and document an obstetric history are

- ***Gravid***—the state of being pregnant
- ***Gravida***—a pregnant woman; gravid I (first time pregnant); gravid II (second time pregnant), and so on
- ***Para***—the number of deliveries after 20 weeks' gestation a woman has completed, regardless of whether the newborn is born alive or dead (multiples count as one pregnancy)
- ***Nullipara*** (para 0)—a woman who has not produced a viable offspring
- ***Primipara*** (para I)—a woman who has given birth once after a pregnancy of at least 20 weeks; commonly referred to as a ***"primip"***

Other systems may be used to document a woman's obstetric history. These systems often break down the category of para more specifically, such as

TPAL = **T** Term pregnancies delivered (over 37 weeks' gestation)

P Preterm pregnancies delivered (between 20 and 37 weeks' gestation)

A Abortions (less than 20 weeks' gestation; can be spontaneous or elective)

L Number of children currently living

Objective C: To Understand the Components of the Physical Exam

6.7 Physical Exam

After obtaining a thorough history, the patient is asked to undress and put on a gown in preparation for a physical exam. The patient is asked for a clean catch urine specimen, which is sent to the lab for a urinalysis in order to detect a possible urinary tract infection.

The physical is begun by obtaining vital signs and height and weight. A complete head-to-toe examination is performed next. The pelvic exam follows, which can give specific information about internal and external reproductive organs. Fundal height measurement, fetal movement determination, and fetal heart rate measurement are done to assess fetal growth and well-being.

When examining the patient's head and neck, the nurse should look for any previous injuries, limitations in range of motion, enlarged lymph nodes, or swelling. Edema of the nasal mucosa and hypertrophy of gingival tissue in the mouth are typical responses to increased estrogen levels in pregnancy. Slight enlargement of lymph nodes is normal, but marked enlargement may indicate hyperthyroidism, requiring further investigation.

Auscultation of heart sounds is done; a soft systolic murmur may be heard due to the increased blood volume that accompanies pregnancy. An increase in heart rate by 10 to 15 beats per minute (starting between 14 and 20 weeks' gestation) secondary to increased cardiac output and blood volume is normal. The body adapts to the increase in blood volume with peripheral dilation to maintain blood pressure. Progesterone causes peripheral dilation.

Auscultation of breath sounds should be clear. Symmetry of chest movement and thoracic breathing patterns should be noted. Estrogen promotes relaxation of the ligaments and joints with an increase in the anteroposterior diameter of the chest. A slight increase in respiratory rate is normal due to the increased respiratory rate to accommodate the increase in tidal volume and oxygen consumption.

When inspecting and palpating the breasts, it is important to know that increases in estrogen, progesterone, and blood supply make the breasts feel full, more modular, and more tender. Blood vessels become more visible, and striae gravidarum (stretch marks) may be seen in women with large breasts. Pigmentation of the nipple and areola becomes darker, along with enlargement of the Montgomery glands.

The appearance of the abdomen depends on the number of weeks of gestation the woman has completed. The abdomen enlarges progressively as the fetus grows. The abdomen should be rounded and nontender. A decrease in muscle tone due to increased progesterone may be noted. Striae gravidarum or linea negra (dark pigmented line from the symphysis pubis to the umbilicus) may be noted.

Legs should be inspected for dependent edema, pulses, and varicose veins. If edema is present early in pregnancy, further evaluation is warranted to rule out gestational hypertension. The woman should be asked if she has any pain in her calf that increases as she ambulates, which may indicate a deep vein thrombosis (DVT). High levels of estrogen during pregnancy predisposes women to a higher risk of DVT.

After the patient is placed in the lithotomy position, the external genitalia are inspected visually. They should be free of lesions, discharge, hematomas, varicosities, and inflammation. A culture for sexually transmitted infections (STIs) may be taken at this time. Next, the internal genitalia are inspected through a speculum exam. The cervix should be smooth, long, thick, and closed. Because of increased pelvic congestion, the cervix will be softened (***Goodell sign***), the uterine isthmus will be softened (***Hegar's sign***), and there will be a bluish coloration of the cervix and vaginal mucosa (***Chadwick's sign***).

The uterus is pear-shaped and mobile, with a smooth surface. It undergoes cell hypertrophy and hyperplasia so that it enlarges throughout the pregnancy to accommodate the growing fetus. During the pelvic examination, a Pap smear is obtained. Additional cultures, such as for gonorrhea, chlamydia, and group B strep may also be obtained. Once the examination of the internal genitalia is completed, a bimanual examination of the uterus is performed to estimate the size of the uterus to confirm dates and to palpate the ovaries. The ovaries should be small, nontender, and without masses. The health care provider will also do a rectal exam to assess for lesions, masses, prolapse, or hemorrhoids.

Pelvic shape is classified as one of four types, the gynecoid pelvis being the most optimal for safe vaginal delivery. Three pelvic measurements are assessed: the diagonal conjugate, true conjugate, and ischial tuberosity. Taking internal pelvic measurements determines the actual diameters of the inlet and outlet through which the fetus will pass.

The contour, size, and muscle tone of the abdomen should be assessed. Fundal height should be measured if the fundus is palpable above the symphysis pubis. The bladder should be emptied prior to taking this measurement. Fundal height is the distance (in centimeters) measured with a tape measure from the top of the pubic bone to the top of the uterus (fundus) with the patient lying on her back with knees slightly flexed. Measurement in this way is termed ***McDonald's method.*** Fundal height increases as the pregnancy progresses. It provides a gross estimate of fetal growth for the duration of the pregnancy. Between 12 and 14 weeks' gestation, the fundus can be palpated above the symphysis pubis. The fundus reaches the level of the umbilicus at 20 weeks' gestation and measures 20 cm. Fundal measurement should approximately equal the number of weeks of gestation until 36 weeks. After 36 weeks, the fundal height then drops due to lightening and may no longer correspond with the week of gestation.

If fundal height is higher or lower than what is expected for the weeks of gestation, additional assessment is necessary to investigate the discrepancy. The cause may be an error in the estimated date of conception, a variation in the amount of amniotic fluid present, or an abnormality in fetal growth. Ultrasound may be performed to obtain further information.

Fetal movement is usually first perceived by the patient between 16 and 20 weeks' gestation. Fetal movement is a gross indicator of fetal well-being. The patient should be instructed to take note of fetal movement. Although there is no established number of fetal movements that indicate fetal well-being, the woman should be instructed to report a count of fewer than three fetal movements within an hour.

Fetal heart rate measurement is an integral part of the prenatal exam throughout the pregnancy. Auscultation of the fetal heart rate is done with a handheld Doppler at each prenatal visit, which helps confirm that the intrauterine environment is still supportive of the growing fetus. The purpose of assessing the fetal heart rate is to determine the rate and rhythm. The fetal heart rate should be 110 to 160 beats per minute.

6.8 Laboratory Tests Commonly Done at the First Prenatal Visit

Blood grouping—to determine blood type and Rh; identifies possible causes of incompatibility with the fetus that may cause jaundice.

Hemoglobin (Hgb) and hematocrit (Hct)—to detect anemia; often checked several times during pregnancy. Hgb ≤11 g/dL in the first and third trimesters or ≤1.5 g/dL in the second trimester may indicate a need for additional iron supplementation.

Hemoglobin electrophoresis—to screen for sickle cell trait if the patient is of African-American descent. If the mother is positive, check the partner; the infant is at risk only if both parents are positive.

Complete blood count—to detect infection, anemia, or cell abnormalities; 12,000/mm or more white blood cells or decreased platelets require follow-up.

Rh factor and antibody screen—to check for possible maternal-fetal blood incompatibility. If the mother is Rh negative, and the father is Rh positive or antibodies are present, additional testing and treatment are required; if Rh- and unsensitized, RhoGAM will be given at 28 weeks.

Venereal Disease Research Laboratory (VDRL) test or rapid plasma regain—to screen for syphilis; treat if test is positive; retest at 36 weeks.

Rubella titer (to determine immunity)—if titer is 1:8 or less, mother is not immune; immunize postpartum if not immune (live virus that cannot be given during pregnancy).

Hepatitis B screen—to detect the presence of antigens in maternal blood; if present, infants should be given hepatitis immune globulin and vaccine soon after birth.

Skin test—to screen for tuberculosis; if results are positive, refer for additional testing or therapy.

Human immunodeficiency virus (HIV)—test, often mandated by law, to be done at first prenatal visit to detect HIV antibodies; positive results require retesting, counseling, and treatment to lower infant infection.

Urinalysis—to detect renal disease or infection; requires further assessment if positive for more than trace protein or bacteria.

Papanicolaou (Pap) test—to screen for cervical neoplasia; treat and refer if abnormal cells are present.

Cervical culture—to detect group B streptococci and sexually transmitted infections; treat and retest as necessary, and treat group B streptococci during labor.

Other common tests include the following:

Between 16 and 18 weeks (multiple marker screen)—maternal serum alpha fetoprotein, hCG, and estriol; abnormal results may indicate Down syndrome or neural tube defects

Between 24 and 28 weeks—blood glucose level is screened; if the result is high, the patient is sent to have a 3-hour glucose challenge test to determine whether she has gestational diabetes

Ultrasound—the test is often performed initially at the first prenatal visit and again at 12 to 20 weeks' gestation; helps to determine gestational age, show some fetal anomalies, and determine the gender

Objective D: To Understand the Need for Assessments Done at Subsequent Prenatal Visits

6.9 Subsequent Prenatal Visits

Ongoing antepartum care is essential to the successful outcome of a pregnancy. The usual schedule for prenatal assessment in a normal pregnancy is as follows:

- Conception to 28 weeks: every 4 weeks
- 29 to 36 weeks: every 2 to 3 weeks
- 37 weeks to birth: weekly

Vital signs should be taken at every prenatal visit. The blood pressure should be measured in the same arm with the mother in the same position every time.

Weight should be recorded to document that weight gain is progressing as expected. The recommended weight gain is 25 to 35 lb in a normal-weight woman. Inadequate weight gain may signify that the pregnancy is not as advanced as was thought or that the fetus is not growing as expected. Sudden, rapid weight gain may indicate excessive fluid retention.

Urine is tested at each visit for the presence of protein, glucose, ketones, and bacteria. A woman may need a culture done if the woman has a history of symptoms of urinary tract infection or if a dipstick indicates the presence of bacteria.

Fundal height is measured at each antepartum visit. It is one method of assessing fetal growth and confirming gestational age.

Fetal heart rate is auscultated at each antepartum visit. The location of the fetal heart sounds provides information that helps determine the position in which the fetus is entering the pelvis. The fetal heart should be counted over 1 full minute.

Leopold's maneuvers provide a systematic method for palpating the fetus through the abdominal wall during the later part of pregnancy. These maneuvers provide valuable information about the location and presentation of the fetus.

Fetal movements (quickening) are usually first noticed by the expectant mother at 16 to 20 weeks' gestation and gradually increase in frequency and strength. In general, fetal activity indicates a physically healthy fetus. In the last trimester a woman may be asked to count fetal movements, commonly called kick counts.

The woman should be asked about the **signs of labor** at each visit. A discussion of contractions, bleeding, and rupture of membranes will help the woman learn how to identify preterm labor. She should be cautioned to call the health care provider or go to the hospital if she thinks any of these signs are occurring.

Objective E: To Understand Common Discomforts of Pregnancy

6.10 Common Discomforts of Pregnancy

Many women experience discomforts of pregnancy that are not serious but detract from the woman's feeling of comfort and well-being. The nurse needs to discuss these discomforts with patients so they know that the discomforts they are experiencing are normal, along with how to overcome these discomforts.

The nausea and vomiting of pregnancy are frequently called "***morning sickness***," because these symptoms are more acute on arising. However, they can occur at any time and may continue throughout the day. Morning sickness occurs in ~75% of pregnant women. For most women, it is self-limiting, and although it is distressful, it does not cause harm to the woman or fetus. However, morning sickness must be distinguished from ***hyperemesis gravidarum***, a condition in which severe vomiting, weight loss, dehydration, electrolyte imbalance, and ketosis can occur. Although the cause is unknown, it is believed to be related to increased levels of hCG and estrogen. Nausea usually ends by the second trimester.

Several antihistamines may be prescribed safely. Various nonpharmacologic remedies may be used, such as crackers or ginger, but should be discussed with the health care provider before use.

Heartburn, an acute burning sensation in the epigastric and sternal regions, occurs in two thirds of pregnant women. Heartburn occurs when reverse peristaltic waves cause regurgitation of acidic stomach contents into the esophagus. The underlying causes are diminished gastric motility and displacement of the stomach by the enlarging uterus. Heartburn can often be relieved by eating small meals, not eating prior to sleeping, or taking calcium/antacid tablets.

Backache is a common complaint during the third trimester. The expanding uterus and the hormone relaxin result in progressive changes that can lead to muscle strain and backache during the last trimester. Prevention of backache with correct posture and body mechanics is a primary focus of teaching.

Round ligament pain is a sharp pain in the side or inguinal area that results from softening and stretching of the ligament from hormones and uterine growth.

Urinary frequency is a common complaint of women during the first and third trimesters, from the growing uterus pressing on the bladder. The condition is usually manageable by women without undue stress, although some may use Kegel exercises to maintain bladder control.

Varicosities occur in 40% of pregnancies and most often occur in those with a family history of them, those who are obese, and in multiparas. During pregnancy the weight of the growing uterus partially compresses the veins returning blood from the legs. As blood pools in the legs, in time the veins may become engorged, inflamed, and painful. Varicose veins are exacerbated by prolonged standing during which the force of gravity makes blood return more difficult. Although varicosities tend to be in the legs, they may also involve the veins of the vulva or rectum (hemorrhoids).

Hemorrhoids may be external (outside the anus) or internal (above the anal sphincter). Some common causes of hemorrhoids are vascular engorgement of the pelvis, constipation, straining at stool, and prolonged standing or sitting. Pushing during the second stage of labor may aggravate the problem, and they may continue into the postpartum period. Topical anesthetic ointments or astringents (witch hazel pads) are measures used for comfort. The patient can try to prevent hemorrhoids by avoiding standing or sitting for long periods when blood in the lower extremities can pool.

Occasional ***constipation*** is not harmful but can cause discomfort by causing feelings of abdominal fullness and flatulence, and can aggravate hemorrhoids. Intestinal motility is decreased during pregnancy and may result in decreased frequency of bowel movements and/or dry, hard stools. Iron supplementation may increase constipation.

Leg cramps are experienced by many women, often during sleep. Leg cramps may be caused by an imbalance of serum calcium and phosphorus, although this has not been proven. Low magnesium levels may also be a cause, and magnesium supplementation may be helpful. Venous congestion in the legs during the third trimester also contributes to leg cramps.

Fatigue is experienced by many pregnant women during the first trimester. The direct cause is unknown but is thought to be from changes in hormones.

Review Exercises

True/False

1. _______ Probable indicators of pregnancy are objective findings that can be documented by an examiner.

2. _______ Fetal movements are usually first noticed by pregnant women at 16 to 20 weeks' gestation.

3. _______ Pregnancy causes a predictable pattern of uterine growth.

4. _______ The pregnant woman may feel fatigue during the first trimester of pregnancy.

5. _______ The recommended weight gain for a normal-weight woman is 40 to 50 pounds.

6. _______ Urinary frequency is a common discomfort of pregnancy during the second trimester.

7. _______ The usual schedule for antepartum visits during the last month of pregnancy is twice weekly.

8. _______ The uterine fundus should be at the level of the umbilicus at 20 weeks' gestation.

9. _______ If a pregnant woman is determined to be rubella nonimmune, she will be given the rubella vaccine as soon as possible.

10. _______ Serum alpha fetoprotein should be done at 24 weeks' postpartum.

11. _______ The 3-hour glucose challenge test is given to every pregnant woman between 24 and 28 weeks' gestation.

12. _______ High levels of progesterone predisposes a pregnant woman to deep vein thrombosis (DVTs).

13. _______ The bluish discoloration of the cervix in pregnancy is called Chadwick sign.

14. _______ Goodell sign is the softening of the cervix that occurs in pregnancy.

15. _______ Infants born to hepatitis-positive mothers need to be given hepatitis immune globulin.

Calculations

Calculate the following due dates:

1. Last menstrual period (LMP) 2/14/11 _______________
2. LMP 8/29/10 _______________
3. LMP 7/24/10 _______________
4. LMP 12/30/10 _______________
5. LMP 11/3/10 _______________

Determine gravida and parity:

6. Ms. Smith is 34 weeks' pregnant with her first baby: _______________
7. Ms. Troy has three children at home and is in labor at the hospital: _______________

Determine TPAL:

8. Ms. Cruz had one elective abortion, one miscarriage at 13 weeks, one full-term delivery, and is 39 weeks' pregnant now: _______________
9. Ms. Ryan is 38 weeks' pregnant now with twins, had two elective abortions, and had two full-term deliveries: _______________
10. Ms. Jones had two miscarriages, one delivery at 32 weeks' gestation (boy now 3 years old), and is now pregnant at 40 weeks' gestation: _______________

Answers

True/False

1. True
2. True
3. True
4. True

5. False. The recommended weight gain is 25 to 35 pounds.

6. False. Urinary frequency experienced by pregnant women is usually during the first and third trimesters.

7. False. Antepartum visits during the last month of pregnancy are usually once weekly.

8. True

9. False. Rubella vaccine has to be given postpartum because it is a live virus and cannot be given during pregnancy.

10. False. Serum alpha fetoprotein is done between 16 and 18 weeks' gestation.

11. False. Only women who have high 1-hour glucose results are sent for further testing with the 3-hour glucose challenge test.

12. True

13. True

14. True

15. True

Calculations

1. 11/21/11 (February 14, 2011 – 3 months = November 14, 2010 + 7days = November 21 + next year)

2. 6/5/11 (August 29, 2010 – 3 months = May 29 + 7days = June 5 + next year)

3. 5/1/11 (July 24, 2010 – 3 months = April 24 + 7 days = May 1 + next year)

4. 10/7/11 (December 30, 2010 – 3 months = September 30 + 7 days = October 7 + next year)

5. 8/10/11 (November 3, 2010 – 3 months = August 3 + 7 days = August 10 + next year)

6. G1P0 Patient's first time pregnant, has not delivered

7. G4P3 Patient's fourth time pregnant, has not delivered

8. T2P0A2L1 = 1 full-term child (delivered), and pregnant now (full-term); P = 0 (no preterm births after 20 weeks' gestation); A = 2 (1 elective abortion, 1 miscarriage [spontaneous] at 13 weeks); L = 1 (1 child living)

9. T2P0A2L2 = 3 (2 full-term pregnancies delivered and now pregnant [full-term]); no premature deliveries; A = 2 (2 elective abortions); L = 2 children alive

10. T1P1A2L1 = 1 (her pregnancy now is full-term); P = 1 (her 3-year-old was born prematurely at 32 weeks); A = 2 (2 miscarriages); L = 1 (1 child living)

Genetics and Fetal Development

Objective A: To Understand Basic Concepts of Inheritance

7.1 Basic Concepts of Inheritance

Hereditary factors influence a person's development from before conception until death. ***DNA*** (deoxyribonucleic acid) is the fundamental unit, or building block, of genes and chromosomes. It is made up of three units: a sugar (deoxyribose), a phosphate group, and one of four nitrogen bases (adenine, thymine, guanine, or cytosine).

DNA resembles a spiral ladder, with a sugar and a phosphate group forming each side of the ladder and a pair of nitrogen bases forming each rung. The four bases of the DNA molecule pair in a fixed way, allowing the DNA to be accurately duplicated during each cell division. The DNA also directs the manufacture of proteins needed for cell function.

The fundamental unit of heredity in humans is a linear sequence of working subunits of DNA called ***genes.*** DNA carries the instructions that allow cells to make proteins and transmit hereditary information from one cell to another. Most genes are located on chromosomes found in the nucleus of cells. Genes occupy a specific location along each chromosome. Genes come in pairs, with one copy inherited from each parent. Many genes come in a number of variant forms, known as alleles. Different alleles produce different characteristics, such as hair color and blood type. One form of the allele (dominant) can be more greatly expressed than the other one (recessive).

All normal somatic (body) cells contain 46 chromosomes that are arranged as 23 pairs of homologous, or matched, chromosomes. One chromosome of each pair is inherited from each parent. Twenty-two of the pairs are autosomes (nonsex chromosomes that are common to both female and males), and there is one pair of sex chromosomes that determines gender. The autosomes are involved in the transmission of all genetic traits and conditions other than those associated with the sex-linked chromosome.

The large ***X chromosome*** is the female chromosome; the small male chromosome is the ***Y chromosome.*** The presence of a Y chromosome causes the embryo to develop as a male; in the absence of a Y chromosome, the embryo develops as a female. Thus, a normal female has a 46 XX chromosome constitution; a normal male has a 46 XY chromosome constitution. The two distinct sex chromosomes carry the genes that transmit sex-linked traits and conditions. Because the chromosomes are paired, there are two copies of each gene. If the gene pairs are identical, they are homozygous; if they are different, they are heterozygous. In the heterozygous state, if one allele is expressed over the other, that allele is considered dominant. Recessive traits can be expressed when the allele responsible for the trait is found on both chromosomes.

The sex of the embryo is determined at fertilization and is dependent on the sperm (X or Y) that fertilizes the ovum. The union of these highly specialized cells marks the beginning of each unique human being. In practice, estimation of pregnancy is calculated from the first day of a woman's last menstrual period, although fertilization usually occurs approximately 2 weeks after the beginning of the woman's last normal menstrual period. ***Gestation*** is defined as the length of time from conception to birth. In humans, the gestational period ranges from 259 to 287 days.

7.2 Inherited Malformations

Heritable characteristics describe those that can be passed on to offspring. The manner in which genetic material is transmitted to the next generation is dependent on the number of genes involved in the expression of the trait.

The majority of congenital malformations result from ***multifactorial inheritance,*** a combination of genetic and environmental influences. They may range from mild to severe depending on the number of genes for the particular defect and the amount of the environmental influence. Examples of these malformations include cleft lip and palate, neural tube defects, and pyloric stenosis.

Unifactorial, **or** ***single-gene, inheritance*** describes a pattern of inheritance that results when a specific trait or disorder is controlled by a single gene. There are many more single-gene disorders than chromosomal abnormalities. They can be autosomal dominant, autosomal recessive, X-linked dominant, or X-linked recessive.

Autosomal dominant inheritance disorders are caused by a single altered gene along one of the autosomes. In most situations, the affected individual comes from a family of multiple generations that have the disorder. The variant allele may also arise from a mutation (a spontaneous, permanent change in the normal gene structure). In this case, the disorder occurs for the first time in the family. An affected parent has a 50% chance of passing the variant allele to each offspring.

Autosomal recessive inheritance disorders are expressed in an individual when both members of an autosomal gene pair are altered. Although each parent carries the recessive altered gene, neither is affected by the disorder because each is heterozygous for the trait, and the altered gene is not expressed. Each parent, or carrier, of the autosomal recessive disorder has a 25% risk of passing the disorder to each offspring, who will then have no normal gene to carry out the necessary function. Because parents must pass the same altered gene for expression of the disorder to occur in their children, an increased incidence of the disorder occurs in closely related parents and in certain populations. Examples include sickle cell disease, phenylketonuria (PKU), and galactosemia.

X-linked autosomal dominant inheritance disorders are the results of an alteration in a gene located along an X chromosome. Because females have two X chromosomes, these disorders occur twice as frequently in females than in males. When the gene is dominant, it need be present on only one of the X chromosomes for symptoms of the disorder to be expressed. X-linked dominant disorders are passed from an affected male to all of his daughters, because daughters receive the father's altered X chromosome. Conversely, none of the sons are affected because they receive only the father's Y chromosome.

A female with an X-linked dominant disorder has a 50% chance of passing the altered genes to her offspring. Each child of a female with an X-linked dominant disorder has a 1 in 2 chance of expressing the disorder. Examples of X-linked dominant disorders include hypophosphatemia and cervico-oculo-acoustic syndrome.

X-linked recessive inheritance disorders are more common than X-linked dominant disorders and occur more frequently in males because males have a single X chromosome, and the single Y chromosome carries the altered gene. When the male receives a single altered gene, the disorder is expressed. For the disorder to be expressed in females, the altered gene must be present on both X chromosomes.

A female who is a carrier of a gene that causes an X-linked recessive disorder has a 50% risk of passing the abnormal gene to her male offspring. Each son has a 1 in 2 chance of expressing the disorder. The female carrier also has a 50% chance of passing the altered gene to her female offspring, who will have a 1 in 2 chance of becoming carriers of the altered gene. A son who is affected by the X-linked disorder has a 100% chance of passing the variant X to his daughters, as the affected father has only one X to pass on. Fathers cannot transmit the altered gene to their male offspring because they transmit the Y instead of the X chromosomes to their sons. Examples of X-linked recessive disorders include color blindness, hemophilia A, and muscular dystrophy.

Objective B: To Understand Cellular Division

7.3 Cellular Division

Human cells can be categorized as either gametes (sperm and eggs) or somatic cells (any body cell that contains 46 chromosomes in its nucleus). Cells reproduce through either meiosis or mitosis. ***Meiosis*** is a process of cell division that leads to the development of sperm and ova, each containing half the number of chromosomes as normal cells. Mitosis is the process of the formation of two identical cells that are exactly the same as the original cell and have the normal amount of chromosomes.

Meiosis occurs during gametogenesis, the process by which cells, or gametes, are produced. During cell division, the genetic complement of the cells is reduced by one half. During meiosis, a sex cell containing 46 chromosomes divides into two, and then four, cells, each containing 23 chromosomes. The resulting cells are exactly alike, but they are all different from the original cell.

In the second division, each chromosome divides, and each half moves to the opposite sides of the cell. The cells divide to form four cells containing 23 single chromosomes each. When the female and male gametes unite to form a fertilized ovum (zygote), the normal number of 46 chromosomes is reestablished. The entire process results in the creation of four gamete cells from one sex cell.

Objective C: To Understand the Process of Fertilization

7.4 Fertilization

Fertilization is a complex series of events. Transportation of the gametes must occur to allow the oocyte and the sperm to meet. This meeting most often occurs in the fallopian tube, in the ampulla. After the first meiotic division, the oocyte is expelled from the ovary during ovulation and passes to the ampulla. With an ejaculation, up to 600 million sperm are deposited around the external cervical os and in the fornix of the vagina. During ovulation, the cervical mucus increases and becomes less viscous and more favorable for sperm penetration. The sperm swim upward through the fallopian tubes. Fusion of the pronuclei of both the oocyte and sperm create a single zygote. The zygote is genetically unique in that it contains half of its chromosomes from the mother and half from the father.

Objective D: To Understand the Process of Implantation and Placental Development

7.5 Implantation and Placental Development

The preembryonic period is the first 2 weeks after conception. Around the fourth day after conception, the fertilized ovum, now called a ***zygote,*** enters the uterus. After several divisions, the cells become tightly compacted and become known as the ***morula***. The outer cells of the morula secrete fluid, forming a ***blastocyst,*** a sac of cells with an inner mass placed off the center within the sac. The inner cell mass develops into the fetus. Part of the outer layer of cells develops as the placenta and fetal membranes.

When the blastocyst contains 100 cells or so, it enters the uterus. It lingers in the uterus 2 to 4 days before it implants itself into the uterus. Normal implantation occurs in the upper uterus, often on the posterior wall of the uterus. This process is called ***nidation.*** The upper uterus is the best area for implantation because

1. The upper uterus is richly supplied with blood for optimal fetal nutrition and gas exchange.
2. The uterine lining is thick in the upper uterus, preventing the placenta from attaching too deeply into the uterine muscle and facilitating easy expulsion after delivery.
3. Implantation in the upper uterus limits blood loss after birth because strong interlacing muscle fibers in this area compress the open endometrial vessel after the placenta detaches.

Enzymes produced by the ***conceptus,*** or the product of the union of oocyte and spermatozoon, erode the decidua and tap into maternal sources of nutrition by diffusion because the circulatory system is not yet established. Chorionic villi are small projections on the surface of the conceptus extending into the endometrium and (later form the fetal side of the placenta). The conceptus is fully implanted within the mother's uterus by 10 days.

The ***placenta*** is a thick, disk-shaped organ. The placenta has two parts: maternal and fetal. It is involved in metabolic, transfer, and endocrine functions. The fetal side is smooth (also known as "shiny Schultz"), with branching vessels over the membrane-covered surface. The maternal side is rough (also known as "dirty Duncan"), where it attaches to the uterus. The umbilical cord is normally inserted on the fetal side of the placenta, near the center. However, it may insert off center or even out on the fetal membranes.

When conception occurs, cells of the mother's endometrium undergo changes that promote early nutrition of the embryo and enable most of the uterine lining to be shed after birth. These changes convert endometrial cells into the ***decidua.*** In addition to providing nourishment for the embryo, the decidua protects the mother from uncontrolled invasion of the placenta into the uterine wall. The three decidual layers are the decidua basalis, which underlies the developing embryo and forms the maternal side of the placenta; the decidua capsularis, which overlies the embryo; and the decidua parietalis, which lines the rest of the uterine cavity. By 22 weeks' gestation, the decidua capsularis fuses with the decidua parietalis and fills in the uterine cavity.

Maternal and fetal blood do not mix in pregnancy, although they do flow closely to each other. Exchange of substances between mother and fetus occurs within the intervillous spaces of the placenta. The fetal side of the placenta develops from the outer cell layer of the blastocyte at the same time the inner cell mass develops into the embryo and fetus. The chorionic villi are the structures that eventually form the fetal side of the placenta. Maternal blood spills into the intervillous spaces through arteries in the decidua. After oxygenated and nutrient-rich blood washes over the chorionic villi containing the fetal vessels, it returns to the maternal circulation through the endometrial veins for elimination of fetal waste products.

The fetal side of the placenta develops from the outer cell layer of the blastocyst at the same time the inner cell mass develops into the embryo and fetus. The chorionic villi are the initial structures that eventually form the fetal side of the placenta. Two umbilical arteries and one umbilical vein transport blood between the fetus and the fetal side of the placenta.

Respiration is a key function of the placenta. Oxygen and carbon dioxide pass through the placenta through simple diffusion. The growing fetus requires a constant supply of nutrients from the mother. Glucose, fatty acids, vitamins, and electrolytes pass readily across the placenta. Glucose is the major energy source for fetal growth and metabolic activity. In addition to carbon dioxide, urea, uric acid, and bilirubin are readily transferred from fetus to mother for disposal.

Many of the immunoglobulin G (IgG) class of antibodies are passed from mother to fetus through the placenta. This confers passive immunity to the fetus against disease that is beneficial to the newborn, which will not produce antibodies against disease for several months after birth.

The placenta produces several hormones necessary for normal pregnancy. Human chorionic gonadotropin (hCG) causes the corpus luteum (site of the ovarian follicle that releases an egg during ovulation) to persist for the first 6 to 8 weeks of pregnancy and secretes estrogen and progesterone. As the pregnancy progresses, it takes over the production of estrogen and progesterone, and the corpus luteum regresses. Human placental lactogen is also produced, promoting normal nutrition and growth of the fetus and maternal breast development for lactation.

Objective E: To Understand the Fetal Membranes and the Function of the Amniotic Fluid

7.6 Fetal Membranes and the Amniotic Fluid

The two fetal membranes are the amnion and chorion. The ***amnion*** is continous with the surface of the umbilical cord, joining the epithelium of the fetus's abdominal skin. Chorionic villi proliferate over the entire surface of the gestational sac for the first 8 weeks after conception. As the embryo grows, it bulges into the uterine cavity. The villi on the outer surface eventually atrophy and become the ***chorion.*** The remaining villi will branch out and enlarge to form the fetal side of the placenta.

Amniotic fluid is derived from two sources: fetal urine and fluid transported from the maternal blood across the amnion. Amniotic fluid protects the fetus by cushioning against impacts to the maternal abdomen and thermoregulation.

Amniotic fluid promotes fetal growth by allowing symmetric development as the major body surfaces fold toward the midline, allows room and buoyancy for fetal movement, and prevents membranes from adhering to developing fetal parts.

The water of the amniotic fluid changes by absorption across the amnion, returning to the mother. The fetus also swallows amniotic fluid and absorbs it in the digestive tract. Waste products are returned to the placenta through umbilical arteries.

The volume of amniotic fluid increases during pregnancy. An abnormally low amount of fluid is called ***oligohydramnios*** and may be associated with poor placental blood flow, preterm rupture of the membrane, failure of fetal kidney development, or blocked urinary excretion. ***Hydramnios,*** also called ***polyhydramnios,*** is an extra amount of amniotic fluid and is associated with poorly controlled maternal diabetes; imbalanced water exchange among mother, fetus, and placenta; or malformation of the central nervous system (CNS), cardiovascular system, or gastrointestinal tract that interferes with normal fluid ingestion, metabolism, or excretion.

Objective F: To Understand Embryonic Period of Development

7.7 Embryonic Period of Development

The embryonic period of development extends from the beginning of the third week after conception through 8 weeks after conception. Basic structures of all major body organs are completed during the embryonic period.

The embryo progresses from undifferentiated cells with essentially identical functions to differentiated, specialized body cells. Development of these specialized structures is controlled by three factors: genetic information in the chromosomes received from the parents, interaction between adjacent tissues, and timing.

During the embryonic period, structures are vulnerable to damage from teratogens because they are developing rapidly. Teratogens (drugs, radiation, and infectious agents) can cause developmental or structural anomalies in the embryo, and a variety of internal and external developmental events may cause structural and functional defects. Normal development of one structure often requires normal and properly timed development of another structure.

Development of the embryo and fetus proceeds in a cephalocaudal and central-to-peripheral direction. Generalized to specific development continues with refinement of organs, such as development of bones, joints, muscles, and tendons of the arm and hand.

By week 2, implantation (nidation) is complete. The most growth occurs in the outer cells, which eventually becomes the fetal part of the placenta. The inner cell mass will develop into the baby.

In week 3, the CNS begins developing. Early heart development begins, and the primitive heart begins beating at 22 or 23 days, resulting in a wavelike flow of blood. Primitive blood cells arise from the endoderm lining the distal blood vessels.

The shape of the embryo changes during the fourth week after fertilization. It folds at the head and tail end, resembling a C-shaped cylinder. The neural tube closes during the fourth week. Formation of the face and upper respiratory tract begins. The upper extremities appear as buds on the lateral body walls. Partitioning of the heart into four chambers begins. The trachea branches to form the left and right bronchi.

During the fifth week, the brain grows rapidly. Upper limb buds are paddle-shaped with obvious notches between the fingers, although the lower extremities are not as defined.

During the sixth week, the heart reaches its final four-chambered form. Upper and lower extremities continue to become more defined. Facial development begins with eyes, ears, and nasal pits that are widely separated and aligned with the body walls.

During week 7, general growth and refinement occur. The face becomes more human-looking. The trunk elongates and straightens.

By week 8, the embryo has a definite human form, and refinements to all systems continue. Fingers and toes are clearly defined. The external genitalia begin to differentiate.

Objective G: To Understand Fetal Period of Development

7.8 Fetal Period of Development

The fetal period is the longest period of fetal development. It begins 9 weeks after fertilization and ends with the birth of the baby. All major systems are present in their basic forms. During the period from 9 to 12 weeks, the body begins growing faster than the head, and the crown-rump length more than doubles by the 12th week. The extremities approach their final relative lengths, although the legs remain shorter than the arms. The first fetal movements begin but are too slight for the mother to detect. The fetus begins producing urine during this period and excretes it into the amniotic fluid. Certain developments occur at specific weeks during this period:

- Week 10: The face is recognizably human.
- Week 11: The intestinal contents leave the umbilical cord and enter the abdomen.
- Week 12: Blood formation switches from the liver to the spleen; fetal gender can be determined by the appearance of external genitalia.

During weeks 13 through 16, the fetus grows rapidly in length, so the head becomes smaller than the body. Movements strengthen, and some women may feel fetal movement, referred to as ***quickening.*** The face looks human, with the eyes and ears in alignment with each other. Ossification of the skeleton takes place, and the bones become clearly visible on ultrasound examination.

During weeks 17 through 20, fetal movements feel like fluttering. Changes in skin and hair are evident. Vernix caseosa, a cheeselike coating, covers the skin to protect it from constant exposure to amniotic fluid. Lanugo, a fine down hair, covers the fetal body and helps the vernix adhere to the skin. Both vernix and lanugo diminish as the fetus reaches term. Eyebrows and head hair also appear. Brown fat is deposited at the back of the neck, behind the sternum, and around the kidneys. This heat-producing fat helps the newborn maintain temperature stability after birth.

During weeks 21 through 24, the lungs begin to produce ***surfactant,*** a surface-active lipid substance that facilitates lung expansion and makes it easier for the baby to breathe after birth. Surfactant reduces tension in the lung alveoli and prevents them from collapsing with each breath. The skin appears pink or red as blood is now visible in the capillaries. Rapid eye movements begin. By the 24th week, the fetus has fingernails.

Weeks 25 through 28 are important because if the fetus is born at this time, it is likely to survive because of maturation of the lungs, pulmonary capillaries, and CNS. Blood formation shifts from the spleen to the bone marrow. The fetus usually assumes a head-down position during this time, which is more favorable for birth.

During the period of weeks 29 through 32, the skin is pigmented according to race and is smooth. Larger blood vessels can be seen over the abdomen. Fingernails and toenails are present. The fetus has more subcutaneous fat, which rounds the body contours.

During weeks 33 through 40, the rate of growth slows as full term approaches. A well-nourished term fetus has abundant subcutaneous fat. The pulmonary system matures to enable efficient breathing after birth. The testes are in the scrotum, and breast buds are enlarged. The fetus has a strong hand grasp reflex and orientation to light. At 38 to 40 weeks' gestation, the average fetus weighs 6.6 to 8.4 ounces (3000–3800 g) and is 17.3 inches to 19.2 inches (40–50 cm) long.

Objective H: To Understand Fetal Circulation

7.9 Fetal Circulation

The course of fetal circulation is from the fetal heart, to the placenta for exchange of oxygen, nutrients, and waste products, and back to the fetus for delivery to fetal tissues. The umbilical cord contains two arteries that carry deoxygenated blood and waste products away from the fetus to the placenta, where these substances are transferred to the mother's circulation. The umbilical vein carries freshly oxygenated and nutrient-laden blood from the placenta back to the fetus. The cord is cushioned with Wharton's jelly to prevent obstruction resulting from pressure. Because the fetus does not breathe air, several alterations of the postnatal fetal circulatory route are needed. The liver also does not have the metabolic functions that it will have after birth.

Three shunts in the fetal circulatory system allow blood with the highest oxygen concentration to be sent to the fetal heart and brain: the ductus venosa, foramen ovale, and ductus arteriosus. At birth, the infant's lungs oxygenate the blood, the placenta is removed from the circulatory path, and the liver must perform its metabolic functions. The path of the fetal circulatory system is

1. Oxygenated blood from the placenta enters the fetal body through the umbilical vein.
2. About two thirds of the blood goes through the liver, and the rest bypasses the liver and enters the inferior vena cava through the first shunt, the ductus venosus.
3. The blood then enters the right atrium and mixes with deoxygenated blood from the lower body and head.
4. Most of the blood passes through the left atrium through the second shunt, the foramen ovale, where it mixes with the small amount of blood returning from the lungs.
5. Blood is pumped from the left ventricle into the aorta to nourish the body.
6. A small amount of blood from the right ventricle is circulated to the lungs and the lung tissue.
7. The rest of the blood from the right ventricle joins oxygenated blood in the aorta through the third shunt, the ductus arteriosus.
8. The head and upper body receive the greatest amount of oxygenated blood.

The wall of the right ventricle of the fetal heart is thicker than that of the left because resistance to blood flow through the uninflated lungs is high, similar to the resistance in other parts of the fetal body When the infant begins breathing at birth, resistance to pulmonary blood flow from the right ventricle falls, whereas resistance to systemic flow from the left ventricle rises. The thickness of the wall of the left ventricle increases to meet greater resistance to systemic outflow. The thickness of the right ventricle shows little change. As cardiac growth progresses throughout childhood, the thickness of the left ventricle remains greater than that of the right ventricle.

Fetal circulatory shunts are not needed after birth because an infant oxygenates blood in the lungs and is not circulating blood to the placenta. As the infant breathes, blood flow to the lungs increases, pressure in the right side of the heart falls, and the foramen ovale closes. The ductus arteriosus constricts as the arterial oxygen level rises. The ductus venosus constricts when the flow of blood from the umbilical cord stops.

Transition to the postnatal circulatory pattern is gradual. Functional closure begins when the infant breathes and the cord is cut, removing the placenta from the circulation. The foramen ovale and ductus venosus are permanently closed as tissue proliferates in these structures. The ductus venosus becomes a ligament, as do the umbilical vein and arteries.

Objective I: To Understand Genetic Counseling

7.10 Genetic Counseling

The purpose of genetic counseling is to educate individuals or families with accurate information so that they can make informed decisions about reproduction and appropriate care for affected members. Genetic counseling is often available through facilities that provide maternal-fetal medicine services. State departments of mental health, mental retardation, and rehabilitation services also may provide counseling services.

Individuals or families may request genetic counseling before or during a pregnancy or after a child has been born with a defect. Genetic counseling services may be a slow process, with many visits needed over time. Multiple family members may be needed for evaluation. Typically, a genetic evaluation consists of a complete medical history of the individuals involved, whether it be a preconception couple or a family with a member with a defect; the medical history of other family members; laboratory, imaging, and other studies; physical assessment of the child with the birth defect and other family members as needed; and construction of a genogram to identify relationships among family members and their relevant medical history.

If a diagnosis is established, genetic counseling educates the family about what is known about the disorder, the natural cause of the disorder, the likelihood that the disorder will occur or recur in other family members, the availability of prenatal diagnosing, and the availability of services and treatment for the person with the disorder.

Genetic counseling is nondirective; the counselor educates the individual/family so they can make informed decisions. Comprehensive genetic counseling includes services of professionals from many disciplines, such as biology, medicine, nursing, social work, and education.

Objective J: To Understand Factors that May Adversely Affect Embryonic and Fetal Development

7.11 Factors that May Adversely Affect Embryonic and Fetal Development

Damage to the developing fetus/embryo may result from genetic factors or from maternal exposure to various environmental factors. In most circumstances, the uterus provides a stable environment for the developing embryo and fetus.

Genetic defects and congenital anomalies usually result from genetic factors, environmental hazards, or a combination of both. However, the exact cause of anomalies is unknown in ~50% of cases. Congenital anomalies may occur singularly or in combination with other defects. Single, minor anomalies occur in ~14% of newborns. Major developmental defects are more common in embryos that are usually spontaneously aborted. It is estimated that approximately one third of all birth defects are caused by genetic factors.

Damage may have already occurred to the chromosomes of one or both parents before fertilization, or one or both may carry a defective gene inherited from their own parents. The extent of teratogenic effect depends on the developmental timing, duration, and dosage of exposure, as well as the maternal genetic susceptibility. Greater exposure during early gestation is associated with more severe defects, which demonstrates the need for preconceptual care for young adults of childbearing age.

The period of ***organogenesis*** lasts from approximately the 2nd through the 11th week of gestation, during which the embryo undergoes rapid growth and differentiation. During this period the embryo is extremely vulnerable to teratogens, such as medications, alcohol, tobacco, caffeine, illegal drugs, radiation, and maternal (TORCH) infections. Structural defects are most likely to occur during this period because exposure to teratogens during this critical period of development of an organ can cause a malformation.

After 11 weeks the fetus becomes more resistant to damage from teratogens because the organ systems have been established. However, insults that occur later in fetal life or early infancy may cause mental retardation, blindness, hearing loss, deafness, or malignancy.

The most critical time for brain development is between 3 and 16 weeks of development; however, the brain tissue continues to grow rapidly until at least the first 2 years of life. Diet and nutrition play an important role during this time. Amino acids, glucose, and fatty acids are considered the primary dietary factors in brain growth and are needed in proper concentrations during this critical period.

As for medications and other substances, many women unintentionally take medications during pregnancy when they do not know yet that they are pregnant. A small number of medications and other substances are strongly suspected to be human teratogens. These include fat-soluble vitamins, alcohol, tobacco, caffeine, cocaine, opiates, anticonvulsants, warfarin, cardiovascular agents, retinoids, certain hormones, antineoplastic agents, certain anti-infective agents, thalidomide, and methyl mercury. Both high and low doses of vitamin A can cause fetal malformations that include anomalies of the CNS, microtia, and clefts. Vitamin D deficiency may cause poor fetal growth, neonatal hypocalcemia, rickets, and poor tooth enamel. High doses of vitamin E may increase the risk of bleeding problems.

Alcohol is one of the most potent teratogens known. A safe threshold for the use of alcohol during pregnancy has never been established. Current data suggest that children of mothers who chronically ingested large amounts of alcohol or who engaged in binge drinking (five or more drinks on one occasion) during pregnancy are at greatest risk for permanent damage.

Cigarette smoking during pregnancy is associated with overall reduction in fetal growth, cleft lip anomalies, impaired infant neurobehavior, and decreased babbling in infants. Nicotine causes vasoconstriction of the uterine blood vessels, resulting in a decreased flow of nutrients and oxygen to the fetus. Smoking doubles the risk of having low birth weight babies.

Caffeine stimulates the CNS and cardiac function and produces vasoconstriction and mild diuresis. The half-life of caffeine is tripled during pregnancy. Although caffeine readily crosses the placenta during pregnancy, it is not known to be a teratogen. However, there is no assurance that maternal consumption of large quantities of caffeine is safe for the developing fetus.

Marijuana passes through the placenta and may remain in the fetus for 30 days. For pregnant women, it increases the risk of combination drug use (cocaine and alcohol), anemia, and low weight gain. For the fetus, marijuana may cause intrauterine growth restriction, adverse effects on neonatal neurobehavior (irritability, tremors, and photosensitivity), and can affect cognitive and language development in infants up to 48 months of age.

Cocaine and ***crack*** use during pregnancy causes vasoconstriction of the uterine vessels and adversely affects blood flow to the fetus. Cocaine use during pregnancy is associated with spontaneous abortion, abruption placentae, stillbirth, intrauterine growth restriction, fetal distress, meconium staining, and preterm birth. Manifestations in children of mothers who used cocaine during their pregnancy include altered neurologic and behavioral disturbances.

The ***opiates*** morphine, heroin, and methadone are sometimes used by pregnant women. Neonatal withdrawal syndrome, characterized by hyperirritability, gastrointestinal dysfunction, respiratory distress, and autonomic disturbances, are associated with infants born to opiate-dependent mothers.

Sedatives, including barbiturates and tranquilizers, are associated with withdrawal syndrome, seizures, and delayed lung maturity in the neonate.

Amphetamines (also known as speed, crystal, or ice) are associated with intrauterine growth restriction, prematurity, cardiac anomalies, cleft palate, and placental abruption. After delivery, affected neonates may exhibit hypoglycemia, sweating, poor visual tracking, lethargy, and difficulty feeding.

High levels of ***radiation*** during pregnancy may cause damage to chromosomes and embryonic cells. Radiation can adversely affect fetal physical growth and cause mental retardation, stunted growth, deformities, abnormal brain function, or the development of cancer later in life.

Lead passes through the placenta and has been found to be associated with spontaneous abortion, fetal anomalies, and preterm birth. The nervous system is the most sensitive target of lead exposure. Fetal anomalies associated with lead exposure include hemangiomas, lymphangiomas, hydrocele, minor skin abnormalities, and undescended testes.

TORCH infections are a group of agents that can infect the fetus or the newborn. These include toxoplasmosis, rubella, cytomegalovirus (CMV), the herpes simplex virus, and other infections.

Toxoplasma gondii is the single-celled parasite responsible for toxoplasmosis. The majority of people infected with this parasite are asymptomatic and unaware of the disease. When symptomatic, symptoms are described as flulike and include swollen lymph nodes, glandular pain, and myalgia. Severe infection can cause damage to the eyes, brain, or organs.

Toxoplasmosis is usually contracted by eating raw or poorly cooked meat contaminated with *T. gondii.* The disease may also be acquired from infected animal feces, most commonly infected cat feces.

Once maternal infection occurs, the organism crosses the placental membranes and infects the fetus, causing damage to the eyes and brain. If the infection is acquired very early in the gestation period, death can occur to the fetus.

Other infections known as teratogens are varicella zoster virus (chicken pox), human immunodeficiency virus (HIV), and syphilis.

The ***varicella zoster virus,*** a member of the herpes virus family, causes chickenpox and shingles. Infection with this virus during the first four months of pregnancy is associated with a number of congenital anomalies including muscle atrophy, limb hypoplasia, damage to the eyes and brain, and mental retardation.

HIV may be transmitted to the fetus through the placenta. Without maternal medical intervention, the risk of perinatal transmission of HIV is ~25%, but with appropriate treatment, the risk can be reduced to ~2%.

Treponema pallidum, the microorganism that causes ***syphilis,*** also readily crosses the placenta. The fetus may become infected at any time during gestation. The organism can be destroyed with proper treatment and can prevent placental transmission to the fetus. Left untreated, only 20% of women infected will give birth to a normal infant. Neonatal manifestations include prematurity, skin rash, hydrops fetalis, failure to thrive, hepatosplenomegaly, lymphadenopathy, and bone lesions. Late-onset manifestations include keratitis, deafness, and bowing of the shins.

The ***rubella virus*** (also known as German measles) can also cause damage to the developing fetus. The earlier in the pregnancy it is contracted, the greater the risk to the developing fetus. Birth defects associated with congenital rubella syndrome include hearing loss, eye defects, blindness, heart defects, and mental retardation.

CMV produces no signs or symptoms of infection in the majority of affected individuals. Up to 80% of adults have antibodies to the virus. CMV can cause disease in unborn babies or in persons with weakened immune systems.

Spontaneous abortion (miscarriage) may result from maternal infection in the first trimester. Infection that occurs later in the pregnancy may result in fetal growth restriction, microphthalmia, chorioretinitis, blindness, microcephaly, cerebral calcification, mental retardation, deafness, cerebral palsy, and hepatosplenomegaly. In the neonate, CMV infections are often associated with audiological, neurologic, and neurobehavioral disturbances.

Spontaneous abortion is increased threefold if maternal infection occurs in early pregnancy. Infection after the 20 gestational week is associated with an increased risk of prematurity.

Congenital anomalies associated with the ***herpes simplex virus*** include dermatologic scarring, micrencephaly, hydrencephaly, encephalitis, microphthalmia, chorioretinitis, and hepatosplenomegaly.

Objective K: To Understand the Nursing Role in Genetic Counseling

7.12 The Nursing Role in Genetic Counseling

Nurses have an important role in helping families who are concerned about birth defects. They may be in a position to identify those who need referrals, do teaching, coordinate services, and offer emotional support to those families seeking genetic counseling.

It is important for the nurse to also be knowledgeable of various cultural practices and beliefs that may have an impact on the development of the fetus. Culture influences every aspect of individuals' lives and how they care for themselves and their families. Women from ethnic groups may choose to visit health healers and lay midwives throughout pregnancy.

The nurse should maintain an unbiased and accepting attitude when working with patients from populations with different beliefs and practices. Recognizing that cultural values and experiences shape an individual's likelihood to continue or discontinue familial beliefs and practices helps the nurse to develop a more accepting attitude, keeps the lines of communication open with the patient, and helps deliver appropriate care in a culturally sensitive manner.

Review Exercises

True/False

1. ________ DNA is composed of a sugar and a nitrogen base.
2. ________ The fundamental unit of heredity is a gene.
3. ________ Chromosomes are named Y for female and X for male.
4. ________ A normal female has 46 XX chromosomes.
5. ________ A normal male has 46 YY chromosomes.
6. ________ A female gamete is called an ovum.

7. _______ DNA carries instructions to allow cells to make proteins and to transmit hereditary information from one cell to another.

8. _______ The sex of an embryo is determined at fertilization.

9. _______ Gestation is defined as the length of time from conception to birth of the baby.

10. _______ In humans the gestational period ranges from 259 to 287 days.

11. _______ The majority of congenital malformations result from multifactorial inheritance.

12. _______ Autosomal dominant inheritance disorders are caused by several altered genes along one of the autosomes.

13. _______ Each parent of an autosomal recessive disorder has a 50% chance of passing the disorder to each offspring.

14. _______ The preembryonic period of gestation is the first 3 weeks after conception.

15. _______ Mitosis is the process of forming two identical cells.

16. _______ TORCH infections include toxoplasmosis, other infections, rubella virus, cytomegalovirus, and herpes simplex virus.

17. _______ Infection after the 20th week of gestation with the herpes simplex virus is associated with the risk of prematurity.

18. _______ With appropriate treatment, the risk of HIV transmission to the fetus is 25%.

19. _______ The risk of spontaneous abortion is doubled in mothers who are infected with the herpes simplex virus in the first trimester.

20. _______ Crack use during pregnancy adversely affects blood flow to the fetus.

21. _______ Radiation during pregnancy can lead to the risk to the fetus of developing cancer later in life.

22. _______ The heart is the most sensitive organ affected in the fetus as a result of a mother's exposure to lead during pregnancy.

23. _______ The use of sedatives by the pregnant mother can result in delayed lung maturity in the fetus.

24. _______ The exact cause of congenital anomalies is unknown, but they are seen in ~50% to 60% of cases.

25. _______ Greater exposure to teratogens during early pregnancy is associated with more severe birth defects.

Completion

1. The fertilized ovum is called a _________________________.

2. Normal implantation of the zygote occurs in the _____________________.

3. The conceptus is fully implanted in the mother's uterus in ____________.

4. The placenta has ____________ parts.

5. ____________ is the major energy source for fetal growth and metabolic activity.

6. Oxygen and carbon dioxide pass through the placenta through simple ____________.

7. The placenta produces several hormones for normal pregnancy, including ____________, ____________, and ____________.

8. The class of antibodies that pass from mother to fetus are ____________.

9. Amniotic fluid is derived from two sources: ____________ and ____________.

10. An abnormally low amount of amniotic fluid is termed ____________.

11. Basic structures of all major body organs are completed during the ____________.

12. Nidation is completed by the ____________ week of fetal development.

13. ____________ is the surface-active lipid substance that facilitates lung expansion and makes it easier for the baby to breathe after birth.

14. The umbilical cord contains ____________ artery (arteries) and ____________ vein (veins).

15. Functional closure of the three shunts begins when the infant ____________ and ____________.

16. Brown fat is deposited on the neck, sternum, and kidneys during the ____________ week of fetal development.

17. The ____________ period is the longest period of fetal development.

18. Quickening felt by the mother occurs during the ____________ weeks of fetal development.

19. The central nervous system (CNS) begins developing during the ____________ week of fetal development.

20. Exchange of substances between mother and fetus occurs within the ____________ of the placenta.

21. ____________ is needed for heat production in the newborn.

22. Vitamin ____________ deficiency is associated with poor tooth enamel.

23. The crown-rump length of the fetus doubles by the ____________ week of gestation.

24. The human face becomes recognizable during the ____________ week of gestation.

25. ____________ is one of the most potent teratogens known to the fetus.

Answers

True/False

1. False. DNA is composed of sugar, a nitrogen base, and a phosphate group.
2. True
3. False. The female chromosome is X, and the male chromosome is Y.
4. True
5. False. The normal male chromosome is composed of an X and Y.
6. True
7. True
8. True
9. True
10. True
11. True
12. False. Autosomal dominant inheritance disorders are caused by a single altered gene along one of the autosomes.
13. False. Each parent of an autosomal recessive disorder has a 25% chance of passing the disorder to each offspring.
14. False. The preembryonic period is the first 2 weeks after fertilization.
15. True
16. True
17. True
18. False. With appropriate treatment, the risk of HIV transmission to the fetus can be reduced to 2%.
19. False. The risk of spontaneous abortion is tripled during early pregnancy.
20. True
21. True
22. False. The CNS is the most vulnerable system of the fetus after maternal lead exposure.
23. True
24. True
25. True

Completion

1. Zygote
2. Upper uterus
3. 10 days
4. 2
5. Sugar
6. Diffusion
7. Human chorionic gonadotropin (hcG), estrogen, progesterone
8. Immunoglobulin G (IgG)
9. Mother's blood, fetal urine
10. Oligohydramnios
11. 12 weeks
12. 2 weeks
13. Surfactant

14. Two arteries, one vein
15. Breathes, cord is cut
16. 17 to 20 weeks
17. Fetal period
18. 16 to 20 weeks
19. Third week
20. Intervillous spaces through arteries in the decidua
21. Brown fat
22. Vitamin D
23. 12th week
24. 10th week
25. Alcohol

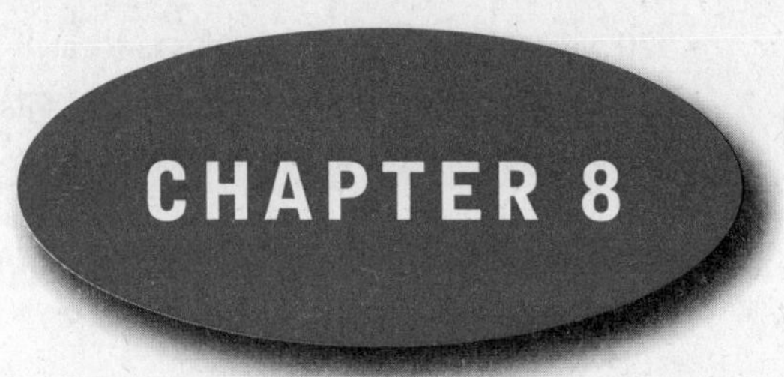

Maternal Adaptation to Pregnancy

Objective A: To Understand What Is Involved in Nursing of the Woman During a Pregnancy

8.1 Pregnancy and the Nursing Role

From the moment of conception, changes occur in the pregnant woman's body that help nourish the fetus, prepare the woman for pregnancy and lactation, maintain the woman's health, and prepare the woman to become a mother.

Women are often puzzled by the changes and unprepared for the physical discomforts that may occur as the result of the pregnancy. Many rely on nurses to provide accurate information and compassionate guidance throughout the pregnancy. Nurses need to understand the physiologic and psychological changes during a pregnancy, especially how these changes affect the daily lives of expectant mothers. Nurses also need to be aware of how cultural beliefs and practices affect the childbearing family in order to provide effective, safe care.

Objective B: To Understand Changes in Body Systems

8.2 Changes in Body Systems

The most dramatic change during pregnancy occurs in the uterus, which before conception is a small, pear-shaped organ entirely contained in the pelvic cavity. Growth is caused by stimulation by estrogen and growth factors and stretching as the embryo grows. During the second and third trimesters, uterine growth of muscle fibers stretching in all directions occurs. Also, fibrous tissue accumulates in the outer muscle layer of the uterus, and the amount of elastic tissue increases.

The uterus grows in a predictable pattern that provides information about fetal growth and helps to confirm the estimated day of delivery. The following developments occur at a particular week of gestation:

- 12 weeks' gestation: the uterus extends out of the maternal pelvis and can be palpated above the symphysis pubis.
- 16 weeks' gestation: the fundus reaches midway between the symphysis pubis and the umbilicus.

- 20 weeks' gestation: the fundus is located approximately at the level of the umbilicus.
- 36 weeks' gestation: the fundus reaches its highest level at the xiphoid process. It pushes against the diaphragm, and the expectant woman may experience shortness of breath, even at rest.
- 40 weeks' gestation: the fetal head descends into the pelvis, and the uterus sinks to a lower level. This descent of the fetal head is called ***lightening,*** because it reduces pressure on the diaphragm and makes breathing easier.

Throughout pregnancy, the uterus undergoes irregular contractions called ***Braxton Hicks contractions***. During the contractions the uterus temporarily tightens, becomes firm, and returns to its original state. During the first two trimesters, the contractions are mild and often are not noticed by the woman. During the last trimester, they become stronger and are often mistaken for the early onset of labor.

As the uterus enlarges, an increase in the size and number of blood vessels expands blood flow dramatically. As pregnancy progresses, the delivery of materials needed for fetal growth and the removal of metabolic wastes depend on adequate perfusion of the placental intervillous spaces. Maternal blood carried by the myometrial arteries enters the intervillous spaces, where oxygen and nutrients are transferred to the chorionic villi and then to the fetus. Metabolic wastes from the fetus diffuse into venous structures of the mother.

The cervix also undergoes significant changes after conception. The most obvious changes occur in color and consistency. In response to rising levels of estrogen, the cervix becomes congested with blood, resulting in the characteristic bluish purple color, referred to as ***Chadwick's sign***. The cervix also softens, which is referred to as ***Goodell sign***.

A less obvious change occurs as the cervical glands proliferate during the pregnancy and the glandular walls become thin; mucus from the cervical glands forms the mucus plug. This plug blocks the ascent of bacteria from the vagina into the uterus and protects the fetus and membranes from infection. The mucus plug remains in place throughout the pregnancy until the onset of labor, when the cervix begins to thin and dilate, allowing the mucus plug to be expelled. One of the earliest signs of labor may be "bloody show," which consists of the mucus plug and a small amount of blood produced by disruption of the cervical capillaries.

Changes in the vagina result from increased vascularity; the walls of the vagina become bluish and soften. Vaginal cells contain an increasing amount of glycogen and favor the growth of *Candida albicans*. Because of this, recurrent yeast infections are common in pregnancy.

Increased vascularity, edema, and connective tissue changes make the tissues of the vulva and perineum more pliable. Pelvic congestion during pregnancy can lead to heightened sexual interest and increased orgasms.

Once conception occurs, the major function of the ovaries is to secrete progesterone for the first 6 to 7 weeks of pregnancy. The corpus luteum secretes progesterone until the placenta is developed and then regresses. ***Progesterone*** is called the ***"hormone of pregnancy"*** because it is needed to maintain a pregnancy. Progesterone helps suppress contractions of the uterus and may also help prevent tissue rejection of the fetus.

Ovulation during pregnancy ceases because the high levels of estrogen and progesterone inhibit the release of follicle-stimulating hormone (FSH) and luteinizing hormone (LH), which are necessary for ovulation.

Breasts change in size and appearance. Estrogen stimulates the growth of mammary ductal tissue, and progesterone promotes the growth of lobes, lobules, and alveoli. The breasts become highly vascular, and veins are often visible just under the surface of the skin. If the increase in breast size is extensive, "stretch marks" (striations) may become evident. The nipples increase in size and become more erect, and the areola becomes more pigmented. Sebaceous glands called Montgomery tubercles (Montgomery glands) become more prominent and secrete a substance that lubricates the nipples. In addition, a thick, yellowish breast fluid, ***colostrum,*** is present beginning in the second trimester and can be readily expressed in the third trimester. Colostrum is the first milk the newborn receives from his or her breastfeeding mother. It is rich in immunoglobulins and gives passive immunity to the infant from the mother.

8.3 Cardiovascular System

Cardiac changes are minor and reverse soon after childbirth. The muscles of the heart enlarge slightly because of the increased workload during pregnancy. The heart is pushed up and toward the left as the uterus elevates the diaphragm during the third trimester. During pregnancy, some heart sounds may be altered and would usually be considered abnormal outside of pregnancy. The changes are first heard between weeks 12 and 20 and continue for up to 4 weeks postpartum. The most common variation in heart sounds are splitting of the first heart sound and a systolic murmur that is found in 90% of pregnant women. Many women have a third heart sound because of rapid filling during diastole.

Plasma volume begins to increase at 6 to 8 weeks of pregnancy, and total blood volume increases ~40% to 50%. The increased volume is needed for two reasons: to transport nutrients and oxygen to the placenta, where they become available to the growing fetus, and to meet the demands of the expanded maternal tissue in the uterus and the breasts. This hypovolemic effect serves to provide a reserve to protect the woman from the adverse effects of blood loss that occurs during childbirth.

The red blood cell (RBC) mass increases by ~25% to 33% above pre-pregnancy values. Although both RBC volume and plasma volume expand, the increase in plasma occurs much earlier. The resulting dilution of the RBC mass causes a decline in maternal hematocrit. This condition is referred to as ***"physiologic anemia"*** because it reflects dilution of RBCs in greatly expanded plasma volume rather than an actual decline of RBCs and does not indicate true anemia.

The blood components erythrocytes, leukocytes, and clotting factors increase during pregnancy. Erythrocytes increase by 25% to 33%, which in turn increases the maternal need for iron that is necessary for hemoglobin formation. Sufficient iron is not always obtained through the woman's diet, so iron supplementation is necessary to prevent the development of iron-deficiency anemia.

Leukocytes increase during pregnancy, during labor, and through the early postpartum period. The level can reach as high as 30,000 cells/mm^3 before infection is ruled out. Pregnancy is a hypercoagulable state in which clotting factors cause an increased ability to form clots. Plasma fibrinogen (factor I) rises ~50%, and plasma fibrin increases by ~40%.

Levels of factors II, VII, VIII, X, and XII are also increased. Fibrolytic activity (breaking down of clots) decreases during pregnancy. These changes offer protection from hemorrhage during childbirth but also increase the risk of clot formation. The risk is of particular concern for women who work standing or sitting for long periods of time.

A major consequence of the expanded blood volume of pregnancy is an increase in cardiac output. Cardiac output is the amount of blood discharged from the heart each minute. Cardiac output rises sharply during the first trimester and increases 30% to 50% by the third trimester. The heart rate also rises 10 to 20 beats per minute by 32 weeks' gestation.

Peripheral vascular resistance falls during pregnancy, most likely due to smooth muscle relaxation in vessel walls, resulting from the effects of progesterone; the addition of the uteroplacental unit; fetal heat production, which may produce vasodilation; synthesis of prostaglandins that causes resistance to circulating vasoconstrictors (angiotensin II and norepinephrine); and increased nitric oxide levels that cause vasodilation.

The effect of peripheral vascular resistance is that blood pressure remains stable during pregnancy despite the increase in blood volume. Systolic pressure remains largely unchanged or decreases slightly if it is measured when the woman is sitting or standing. Diastolic pressure shows a decrease (~10–15 mm Hg) that is greatest at 24 to 32 weeks' gestation. Blood pressure returns to normal by term. When the pregnant woman is in a supine position, particularly in the second and third trimesters, the weight of the pregnant uterus partially occludes the vena cava and the aorta. The occlusion impedes return blood flow from the lower extremities and reduces cardiac return. Some women experience a drop in blood pressure known as ***supine hypotensive syndrome,*** with symptoms of faintness, lightheadedness, dizziness and agitation, especially if lying supine. Blood flow through the placenta is decreased if a woman is supine for a prolonged time, which could result in fetal hypoxia. A lateral recumbent position alleviates the pressure on blood vessels and quickly corrects supine hypotension.

During pregnancy, blood flow is altered to include the uteroplacental unit; ~50% more blood circulates through the kidneys to remove the increased metabolic wastes generated by the mother and the fetus. Additionally, the woman's skin requires increased circulation to dissipate heat generated by increased metabolism during pregnancy; blood flow to the breasts is increased 2 to 3 times by the end of the pregnancy, resulting in engorgement and dilated veins; and the weight of the expanding uterus on the inferior vena cava and iliac veins partially obstructs blood flow from the legs, and blood pools in the deep and superficial veins of the legs. The resulting stasis of blood exerts pressure on the veins and causes them to be distended. Prolonged engorgement of the veins of the lower legs may lead to varicose veins of the legs, vulva, or rectum (hemorrhoids).

8.4 Respiratory System

Respiratory consumption increases ~15% to 20% during pregnancy. Half the oxygen is used by the fetus and placenta, and the rest is consumed by the breasts, uterus, and increased maternal respiratory and cardiac demands. To compensate for the increased need for oxygen, progesterone causes the woman to hyperventilate slightly by breathing more deeply, although her respiratory rate remains unchanged.

Progesterone is a major factor in the respiratory changes that occur in pregnancy. Besides causing mild hyperventilation, progesterone, along with other prostaglandins, helps decrease airway resistance by relaxing the smooth muscle in the respiratory tract. It is also thought to increase the sensitivity of the respiratory center. Estrogen causes increased vascularity of the mucous membranes of the upper respiratory tract. As the capillaries become engorged, edema and hyperemia develop within the nose, pharynx, larynx, and trachea. This congestion manifests itself in different conditions commonly seen during pregnancy—nasal and sinus stuffiness, epistaxis (nosebleeds), and changes in the voice, fullness in the ears, or earaches.

8.5 Gastrointestinal System

The gastrointestinal system undergoes changes that are clinically significant because they may cause discomfort for the pregnant woman. Initially, many women experience nausea/vomiting. Although the exact cause is unknown, it is thought to be due to increasing levels of human chorionic gonadotropin (hCG) and estrogen and the relaxation of the smooth muscles of the stomach. Although the condition is known as ***"morning sickness,"*** it can occur at any time of the day. Later in pregnancy, the woman's appetite is often increased. This helps the woman ingest the extra calories she needs to support the pregnancy.

Elevated levels of estrogen cause hyperemia of the tissues of the mouth and gums and may lead to gingivitis and bleeding gums. These conditions regress spontaneously after childbirth. Some women experience ***ptyalism,*** or excessive salivation. Small, frequent meals and chewing gum may offer some relief for women. Many women think that pregnancy adversely affects the teeth. However, the teeth do not lose minerals to the fetus and remain unaffected by the pregnancy. Women should be encouraged to continue regular checkups with the dentist, as most dental treatment is not harmful to the mother or fetus.

The lower esophageal sphincter tone decreases during pregnancy, primarily because of the relaxant activity of progesterone on the smooth muscles. This allows gastroesophageal reflux of acidic stomach contents into the esophagus and produces heartburn.

Elevated levels of progesterone lead to decreased tone and motility of the gastrointestinal tract. The effect on emptying time of the stomach is unclear, with some studies showing a decrease and others showing no change during pregnancy. The small intestine takes longer to empty during pregnancy, which may cause bloating and distention. Decreased motility in the large intestine allows more time for water to be absorbed, which tends to make the stools hard and may lead to constipation.

The gallbladder becomes hypotonic, and emptying time is prolonged. The bile becomes thicker, and cholesterol crystals may be retained, predisposing to the development of gallstones. Reduced gallbladder tone also leads to a tendency to retain bile salts, which may cause pruritis (itching).

8.6 Urinary System

During pregnancy the kidneys change in size, shape, and function. These changes facilitate normal waste elimination for the woman and fetus. During the first trimester, the bladder, a pelvic organ, is compressed by the weight of the enlarging uterus. The added pressure, along with progesterone-induced relaxation of the urethra and sphincter musculature, leads to urinary urgency, frequency, and nocturia. In the second trimester, when the uterus becomes an abdominal organ, bladder pressure is relieved. By the third trimester, the fetal head descends into the pelvis again, increasing pressure on the bladder, and symptoms of urgency, frequency, and nocturia return.

Elongation and dilation of the ureters occur. Peristalsis that normally facilitates the movement of urine from the kidneys to the bladder is reduced. This change, coupled with pressure on the ureters from the enlarging uterus, causes an obstruction of urine flow. The stagnant urine becomes an excellent medium for the growth of microorganisms.

The glomerular filtration rate (GFR) and renal plasma flow are increased due to hormonal changes, blood volume increases, the woman's posture, physical activity level, and nutritional intake. During the second trimester, the GFR increases up to 50% in most women. This alteration prompts an increase in renal tubular absorption. As a result, glucose excretion increases in virtually all pregnant women. Although it may be a normal finding, glucose should always be investigated to rule out gestational diabetes.

8.7 Endocrine System

The thyroid gland changes in size and activity during pregnancy. On palpation, the increase in size is appreciated. Enlargement is caused by increased circulation from the progesterone-induced effects on the vessel walls and by estrogen-induced hyperplasia of the glandular tissue. In early pregnancy, elevated levels of thyroxine-binding globulins cause an increase in the total thyroxine (T4) and 3,5,3-triiodothyronine (T3). The levels of total T4 continue to be elevated until several weeks postpartum. These changes in thyroid regulation cause a progressive increase in the ***basal metabolic rate (BMR)*** of up to 25% by term. The BMR is the amount of oxygen consumed by the body over a unit of time (mL/min). Maternal effects of the increase in BMR include heat intolerance and an elevation in pulse rate and cardiac output. Within a few weeks after birth, thyroid function returns to normal levels.

The parathyroid glands, which regulate calcium and phosphate metabolism, increase in size from estrogen-induced hyperplasia and hypertrophy. Maternal concentrations of parathyroid hormone increase as the fetus requires more calcium for skeletal growth during the second and third trimesters. Calcium intake is extremely important for the pregnant woman, whose daily intake should be 1,200 to 1,500 mg.

The anterior lobe of the pituitary gland, stimulated by the hypothalamus, increases in size and weight. Most hormones of the pituitary gland are suppressed, though, during pregnancy. The hormones FSH and LH, which stimulate ovulation in the nonpregnant woman, are unnecessary during pregnancy, and growth hormone also decreases during pregnancy. Prolactin, however, increases to prepare the breasts for milk production. Prolactin may also play a role in fluid and electrolyte shifts across the fetal membranes. The elevated levels of estrogen and progesterone inhibit lactation until close to term.

Oxytocin and vasopressin are produced in the posterior lobe of the pituitary. Oxytocin primarily causes uterine contractions, but high levels of progesterone prevent contractions until close to term. It also stimulates milk ejection from the breasts, or the ***"let down" reflex.*** Vasopressin causes vasoconstriction. Vasoconstriction produces an increase in maternal blood pressure and exerts an antidiuretic effect that promotes maternal fluid retention to maintain circulating blood volume. The increased blood volume occurs during pregnancy, along with changes in plasma osmolarity, which controls the release of vasopressin.

Human placental lactogen (hPL), an insulin antagonist that acts as a fetal growth hormone, increases the number of circulating fatty acids to meet maternal metabolic needs and decreases maternal glucose utilization, which increases glucose availability to the fetus.

Significant changes in the pancreas during pregnancy are the result of alterations in maternal blood glucose levels and consequent fluctuations in insulin production. Blood glucose levels during pregnancy are 10% to 20% lower than before pregnancy, and hypoglycemia may develop between meals and at night as the fetus continuously draws glucose from the mother.

During the second half of pregnancy, maternal sensitivity to insulin begins to decline because of the effects of hormones such as hPL, prolactin, estrogen, progesterone, and cortisol. As a consequence of the tissue resistance to insulin, postprandial blood glucose levels are higher than before pregnancy. The rise in glucose makes it more available for fetal energy needs and stimulates the pancreas of a healthy woman to produce additional insulin. Insulin production more than doubles during meals, and 24-hour levels average 30% higher than usual by the end of the third trimester to meet the increased insulin needs. Inadequate insulin production results in gestational diabetes.

The adrenal glands, located above the kidneys, change little during pregnancy. The adrenal cortex produces ***cortisol,*** a hormone that allows the body to respond to stressors. Cortisol is increased in pregnancy due to decreased renal secretion. It regulates protein and carbohydrate metabolism and stimulates glycogenesis whenever the supply of glucose is inadequate to meet the body's needs for energy. It is also believed to promote fetal lung maturation and stimulate labor at term.

Aldosterone regulates the absorption of sodium from the distal tubules of the kidneys. Production increases very early in pregnancy to maintain the necessary level of sodium in the greatly expanded blood volume and to meet the needs of the fetus. Aldosterone is closely related to water metabolism.

Prostaglandins are lipid substances found in high concentrations in the female reproductive tract and in the uterine decidua during pregnancy. Their exact function in pregnancy is unknown, although they may maintain a reduced placental vascular resistance. A decrease in prostaglandin levels may contribute to hypertension and preeclampsia. At term, an increased release of prostaglandins may contribute to the onset of labor.

In early pregnancy, ***hCG*** is produced by the cells surrounding the embryo. The primary function of hCG in early pregnancy is to prevent deterioration of the corpus luteum so that it can continue producing progesterone until the placenta is sufficiently developed to assume this function. The presence of this hormone produces a positive pregnancy result.

Estrogen is produced by the corpus luteum for the first few weeks of pregnancy, but primarily by the placenta after the 6th or 7th week of pregnancy. Functions of estrogen during pregnancy include stimulating uterine growth; increasing blood supply to the uterine vessels; increasing uterine contractions near term; aiding in the development of the glands and ductal system in the breasts in preparation for lactation; and causing hyperpigmentation, vascular changes in the skin, increased activity of the salivary glands, and hyperemia of the gums and nasal mucous membranes.

Progesterone is produced first by the corpus luteum and then by the fully developed placenta. It is the most important hormone of pregnancy. Its major functions are maintaining the endometrial layer for implantation of the fertilized ovum; preventing spontaneous abortion by relaxing smooth muscles of the uterus; helping to prevent tissue rejection of the fetus; stimulating the development of the lobes and lobules in the breast in preparation for lactation; and facilitating the deposit of maternal fat stores, which provide a reserve of energy for pregnancy and lactation.

Relaxin is produced by the corpus luteum and placenta and is present by the first missed menstrual period. It inhibits uterine activity, softens connective tissue in the cervix, and relaxes the cartilage and connective tissue of the pelvic joints.

8.8 Musculoskeletal System

Musculoskeletal changes during pregnancy are progressive. During pregnancy, fetal demands for calcium increase, especially in the third trimester. Calcium is stored to meet the needs of the fetus. During the third trimester, 25 to 30 mg of maternal bone stores are transferred to the fetus, but this amount is small in comparison with the mother's total stores and does not deplete the mother's bones.

Pregnant women often complain of cramping in the lower extremities and calves, especially at night. The cramps, sometime called ***"charley horses,"*** can be extremely painful and are caused by poor circulation to the extremities. They have also been associated with imbalances in calcium and phosphorus. Increasing or decreasing calcium may be helpful.

Relaxin and progesterone initiate gradual softening of the pelvic cartilage and connective tissue during the second trimester to facilitate the passage of the fetus through the pelvis during birth. Loosening and widening of the symphysis pubis and the sacroiliac joints cause pelvic instability and may cause pain at the symphysis pubis and inner thighs. The pregnant woman may assume a wide stance with the ***"waddling" gait of pregnancy,*** which occurs because of muscle fatigue and an effort to compensate for a changing center of gravity.

During the third trimester, as the uterus increases in size, the pregnant woman must lean backward to maintain her balance. This creates a progressive lordosis, or curvature of the lower spine. The strain on the muscles and ligaments of the back often causes backache.

As the pregnancy progresses, the muscles of the abdomen become weaker, and the rectus abdominus muscles separate (***diastasis recti***) to accommodate the growing uterus. Pregnant women often complain of sharp pain in the lower abdominal quadrants or in the groin area. Most often, this pain is caused by stretching and hypertrophy of the round ligaments that support the uterus (***round ligament pain***).

8.9 Neurologic System

The central nervous system seems to be affected by the hormonal changes of pregnancy, although the specific alterations other than those involving the hypothalamic-pituitary axis are less well known. Many women complain of a decreased attention span, poor concentration, and memory lapses during and shortly after pregnancy.

Edema from vascular permeability can lead to a collection of fluid in the wrist that puts pressure on the median nerve lying beneath the carpal ligament. This alteration leads to ***carpal tunnel syndrome,*** a condition that usually develops during the third trimester. It is manifested by pain and paresthesia (a burning, "tingling," or numb sensation) in the hand that radiates to the elbow. The pain can occur in one or both hands and is intensified with attempts to grasp objects. Carpal tunnel usually subsides after the pregnancy has ended.

Syncope (a transient loss of consciousness and postural tone with spontaneous recovery) during pregnancy is frequently attributed to orthostatic hypotension and/or vena cava compression by the gravid uterus. It may also occur as increased abdominal pressure from the growing uterus places pressure on the vagus nerve. Coughing, straining during bowel movements, and upward pressure from the growing fetus can trigger a vasovagal response that produces faintness or loss of consciousness. Lightheadedness, sweating, nausea, yawning, and feelings of warmth are signs that often precede syncope.

8.10 Integumentary System

Estrogen, progesterone, and alpha-melanocyte-stimulating hormones cause many changes in the appearance, structure, and function of the integumentary system. Although these changes are seldom serious, the woman may be negatively affected in relation to body image and self-concept. Circulation to the skin increases during pregnancy and encourages activity of the sweat and sebaceous glands. This helps dissipate excess heat produced by increased metabolism. Pregnant women feel warmer and perspire more, particularly during the last trimester. Accelerated activity by the sebaceous glands fosters the development of facial blemishes or extreme oiliness.

Increased pigmentation occurs in many pregnant women. It may begin as early as the second month of pregnancy and may be the result of estrogen, progesterone, and elevated levels of melanocyte-stimulating hormone. Women with dark hair or skin usually exhibit more hyperpigmentation than women with very light skin. Areas of pigmentation include brownish patches called chloasma ***(chloasma)***, or the ***"mask of pregnancy,"*** which can involve the forehead, face, and bridge of the nose. Chloasma increases with exposure to sunlight, but use of sunscreen can reduce the severity. Although melasma usually resolves after pregnancy when estrogen and progesterone decline, it continues for months or years in some women.

Linea negra, the line that marks the longitudinal division of the midline of the abdomen, may extend from the symphysis pubis to the top of the fundus. Preexisting moles (nevi), freckles, and the areolae, axillae, vulvar area, and perineum become darker as pregnancy progresses. Hyperpigmentation usually disappears after childbirth when levels of estrogen and progesterone decline.

Alterations in hair and nail texture may occur. The nails may become stronger and grow faster. The number of hair follicles in the dormant phase may decrease, and this stimulates new hair growth. Once the infant is born, the process is reversed, and there is an increase in hair shedding for approximately 1 to 4 months. Although this change may be disconcerting, hair is usually replaced within 6 to 12 months.

Increased adrenal steroid levels cause the connective tissue to lose strength and become more fragile. This change can cause ***striae gravidarum,*** or "stretch marks" on the breasts, buttocks, thighs, and abdomen. Striae appear as reddish, wavy, depressed streaks that will fade to a silvery white color after birth. They do not usually disappear completely.

Increased levels of estrogen during pregnancy may cause angiomas and palmar erythema. ***Angiomas,*** also known as "vascular spiders," are tiny, bluish, end arterioles that can occur on the face, neck, thorax, and arms. ***Palmar erythema*** is a condition characterized by color changes over the palmar surfaces of the hands that present as diffuse, reddish pink mottling of the palms. Increased blood flow, along with high levels of circulating hormones, can produce other skin changes, such as inflammatory pruritis and acne vulgaris, conditions seen primarily in the first trimester.

8.11 Changes in Metabolism

Because a correlation between infant mortality and low birth weight has been documented, women are encouraged to gain an average of 25 to 35 lb (11.3 to 15.9 kg) during pregnancy. The fetus, placenta, and amniotic fluid make up less than half the recommended weight gain. The remainder is found in breasts, increased blood volume, increased interstitial fluid, and maternal stores of subcutaneous fat.

The amount of water needed during pregnancy increases to meet the needs of the fetus, placenta, amniotic fluid, and increased blood volume. Increased GFR, decreased concentration of plasma proteins, and increased progesterone levels all result in an increase in sodium retention. Increased concentrations of cortisol, estrogen, prolactin, and aldosterone all tend to promote the reabsorption of sodium. The net effect of these combined hormonal actions lead to the maintenance of the sodium balance.

Because of hemodilution, colloid osmotic pressure slightly decreases, which favors the development of edema during pregnancy. Edema further increases toward term as the growing uterus presses on the pelvic veins. This process increases venous pressure, resulting in additional fluid shifts from the vascular compartment to the interstitial spaces.

All women, including those without edema, accumulate water during pregnancy to allow for the added fluid needs of the fetus as well as those of the woman. Edema of the feet and ankles are apparent, especially at night if the woman has been standing or sitting for long periods during the day. Dependent edema is clinically insignificant if no other abnormal signs are present.

Objective C: To Understand Psychosocial Adaptations to Pregnancy

8.12 Pyschosocial Adaptations to Pregnancy

The process of becoming a parent starts before conception and involves major changes in the woman, her partner, and the entire family. Although each couple adapts in their own way, by the end of the pregnancy, they should have completed the developmental tasks needed to become parents. Social and cultural factors also influence their adjustment to pregnancy. A woman's psychological response to pregnancy changes over time. During the early weeks the woman is unsure if she is pregnant and tries to confirm it. Reaction to the uncertainty of a pregnancy depends on the individual. She usually seeks confirmation from a health care provider during the first trimester of pregnancy.

Because half of all pregnancies are unintended, most women have conflicting feelings when they confirm they are pregnant. Pregnancy causes permanent life changes for the woman, and she often begins to examine expected changes and how she will cope with them. If it is her first pregnancy, the woman may worry about the added responsibility and feel unsure about her ability to be a good parent. She may be apprehensive about how the pregnancy will affect her relationship with her significant other or her other children. Ambivalence about the pregnancy is usually changed to acceptance by the second trimester.

Throughout the first trimester, the woman's focus is on herself, not the fetus. Early physical responses to pregnancy, such as nausea and fatigue, confirm that something is happening to her, but the concept of the fetus seems vague and unreal. Because she has not gained weight or felt the baby move, she thinks more about being pregnant rather than about the coming baby. Physical changes and increased hormone levels may cause emotional lability (unstable moods), and her partner and family members may find them confusing.

During the second trimester, physical changes occur in the woman that make the fetus feel "real." The uterus grows rapidly, weight increases, and breast changes are obvious. Ultrasound examination allows her to see the fetus, and she may receive an image to show to her family. ***Quickening,*** the feeling of movement by the fetus, occurs during this time. As a result of these changes, the woman now perceives the fetus as a separate entity although entirely dependent. The fetus becomes the primary focus of the pregnant woman. She is now concerned with having a healthy infant. She is often interested in information about diet and fetal development. A feeling of energy and satisfaction is common during the second trimester.

During the second trimester, the woman becomes increasingly concerned about her ability to protect and provide for the fetus. The concern is often manifested as narcissism and introversion. Selecting the right foods to eat or the right clothes to wear may assume more importance than previously. Some women lose interest in their jobs or become less interested in current events. The pregnant woman starts to wonder what her infant will look like. She will look at baby pictures of herself and wonder what life will be like when the baby is born. Because rapid and profound changes in the body take place during the second trimester, some women may feel distressed and have a negative body image. In addition, changes in body function, such as altered balance, reduced physical endurance, and discomfort in the pelvis and lower back, may affect her image of herself.

Sexual interest and activity of pregnant women and their partners are unpredictable and may increase, decline, or remain unchanged. The woman's physical comfort and sense of well-being are closely linked to her desire for sexual activity. During the first trimester, freedom from the use of contraceptives may make the couple more at ease and may enhance sexual interest for both partners. Fear of miscarriage may cause couples to avoid intercourse, particularly if the woman has previously lost a pregnancy. The couple can be reassured that no evidence has been found that shows intercourse is related to early pregnancy loss when no other complications are present. During the second trimester, women experience increased sensitivity of the labia and clitoris and increased vaginal lubrication as a result of pelvic vasocongestion. Orgasm may occur more frequently and with greater intensity because of these changes.

During the third trimester, the discomforts of pregnancy may make the woman reluctant to engage in sexual activity. As they become larger, some women believe their bodies are no longer attractive, and they may worry about their partners' reactions to their increased size. Sexual response varies among men. Some men report feelings of heightened sexual interest, but others perceive the woman's body late in pregnancy to be unattractive, and erotic feelings decrease. In addition, fear of harming the fetus or causing discomfort during pregnancy may interfere with sexual activity. The couple should be made aware of the normal changes in sexual desire that may occur during pregnancy and reassured that their feelings are normal.

The sense of well-being and contentment that dominates the second trimester gives way to increasing feelings of vulnerability that peak during the seventh month. Many pregnant women have fears or nightmares about having a deformed baby or harm coming to the infant and become very cautious as a result. They need reassurance that their fears are not unusual in pregnancy. They also become more dependent on their partners in the last weeks of pregnancy. Women often have fears about the safety of their partners and that something will happen to them. Their need for love and attention from their partners is even more pronounced in late pregnancy. Women may rely on their partners and family members more during this time. Partners need to be sympathetic.

In the few weeks prior to the birth, feelings of vulnerability decrease, and the woman comes to terms with her situation. She becomes worried about getting to the hospital in time. Women often say that they are tired of being pregnant and want the pregnancy to be over. During the last trimester, the woman prepares for the infant, if that is appropriate in her culture. ***"Nesting"*** behavior begins, with the woman arranging a place for the infant to sleep, obtaining clothing, cleaning, and preparing the home in order to bring the infant home.

Objective D: To Understand Maternal Role Tasks of Pregnancy

8.13 Maternal Role Tasks of Pregnancy

The transition into mothering begins during pregnancy and increases with gestational age. Some aspects of this transition must be accomplished before the woman moves on to the next step in the process. To become mothers, pregnant women spend a lot of time and energy learning new behaviors. As the woman works at establishing a relationship with her infant, she must also reorder her relationship with her partner and family.

The psychological work of pregnancy has been grouped into four maternal tasks:

1. Seeking safe passage for herself and the baby through pregnancy, labor, and childbirth
2. Securing acceptance of herself and the baby from her partner and family
3. Learning to give of herself
4. Developing attachment and interconnection with the unknown child

Seeking safe passage for herself and the baby is the woman's priority. During this time she is concerned with prenatal care and taking care of herself with diet, vitamins, and rest. She may also be concerned with cultural beliefs and practices during this time.

Securing acceptance is a process that begins in the first trimester and continues throughout the pregnancy. This process involves reworking relationships so that the important persons in the family accept the woman in the role of a mother so that the baby will be accepted into the family. Support and acceptance from the woman's own mother are especially important at this time. Many pregnant women gain a sense of increased closeness with their mothers, and previous conflicts may be resolved at this time.

Giving is one of the most idealized but essential components of motherhood. Learning to give to the infant begins in pregnancy when the woman allows her body to give space and nurturing to the fetus. This involves considering the benefits and costs of motherhood in terms of the effect on her lifestyle. The woman observes giving by others and begins to test her own ability to derive pleasure from giving. Pregnant women also learn to give by receiving. Baby showers are an example of how the pregnant woman confirms the continued interest and commitment from family and friends and enhances the woman's ability to give. Intangible gifts from others, such as companionship, attention, and support, help increase her energy and affirm the importance of giving.

The process of attachment begins in early pregnancy when the woman accepts the idea that she is pregnant, even though the baby is not real to her yet. During the second trimester, the baby becomes real when quickening occurs and feelings of love and attachment surge.

Women report feedback from their unborn infants' sleep-wake cycles, temperament, and communication. Love of the infant becomes progressive. The pregnant woman becomes comfortable with herself as a mother and derives pleasure from contemplating her new role.

Objective E: To Understand Paternal Adaptation

8.14 Paternal Adaptation

Expectant fathers do not experience the biologic processes of pregnancy, but they also must make major psychosocial changes to adapt to a new role. Wide variations exist in paternal responses to pregnancy. Some men are emotionally invested and comfortable as full partners in the pregnancy, in childbirth, and in becoming a parent. Others are more task-oriented and view themselves as managers. Still others are more comfortable as observers and prefer not to participate. In some cultures men are conditioned to believe that pregnancy and childbirth are "women's work" and may not be able to express their true feelings about childbirth and fatherhood.

Readiness for fatherhood is more likely in the presence of a stable relationship with the expectant mother, financial security, and a desire for parenthood. Additional factors are the man's relationship with his own father, his previous experience with children, and his perception of his ability to care for the infant.

Three developmental processes have been identified that an expectant father must address:

1. Grappling with the reality of pregnancy and the new child
2. Struggling for recognition as a parent from his family and peers
3. Making an effort to be seen as part of the childbearing process

The term ***couvade*** refers to pregnancy-related symptoms and behaviors in expectant fathers. Men sometimes experience physical symptoms similar to the expectant mother—nausea and vomiting, headache, loss of appetite, fatigue, and weight gain. These may be caused by stress, anxiety, or empathy for the pregnant partner. Symptoms are more likely to occur earlier in pregnancy and lessen as the pregnancy progresses. They are usually harmless but may persist and result in nervousness, anxiety, insomnia, restlessness, and irritability.

Objective F: To Understand Adaptation of Grandparents to the Birth of a New Baby

8.15 Adaptation of Grandparents

The initial reaction of grandparents depends on several factors, such as their ages, the number of other grandchildren, and their perceptions of the role of grandparents. By the time some individuals become grandparents, they have already dealt with their feelings about aging and react with joy when they find out they are going to be grandparents. They look forward to having grandchildren, who signify the continuity of life and family. Younger grandparents may have an issue with aging and may not be happy with the stereotype of grandparents as being "old." They may have career responsibilities and may not be available because of the continuing demands on their own lives.

If grandparents have other grandchildren, another will be welcomed, but the excitement is often less than for the first grandchild. This reaction may be disappointing to the couple who expected the same excited reaction as that given to the first grandchild. Grandparents' beliefs about their importance to grandchildren vary. In the past, grandparents were looked to for advice about childbirth and child rearing, but now professionals have become the "experts," and some grandparents have difficulty with this. Classes are offered widely to teach grandparents about current childbearing practices.

Some grandparents have little time to be actively involved with their grandchildren. Others feel they have raised their own children and do not wish to "raise" grandchildren. This attitude often hurts the parents who want the assistance of their parents during the childbearing and child rearing processes.

Objective G: To Understand Adaptation of Siblings to the Birth of a New Baby

8.16 Adaptation of Siblings

Sibling adaptation to the birth of an infant depends largely on age and developmental level. Very young children (2 years or younger) are unaware of maternal changes occurring during pregnancy and are unable to understand that a new brother or sister is going to be born. Because toddlers have little perception of time, many parents choose to delay letting the toddler know the baby is about to be born until right before delivery. Children 2 years old are not usually welcoming of newborns. Strong feelings such as anger, jealousy, and frustration may be normal for children at this age. Parents need to reassure them that they are loved and that the new baby is not replacing them.

Children from ages 3 to 12 years are more aware of changes in the mother's body that show a baby is to be born. They may be interested in observing the mother's abdomen, feeling the fetus move, and listening to the heartbeat. School-age children are often told about the pregnancy during the second trimester and benefit from being included in the preparations for the new baby. They may wonder how the birth will affect their role in the family. Parents should address these concerns and reassure the children on their importance and special place in the family.

The response of adolescents also depends on their developmental level. Some are embarrassed because the pregnancy confirms the continued sexuality of their parents. They may be repelled by the obvious physical changes of the mother. Many adolescents are immersed in their own developmental tasks involving loosening ties to their parents and coming to terms with their own sexuality. They may actually be indifferent to the pregnancy, as it does not directly affect them or their activities. Other adolescents become very involved and want to help in preparing for the baby's arrival.

Sibling classes are often given at birth facilities. Children as young as 3 years can benefit from such classes. The classes provide an opportunity for them to discuss what newborns are like and what new changes the baby will bring to the family.

Review Exercises

True/False

1. _______ Mothers will lose a tooth with each pregnancy.

2. _______ Maternal nail growth increases during pregnancy.

3. _______ Braxton Hicks contractions are often termed "false labor" when mistaken for the onset of early labor.

4. _______ Softening of the cervix during pregnancy is called the Chadwick's sign.

5. _______ Uterine growth during pregnancy occurs as a result of hyperplasia and hypertrophy.

6. _______ The cervix undergoes significant changes after conception.

7. _______ A major consequence of expanded blood volume during pregnancy is an increase in maternal cardiac output.

8. _______ The effect of decreased peripheral resistance during pregnancy is that blood pressure remains stable despite the increase in blood volume.

9. _______ During the third trimester, the enlarging uterus lifts the diaphragm, preventing the lungs from expanding fully.

10. _______ Heartburn is common in pregnant women.

11. _______ Striae gravidarum disappear after pregnancy.

12. _______ Oxytocin stimulates the milk-ejection reflex after childbirth.

13. _______ Pregnant women are encouraged to gain 25 to 35 lb (11.3 to 15.9 kg) during pregnancy.

14. _______ Estrogen is produced primarily by the placenta after the 7th week of pregnancy.

15. _______ Dependent edema in the pregnant woman is clinically insignificant if no other abnormal signs are present.

16. _______ Persistent yeast infections are common during pregnancy.

17. _______ Pelvic congestion during pregnancy can lead to heightened sexual interest and increased orgasmic experiences.

18. _______ Pregnancy is a hypercoagulable state in which changes in clotting factors cause an increased ability to form clots.

19. _______ Throughout the first trimester of pregnancy, the woman's focus is primarily on herself, not the fetus.

20. _______ Changes in the maternal body during pregnancy may result in a negative body image.

21. _______ The response of siblings to pregnancy depends on their age and developmental stage.

22. _______ Reaction to the uncertainty of pregnancy depends on the individual.

23. _______ Narcissism and introversion usually occur during the second trimester of pregnancy.

24. _______ The waddling gate of pregnancy occurs because of muscle fatigue and an effort to compensate for a changing center of gravity.

Completion

1. ________________ is the "hormone of pregnancy."

2. Carpal tunnel syndrome usually resolves itself by ________________.

3. ________________ softens connective tissue in the cervix and relaxes the cartilage and connective tissue of the pelvic joints.

4. At ______________________ gestation, the fundus can be palpated at the level of the umbilicus.

5. The dilution of red blood cell (RBC) mass causing a decline in maternal hematocrit in pregnancy is termed ______________________.

6. Some women experience a drop in blood pressure during pregnancy with symptoms of faintness and lightheadedness. This condition is known as ________________.

7. The clotting factor changes during pregnancy predispose the woman to ____________ and ______________________.

8. Hyperemia of the tissues of the gums and mouth may lead to ____________ and ____________ ____________.

9. Reduced gallbladder tone leads to a tendency to retain bile salts, which may cause ____________ in the pregnant woman.

10. ________________ is common in the pregnant woman because sodium and water are retained when the woman is standing and excreted during the night when she is lying down.

11. Accelerated activity by the sebaceous glands during pregnancy fosters the development of ______________________.

12. The dark line of pigmentation that extends from the symphysis pubis to the top of the fundus is called the ______________________.

13. ________________ prepares the breasts to produce milk.

14. By______________________ gestation, the fundus reaches its highest level at the xiphoid process.

15. The bluish purple discoloration of the cervix, vagina, and labia is referred to as ____________ ____________.

16. ________________ regulates carbohydrate and protein metabolism during pregnancy.

17. The presence of the hormone ________________ produces a positive pregnancy test result.

18. The basal metabolic rate in the pregnant woman increases by ____________ primarily because of metabolic activity of the fetus.

19. ________________ relaxes smooth muscles in the pregnant woman and is associated with decreased motility of the bowel, dilation of the ureters, and increased bladder capacity.

20. ________________ are the least likely age group of children to welcome a new baby into the family.

21. The term ________________ refers to pregnancy-related symptoms and behavior in expectant fathers.

22. During the second trimester, the fetus becomes real as the woman begins to feel fetal movement, also known as ______________________.

23. Although the cause of nausea and vomiting during pregnancy is unknown, it is believed to be related to increased levels of ________________ and ________________.

24. ________________ pain is a sharp pain in the side or inguinal area that results from softening and stretching of the ligaments from hormones and uterine growth.

25. Backache is a common complaint of pregnant women during the ______________ trimester.

26. ______________ is the pigmentation that may develop that covers the pregnant woman's face.

27. Hair loss during pregnancy is usually replaced within ________ to __________ months postpartum.

28. Stretching of the abdominal muscles during pregnancy causes the ______________ muscles to separate.

29. "Charley horses" (leg cramps) during pregnancy are thought to be caused by ______________.

30. The process of attachment begins in ______________ when the woman accepts that she is pregnant.

Answers

True/False

1. False. Teeth are not affected by pregnancy.
2. True
3. True
4. False. Softening of the cervix during pregnancy is called the Goodell sign.
5. True
6. True
7. True
8. True
9. False. The fetus drops in the pelvis, taking pressure off the diaphragm, allowing the lungs to expand more fully, and causing the pregnant woman less discomfort.
10. True
11. False. Striae gravidarum never fully disappear but become fainter in color (silvery).
12. True
13. True
14. True
15. True
16. True
17. True
18. True
19. True
20. True
21. True
22. True
23. True
24. True

Completion

1. Progesterone
2. End of pregnancy
3. Relaxin
4. 20 weeks'
5. Physiologic anemia
6. Syncope
7. Postpartum hemorrhage, blood clots
8. Gingivitis, bleeding gums
9. Pruritis
10. Ankle/feet edema
11. Facial blemishes
12. Linea negra
13. Prolactin

14. 37 weeks'
15. Chadwick sign
16. Cortisol
17. hCG (human chorionic gonadotropin)
18. 25%
19. Progesterone
20. 2-year-old children
21. Couvade
22. Quickening
23. hCG and estrogen
24. Round ligament
25. Third
26. Chloasma
27. 6 to 12 months
28. Diastasis recti
29. Increased or decreased calcium
30. Second trimester

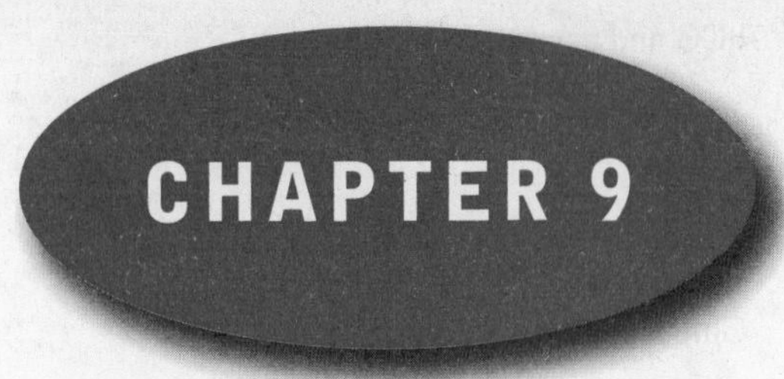

CHAPTER 9

Nursing Management During Pregnancy

Objective A: To Understand the Process of Choosing Childbirth Health Care

9.1 Choosing Childbirth Health Care

Expectant parents face several decisions about their childbirth experience. One of the earliest decisions facing expectant parents is the selection of a health care provider. The nurse can assist the couple by explaining the various options available to them and outlining what can be expected from each. A thorough understanding of educational preparation, skill level, practice style, and general philosophy and characteristics of certified nurse midwives, obstetricians, family practice physicians, and lay midwives is essential. The nurse can encourage the couple to investigate the care provider's credentials, basic and special education and training, fee schedule, availability to new clients, cesarean section rate, and any malpractice claims against the provider. Most of this information can be obtained by calling the provider's office; other information can often be obtained online through looking at public records. The nurse can help the couple develop a list of questions for their first visit to a care provider. Many couples get references from friends and family members when choosing a health care provider.

Expectant couples also need to discuss the qualities they want in a care provider for their newborn. They may want to interview several providers before birth to select someone who will meet their needs and those of their child. Again, most couples seek out a health care provider for their child based on recommendations from their friends and family, or in some cases, by recommendations from their own childbirth health provider who may work with certain pediatric care providers. Couples often seek a pediatric care provider based close to their home for ease of access.

Objective B: To Understand How a Couple Chooses a Birth Setting

9.2 Choosing a Birth Setting

The nurse can assist the couple in choosing a birth setting by suggesting they tour facilities and talk with nurses there, as well as talk with friends and family who are recent parents. The nurse can describe the different options available, including the traditional hospital setting, birthing centers, and home births. Often the choice is made when the couple chooses a health care provider who is affiliated with a certain facility. Some couples choose the type of facility they wish to deliver in and then choose a practitioner.

Whatever decisions they make about a health care provider or birth setting, the nurse should encourage the couple to personalize their birth setting. The couple might plan, for example, to bring extra pairs of warm socks, music, pictures, a pillow, or a favorite blanket. Such measures may give expectant parents enhanced relaxation and a sense of empowerment.

Objective C: To Understand the Decision to Write a Birth Plan

9.3 Birth Plan

In writing a birth plan, expectant parents can identify aspects of the childbearing experience that are most important to them. The birth plan helps identify available options and becomes a tool for communication between the expectant parents and the health care providers at the birth setting. The birth plan can also specify options the couple might wish to avoid.

It is imperative that the couple discuss their preferences with the health care provider before they go to the hospital in labor. The couple needs to know that although most birth experiences are close to those desired, at times expectations cannot be met. This may be because of unavailability of some choices in the community or unexpected problems during pregnancy or birth. It is important for nurses to help expectant parents keep sight of what is realistic for their situation. Maternal satisfaction is important when childbirth outcomes are considered; however, the greater priority is the safety of both mother and child.

Objective D: To Understand Cultural Influences on Childbearing

9.4 Cultural Influences on Childbearing

More distinct cultural groups live in the United States than anywhere else in the world. Each culture has its own health and healing belief system for major life events such as pregnancy and childbirth. The success of health care depends on its ability to fit in with the beliefs of those being served. Therefore, awareness of culturally divergent beliefs will optimize the health care a population receives.

Wide variations of beliefs and practices exist within each culture, and nurses need to be aware that people sharing the same culture may not practice behavior prescribed by their culture. Nurses must be careful not to stereotype people or a certain type of behavior from an individual because of his or her cultural background. Nurses need to be aware that a woman who does not normally follow certain beliefs of her culture may adhere to them when she is pregnant. She may do this to avoid offending or to show respect for family members to whom these beliefs are especially important during pregnancy, or she may feel that some part of the belief may be true after all and that she will harm her baby if she does not follow it.

The predominant culture in the United States treats pregnancy like an illness, with frequent visits to a physician, many laboratory tests, and hospitalization for childbirth with many medical interventions. Many other cultures, however, view pregnancy as a natural condition with little or no need for medical care. Visits to a health care provider often occur later in pregnancy if at all.

Different cultures have various requirements for the pregnant woman for maintaining health during pregnancy. Practices that maintain health may include wearing loose clothing, eating certain foods or avoiding them, and avoiding "unclean" things and strong emotions, such as anger. Concentration, silence, prayer, and meditation to maintain mental and spiritual health are practiced by some cultures. In many cultures, pregnant women must avoid contact with illness and death and may not attend funerals during pregnancy. They must also surround themselves with beautiful things and positive people.

Advance preparation for the baby is also avoided in some cultures, including naming the infant, for fear that it may harm the infant. Practices that prevent illness include use of protective religious objects or charms, such as an amulet. Some women also believe that eating certain foods can prevent illness. For instance, some people in many cultures eat raw garlic or onion or adhere to numerous food taboos. Strict adherence to religious codes, morals, and practices is also believed to prevent illness.

Fear, modesty, and a desire to avoid examination by men may keep a woman from seeking health care during pregnancy. In many cultures, exposure of the genitals to men is considered demeaning. In these cultures, the reputations of women depend on their demonstrated modesty. If necessary, female health care providers can perform examinations. Obtaining permission from the husband may be required before any examination or treatment can be performed.

Traditional ways to restore health include natural folk medicine such as herbs and plants. Women may often use charms, holy words, prescribed acts, and traditional healers before seeking other medical advice. Some cultures may even rely on witchcraft, voodoo, and magic.

Language can be a major barrier to the effective provision of health care. Numerous dialects within many languages can make it difficult for nurses and birth facilities to find competent interpreters. The ideal situation is to have female interpreters in the maternity setting because of the highly sensitive nature of the circumstances. Telephone interpreter services are provided by many agencies. Although this is more awkward than having an interpreter at the bedside, it ensures that both the nurse and the patient receive accurate information.

Styles in communication differ among cultures. When presenting information, the nurse should validate the person's understanding by requesting that the listener repeat it. Some groups engage in "small talk" before bringing up questions they have about their care. Nurses must not dismiss this small talk, as it establishes rapport and often helps to accomplish goals of care.

People in the United States often consider eye contact important to communication and believe it indicates honesty. However, this belief is not held by all cultures. Eye contact between unmarried men and women, for example, is considered seductive by some cultures. In dealing with infants, it is important not to admire a baby too openly, as some cultures fear the *mal ojo*, or evil eye, which can cause harm to the child.

Touch is also an important component of communication. In some cultures, touch by a woman other than the spouse is offensive. In contrast, some cultures find touch supportive and reassuring, and gentle touch is particularly important during labor and birth. Nurses must remain sensitive to the response of the person being touched and should refrain from touching if the person indicates it is not welcomed.

Objective E: To Understand Culturally Competent Nursing Care

9.5 Culturally Competent Nursing Care

Culturally competent nursing care requires an awareness of, sensitivity to, and respect for the clients served. It involves assessment of the family's culture and cultural negotiation when necessary.

Cultural negotiation involves providing information while acknowledging that the family may hold views that are different from those of the nurse and/or birth facility practice. If the family indicates that the information would be helpful, it may be incorporated into the teaching plan. However, while taking cultural practices of clients into consideration, the priority is that the safety of the mother and child must be maintained at all times.

Objective F: To Understand Health Promotion During Pregnancy

9.6 Nutrition and Weight Gain

Nutrition and weight management play an essential role in the development of a healthy pregnancy. Not only does the patient need to have an understanding of the essential nutritional elements, but she must also be available to assess and modify her diet for the developing fetus and her own nutritional maintenance. To facilitate this process, the nurse provides education and counseling concerning dietary intake, weight management, and potentially harmful nutritional practices.

Often pregnant women are told to "eat for two"; however, this is not accurate advice. Practitioners need to evaluate the amount and nutritional value of the food the patient is consuming. Calories are an important consideration when planning the patient's daily food intake. Other essential nutritional elements are protein, water, iron, folic acid, and calcium. Maternal dietary practices must also be assessed because they may exert a negative impact on the pregnancy.

During pregnancy, the recommended daily allowance (RDA) for caloric intake requires only a 300 kcal increase from pre-pregnancy needs (2,400 calories/day). Growth during the first and second trimesters occurs primarily in the maternal tissues; during the third trimester, growth occurs mostly in the fetal tissues. The total recommended weight gain for pregnant women is 25 to 35 lb (11.3 to 15.9 kg).

Pregnant women need to be counseled about healthy ways to incorporate the additional 300 kcal daily into their diets. Adding a serving from each of the major food groups meets this need. It is essential for the nurse to emphasize that the additional calories should not be met with an increased intake of "empty calories," such as soda, concentrated sweets, and simple carbohydrates. Health care providers should caution pregnant women regarding microbial foodborne illnesses. Raw or unpasteurized milk, as well as partially cooked eggs and foods containing raw or partially cooked eggs, should be avoided. Deli meats, luncheon meats, and frankfurters should be heated before consumption. In addition, raw shellfish and fish high in mercury, including shark, swordfish, tilefish, and king mackerel, should be avoided. Tuna, red snapper, and orange roughy contain moderate amounts of mercury, and women who are pregnant should limit their intake to 12 oz (340 g) weekly.

Water is necessary for all body tissues and body system functions. It is essential for the maintenance of life and must be consumed in sufficient quantity to maintain homeostasis. All persons should consume 6 to 8 (8 oz) glasses of water each day, and the pregnant woman needs to consume 8 to 10 (8 oz) glasses of water each day.

Water intake can be in the form of many different types of fluids, including fruit and vegetable juices. Patients need to be cautioned not to consume beverages high in sugar, diet drinks with artificial sweeteners, and caffeinated drinks. Alcohol should be avoided entirely throughout the pregnancy, as no safe amount has been determined.

Women who eat a balanced diet that includes the recommended servings and serving sizes may meet the recommended nutritional needs during pregnancy without vitamin supplementation. However, the need for an increased intake of specific nutrients must be taken into consideration as the pregnant woman plans her diet. Specifically, the daily intake of calcium, iron, and folic acid must be adequate to meet the maternal-fetal needs for adequate growth and development. Most health care providers will prescribe a prenatal vitamin for their patients during the pregnancy. Patients are often encouraged to continue them after they deliver during the first 6 weeks postpartum to aid in tissue healing and for as long as they continue to breastfeed.

The RDA for calcium is 1,000 mg for pregnant and pre-pregnant women. Calcium requirements are increased in pregnant adolescents, who need an intake of 1,300 mg daily. Without supplementation, most women fail to meet the dietary requirements. Calcium is essential for maintaining bone and tooth mineralization and calcification. During pregnancy, calcium must be available to the fetus for the growth and development of the skeleton and teeth. Dairy products, especially milk and milk products, constitute the best sources of calcium. Servings of dairy products are recommended daily for women; in pregnant women, an extra two servings are recommended. Other rich sources of calcium are legumes, dark green leafy vegetables, dried fruits, and nuts. Vitamin D is important in the absorption and metabolism of calcium. All women should be taught about the need for vitamin-D fortified foods or supplements. Most ready-to-eat cereals are vitamin-D fortified. Other good sources of vitamin D are eggs, liver, salmon, and tuna (up to 12 oz per week with limit of 6 oz for albacore tuna) (FDA, 2004).

Maternal iron intake must be increased during pregnancy. The iron RDA for pre-pregnant women is 18 mg but should be increased to 30 mg for pregnant women. Although most other necessary nutrients can be met through a balanced diet, it is almost impossible to meet the maternal daily requirements for iron without a dietary supplement. Sources of dietary iron are found in fortified ready-to-eat cereals, white beans, lentils, spinach, kidney beans, lima beans, soy beans, shrimp, prune juice, red meats, and organ meats.

Maternal iron intake must be increased to maintain the oxygen-carrying capacity of the blood and to provide an adequate number of red blood cells. Fetal iron needs are increased during the last trimester, when iron is stored in the immature liver for use during the first 4 months of life while the liver matures and liver enzymes are being produced. The newborn uses the stored iron to compensate for insufficient amounts of iron in breast milk and non-iron-fortified formula.

Vitamin C (ascorbic acid) is important in tissue formation and enhances the absorption of iron. Most pregnant women are able to meet the RDA requirements of 80 mg to 85 mg by including at least one serving of citrus fruit or juice or other vitamin source, although women who smoke need more. Food sources rich in vitamin C include red and green sweet peppers, oranges, kiwi fruit, grapefruit, strawberries, brussels sprouts, cantaloupe, broccoli, sweet potatoes, tomato juice, cauliflower, pineapple, and kale.

Folic acid (vitamin B_9) is a water-soluble vitamin that is closely related to iron. Working with vitamin B_{12}, folic acid helps to regulate red blood cell development and facilitates the oxygen-carrying capacity of the blood. It is essential in the production of DNA and RNA, helps to maintain normal brain function, and stabilizes mental and emotional health. Folic acid also works with vitamins B_6 and B_{12} to control blood levels of homocysteine, an amino acid that, in elevated amounts, has been linked to heart disease, depression, and Alzheimer disease. Folic acid deficiency is primarily responsible for neural tube defects, including spina bifida, cleft lip and palate, and anencephaly in the newborn. Foods that are rich in folic acid include dark green leafy vegetables, asparagus, brussels sprouts, soybeans, liver, root vegetables, beans, orange juice, and enriched grains. Several factors affect nutrition during pregnancy and may lead to potentially adverse effects. These factors include eating disorders and certain cultural variations.

Pica, the consumption of nonnutritive substances or food, is a common disorder that can affect pregnancy. Substances that are most commonly ingested include clay, dirt, cornstarch, and ice. Causes of pica are believed to include nutritional deficiencies, cultural and familial factors, stress, low socioeconomic status, and biochemical disorders. This practice usually subsides after the birth of the baby.

Anorexia nervosa and ***bulimia nervosa*** are conditions characterized by a distorted body image. Both involve a tense feeling of becoming obese and can have a major impact on a person's physical and psychological health. These disorders are potentially harmful to the developing fetus, as nutrients either are not consumed or are quickly eliminated from the body. Prenatal care should be approached from a team perspective that includes nutritional and psychological counseling, stress management, and active participation in support groups for individuals with eating disorders.

For many cultures and religions, food items have symbolic or special meaning, especially during pregnancy. Persons from different backgrounds need to be encouraged to continue their cultural practices as long as there is adequate nutrition for the patient and her fetus. Food cravings during pregnancy are considered normal by most cultures, although specific foods are culturally influenced. In most cultures, women crave nutritionally acceptable foods. As the woman and her family become more integrated into the dominant culture, cultural influences on food choices lessen.

Most vegetarian diets include vegetables, fruits, legumes, nuts, seeds, and grains. However, there are many variations. Nutritional counseling and ongoing assessment of maternal weight gain and laboratory testing for evidence of anemia are important strategies in ensuring optimal maternal-fetal well-being in vegetarians.

Objective G: To Understand Lifestyle as It Relates to Health Promotion

9.7 Lifestyle and Health Promotion

The demands of daily life can create significant stressors during pregnancy, as well as opportunities for incorporating facets of health promotion into a woman's life. Exercise can provide women who are pregnant with many benefits, whether they are already active in an exercise routine or are just beginning to exercise to facilitate a healthy pregnancy. The exercises practiced during pregnancy should focus on strengthening muscles without rigorous aerobic activity that may cause complications. Muscle strengthening will benefit the woman as she copes with the physical changes of pregnancy, including weight gain and postural changes. Exercise also increases energy level, improves posture, relieves back pain, enhances circulation, increases endurance, decreases muscle tension, and encourages feelings of well-being.

Women should adhere to some basic guidelines when formulating their exercise program. The most important consideration involves monitoring the breathing rate and ensuring that the patient's ability to walk and talk comfortably is maintained during physical activity. She should maintain adequate fluid intake in order to prevent dehydration. Activities that involve balance and coordination should be avoided, especially during later pregnancy when the center of gravity shifts and the joints and ligaments soften and relax. Limiting strenuous aerobic exercise and engaging in low-impact aerobics, swimming, walking, and cycling are strategies to ensure against overheating, increased metabolism, and injury.

Travel is usually safe for the pregnant woman. For automobile travel, seat belts that consist of a combination lap belt and shoulder harness should always be used. The shoulder harness is placed above the gravid uterus and below the woman's neck to avoid irritation. The woman should assume an upright position and ensure the headrest is properly aligned to avoid a whiplash injury. Airline travel does not usually pose any maternal-fetal risk. The metal detectors used at security checkpoints are not harmful to the fetus. Because the plane cabin humidity is typically maintained at a low level, the nurse should advise the pregnant woman to drink plenty of water to remain hydrated throughout the flight. Taking brief walks around the cabin every hour of travel helps minimize the risk of superficial and deep vein thrombophlebitis.

Many women who work discover rather early in pregnancy that they must make decisions regarding the continuation of employment, the safety of the workplace, the demands of the work environment, and plans for maternity leave. The pregnant woman may be advised to reduce the number of hours worked if the job requires heavy lifting, prolonged standing, extensive walking, or physical exertion. When the nature of the work is physically demanding, safety concerns may require that she stop working altogether. The potential for maternal exposure to toxic substances such as chemotherapeutic agents, lead, ionizing radiation, or heavy machinery or other hazardous equipment should prompt reassignment to a different work area. If reassignment is not possible, the woman may need to stop working until the pregnancy is completed.

Women who are currently experiencing pregnancy complications or who have experienced pregnancy complications in the past may also need to stop working until the pregnancy is completed. All women who are employed outside the home should be encouraged to speak with their employers to discuss the options that are provided by the workplace and to determine a satisfactory plan for their leave.

The Family and Medical Leave Act of 1993 guarantees most women, as well as men, 12 weeks of unpaid maternity leave following the birth or adoption of a child. By law, the employer is required to allow the family member to return to his or her job or a similar job with the same salary and benefits, without a reduction in seniority. Family members qualify for this benefit if they work for the federal, state, or local government or if the company has 50 or more employees working within 75 miles of the workplace. In addition, family members must have worked for the employer for at least 12 months or for at least 1,250 hours in the previous year. In 2007, 76.1 million workers were eligible for FMLA leave.

Fatigue and tiredness are common symptoms associated with pregnancy. As the pregnancy progresses from one trimester to the next, the woman's level of fatigue changes, along with the need for rest. Through education, the health care provider can empower the woman throughout the pregnancy to manage her rest demands and cope with fatigue. Planning and making healthy choices concerning rest enable the woman to feel more relaxed and comfortable.

Medication use during pregnancy must be handled very carefully. The needs of the patient and her fetus should always be considered on an individual basis. Nurses need to be aware that patients taking over-the-counter (OTC) medications and herbal preparations often do not readily report this information to the health care provider during the prenatal interview unless specifically asked about them. Therefore, the nurse must ask specific questions regarding the use of these remedies.

Use of alcohol and illicit drugs is contraindicated during pregnancy. Often the effects to the fetus outweigh the effects on the mother. Nurses need to include asking the question of use of these substances during the prenatal interview.

Smoking during pregnancy decreases placental perfusion to the fetus and is associated with intrauterine growth restriction (IUGR), low birth weight, and preterm birth. Patients should be encouraged to go for counseling and tobacco-cessation classes. Many are offered free of charge at local health departments.

Objective H: To Understand the Decisions Involved in Choosing a Method of Infant Feeding

9.8 Choosing a Method of Infant Feeding

Many women decide on a feeding method well before the infant's birth. Some may not have questions about which method is best for them until late in pregnancy. Nurses can help mothers decide on a method and gain confidence in feeding their infants. For women who are undecided, nurses should explain the many benefits of breastfeeding for both the infant and mother. The Healthy People 2020 goals for breastfeeding are for 75% of mothers to initiate breastfeeding at birth, to have 50% of mothers still breastfeeding at 6 months, and to have 25% of mother still breastfeeding at 1 year.

Women choose formula feeding for many reasons. Some women are embarrassed by breastfeeding, seeing the breasts only in a sexual context. Many have few friends or relatives who have had breastfeeding experiences. A woman may feel the need to maintain a strict feeding schedule and may be uneasy not knowing exactly how much milk the infant is getting when breastfeeding. Her partner may not be supportive of breastfeeding. Occasionally, a woman must give formula because she is taking medications that might harm the infant. It may be that the woman will need to return to work soon after giving birth, and she will not have the support and opportunity to pump her breasts at the workplace. Frequently, though, women lack information about the benefits of breastfeeding.

Some patients prefer combination feeding. If the woman chooses combination feeding, the nurse should be supportive so that the infant receives the benefit of breast milk at least part of the time.

Nurses must be sensitive to the woman's feelings about feeding. Although nurses should encourage breastfeeding as the best method in most cases, they should be supportive of each patient's choice once the decision is made. The early days of parenting are a very vulnerable period for women, who may feel that their feeding abilities reflect their mothering abilities.

Objective I: To Understand the Common Discomforts of Pregnancy and Self-Care Relief Measures

9.9 Common Discomforts and Self-Care Relief

Common discomforts experienced during pregnancy are caused by the major hormonal and anatomical changes that take place in the woman's body. As the pregnancy progresses, most patients report at least some of the common discomforts. Anticipatory guidance includes educating the woman about the normal physiologic changes that occur during pregnancy, symptoms that frequently accompany the changes, and strategies for dealing with the discomfort.

Nausea is often one of the first symptoms of pregnancy experienced by the expectant woman. Although commonly known as ***"morning sickness,"*** it can occur at any time of the day or night. While the exact cause of nausea is unknown, it is most probably related to the increased levels of pregnancy hormones. Nausea is primarily noted in the first trimester and usually resolves by 13 to 14 weeks. Nurses can suggest self-care strategies for relief of nausea that include avoiding trigger foods and tight clothing, employing relaxation techniques (deep breathing, mental imagery), eating plain saltine crackers or sucking on peppermint candy before arising, eating small meals, and remaining in an upright position after eating.

Vomiting is often associated with nausea during early pregnancy. It is important to assess for weight loss, dehydration, urine ketones, blood alkalosis, and hypokalemia, which may be indicative of a more serious problem known as hyperemesis gravidarum. Generally, vomiting resolves itself along with nausea, and many of the self-care remedies for nausea are also effective remedies for vomiting.

Ptyalism, or excessive salivation, can be quite distressing for the pregnant woman, who may frequently wipe her mouth or spit in a cup. Although the cause of ptyalism is unknown, it is most likely related to increased hormone levels. While little can be done to reduce the amount of saliva, it is important to rule out dental abnormalities, gastrointestinal problems, and pica. Nurses can counsel patients to consume small, frequent meals, avoid starchy foods, drink plenty of water in small amounts, suck on hard candies, and brush their teeth often.

Fatigue occurs throughout pregnancy and increases progressively over time. This is most likely due to physiologic and hormonal changes. Psychological concerns may also lead to ***insomnia.*** During the third trimester, fatigue is usually related to physical discomfort and an increased inability to sleep because of the discomfort. Nurses should counsel patients to take naps during the day whenever possible, take frequent rest periods, establish a bedtime ritual that includes going to bed at the same time every night, increase daytime exercise, and practice relaxation techniques. If the patient demonstrates signs of increased stress or depression, she should be referred for additional evaluation.

Back pain during pregnancy results from the change in the center of gravity as the uterus enlarges. It is also related to high levels of progesterone, which cause relaxation and softening of the connecting cartilage and joints. Nurses can educate patients in relief measures that include wearing low-heeled, supportive shoes; using proper body mechanics; performing back strengthening and pelvic rock exercises; taking frequent rest periods; sleeping on a firm, supportive mattress; and wearing a well-fitting, supportive bra.

Leukorrhea is a common complaint from pregnant women. High levels of estrogen stimulate vascularity and hypertrophy of the cervical glands, causing an increase in vaginal discharge. The discharge is usually yellow, thin, and more acidic than normal. It is important to rule out vaginal and sexually transmitted infections. Patient self-care teaching would include instructing the patient to wear cotton underwear, avoid tight-fitting clothing, and follow strict hygiene measures to prevent infection. Patients might want to wear a sanitary napkin but should be encouraged to change the pad often to prevent odor and infection.

Urinary frequency is a common complaint of pregnant women, especially in the first and third trimesters. In early pregnancy the enlarging uterus causes pressure on the bladder, and in the third trimester the fetus descends into the pelvic cavity and presses on the bladder. The nurse can suggest relief measures such as drinking an adequate amount of fluids, doing Kegel exercises, using panty liners, voiding frequently, and decreasing fluid intake by several hours before going to bed.

Dyspepsia* or *heartburn results from the reflux of acidic gastric contents into the lower esophagus. Dyspepsia is caused by the progesterone-induced relaxation of the cardiac sphincter and delayed gastric emptying. As the pregnancy advances, the enlarging uterus pushes up on the stomach, causing a reduced capacity. Making changes such as eating smaller meals, maintaining good posture, remaining upright after meals, avoiding greasy and fatty foods, not eating very cold food, and not drinking beverages with meals may help. Drinking milk and using OTC antacids may also be helpful.

Flatulence (excessive gas in the stomach and intestines) is caused by decreased gastric motility that results from elevated levels of progesterone during pregnancy. Patients may find relief by avoiding gas-forming foods, constipation, gum chewing, and consuming large meals.

Constipation is another common complaint during pregnancy. Elevated levels of progesterone relax the smooth muscles, causing decreased contractility of the lower gastrointestinal tract and slowed movements of the stool. As the uterus enlarges, the large intestines become compressed, further slowing the movement of the bowels. Supplemental iron may also contribute to constipation. Patients should be taught to drink plenty of fluids, engage in regular exercise, consume a high-fiber diet, and avoid straining while defecating. The use of mineral and bulk-forming laxatives may also be used when other remedies are unsuccessful.

Dental problems may become an issue during pregnancy. Elevations in pregnancy hormones cause the gums to become edematous and friable, which can lead to bleeding during brushing. Patients should be encouraged to continue with regular dental visits and to maintain meticulous dental hygiene during pregnancy. If dental treatment is indicated, most local anesthetics can be used safely during pregnancy.

The actual cause of ***leg cramps*** is unknown but is thought to be from decreased levels of calcium and phosphorus. For relief of leg cramps, the patient should be advised to engage in regular exercise, maintain good body mechanics, elevate the legs above the heart several times a day, and consume a diet that includes adequate calcium and phosphorus. Dorsiflexion of the foot may help relieve leg cramps.

Edema in the lower extremities is caused by relaxation of the blood vessels and increased pressure on the pelvic veins by the enlarging uterus. The patient should be taught to avoid tight, restrictive clothing, elevate the legs periodically, and assume a side-lying position when resting.

A positive family history, along with the normal physiologic changes of pregnancy, predisposes the patient to the development of ***varicose veins***. Nursing care of the patient with varicose veins includes regular assessment of the lower extremities and peripheral pulses and education. Patients should be advised to elevate legs several times during the day and avoid tight, restrictive clothing. With severe varicosities, the woman may need to be fitted for antiembolism stockings.

Dyspareunia, or painful intercourse, may result from pelvic congestion and impaired circulation caused by the enlarging uterus. Also, as the pregnancy advances, finding a position of comfort for intercourse may become increasingly difficult due to the enlarging abdomen. Unless a medical condition contraindicates intercourse, the patient and her partner should be reassured that intercourse is safe during pregnancy. Education should include suggestions for comfortable positions for intercourse and alternative methods for mutual sexual satisfaction.

Nocturia, or excessive nighttime urination, is more common during the first and third trimesters. Although there is no cure, the patient should be advised to limit her fluid intake in the hours before retiring.

Insomnia may have a variety of causes, including physical discomfort, nocturia, caffeine, and stress. The nurse can suggest strategies to enhance relaxation and comfort before bedtime so the expectant woman can sleep more peacefully.

Round ligament pain is common in pregnant women. As the uterus enlarges, the round ligaments stretch and produce a painful sensation in the lower quadrants. The nurse can advise the patient that taking a warm bath, applying heat, supporting the uterus with a pillow when resting, and using a pregnancy girdle may help alleviate some of the discomfort.

Patients may experience ***shortness of breath*** related to uterine enlargement and the upward pressure on the diaphragm. One suggestion the nurse can make is to tell the patient to avoid rushing, to encourage her to take her time when engaging in any activity, and to take frequent rest periods during the day. ***Hyperventilation*** may occur due to the increase in the amount of carbon dioxide from the increased metabolic activity during pregnancy. Measures that may be helpful include breathing into a paper bag, maintaining good posture, and stretching the arms above the head.

Numbness and ***tingling*** in the fingers may be associated with hyperventilation or from nerve compression in the median and ulnar nerves in the arm. Maintaining good posture, elevating the hands on a pillow while sleeping, or wearing a wrist brace may provide symptomatic relief.

Supine hypotension is caused by pressure of the enlarging uterus on the inferior vena cava while the woman is in the supine position. Vena caval compression impedes venous blood flow, reduces the amount of blood in the heart, and reduces cardiac output, causing dizziness and syncope. The nurse should educate the patient about the causes of supine hypotension and advise the woman to rest on her side and slowly move from a lying, to a sitting, to a standing position to minimize changes in blood pressure.

Objective J: To Understand the Danger Signs of Pregnancy

9.10 Danger Signs of Pregnancy

Complications can occur at any time during the pregnancy, Nurses need to educate pregnant women and their families about danger signs and symptoms so that they know to either contact the health care provider or go straight to a hospital emergency room or labor and delivery unit to be evaluated.

First Trimester

During the first trimester, nausea and vomiting are common discomforts. However, when vomiting becomes severe, weight loss and dehydration can occur and place both the woman and her fetus at risk. The patient needs to contact her health care provider if nausea and vomiting become severe. Dehydration may require hospitalization and intravenous (IV) fluids. Abdominal cramping, vaginal spotting, or bleeding may indicate spontaneous abortion, or miscarriage. Treatment includes bed rest and emotional support. If bleeding and pain are excessive, the patient should contact her health care provider or go to the emergency room.

Second Trimester

Preeclampsia is one of the most common pregnancy complications during the second trimester. It is a pregnancy-specific disorder that is clinically defined as an increase in blood pressure after 20 weeks' gestation accompanied by proteinuria. Early signs of preeclampsia include headache, vision changes, elevated blood pressure, and edema. Patients who exhibit any of these symptoms should promptly notify their health care provider. Bed rest is the first intervention implemented in an effort to reduce blood pressure and alleviate the other problems that can be associated with this disorder.

Premature rupture of the membranes (PROM), which is rupture of the membranes before the onset of labor, can also occur during the second trimester. Patients should be taught to promptly seek advice from their health care provider if vaginal discharge is present. The provider will determine if the patient has increased vaginal secretions, an infection, or true leakage of amniotic fluid. Women who experience premature rupture of the membranes must be closely monitored for signs of infection.

The presence of uterine contractions during the second trimester may indicate ***preterm labor***. Preterm labor is defined as regular uterine contractions before the end of the 36th week of gestation. All women should be taught the signs of preterm labor and instructed to call their health care provider if the symptoms appear. True labor must be differentiated from ***Braxton Hicks contractions,*** which are disorganized tightening of the uterine muscles as they stretch, so that appropriate interventions may be initiated.

During the second trimester, the fetus is assessed for well-being. The fundal height measurement should correlate with weeks of gestation (22–34 weeks). A decreased fundal height may indicate intrauterine growth restriction, whereas increased fetal height is suggestive of multiple gestation, fetal macrosomia, or hydramnios. Further diagnostic evaluation will be done.

A number of other potentially dangerous fetal problems may occur during the second trimester. These include fetal hypoxia from maternal hypertension, irregular or absent heart rate, preterm birth, infection from PROM, and absence of fetal movement after quickening.

If the woman experiences an absence of fetal movement, she should be instructed to call her health care provider. Very often, she will be instructed to do fetal kick counts at home. She will be instructed to drink a large glass of juice and rest on her left side for 1 hour, counting fetal kick counts. She should be able to feel at least 10 fetal movements in an hour. If fewer than 10 fetal movements are noted, she will be instructed to go to the hospital for a nonstress test (NST).

Third Trimester

During the third trimester, the patient may develop the same problems that can occur during the second trimester. Also, ***gestational diabetes*** may develop during this time. Patient care involves education and a team approach that usually includes the obstetrician, internist, endocrinologist, diabetes educator, neonatologist, dietitian, and nurse.

Hemorrhagic disorders may also develop during the third trimester. ***Placenta previa*** is an implantation of the placenta in the lower uterine segment, near or over the internal cervical os. The abnormal location of the placenta can cause painless, bright red vaginal bleeding. Depending on the exact location of the placenta, strict bed rest may have to be maintained, and a cesarean birth may be necessary. ***Abruptio placentae***, or placental abruption, is the premature separation of a normally implanted placenta from the uterine wall. An abruption results in hemorrhage between the uterine wall and the placenta, causing abdominal pain and vaginal bleeding. Interventions may include hospitalization, bed rest, Trendelenburg position, IV fluids, and delivery.

During the third trimester, Leopold maneuvers are used to determine lie, presentation, and position of the fetus. To monitor fetal growth, fundal height is measured and compared with the estimated date of delivery. NSTs may be performed to evaluate fetal well-being.

Objective K: To Understand the Various Diagnostic Tests that Assess Fetal Well-Being

9.11 Diagnostic Tests that Assess Fetal Well-Being

Fetal assessment is an integral component of prenatal care. Careful assessment of fetal well-being enhances perinatal outcome through early identification and intervention for fetal compromise. The goals of antepartum fetal surveillance are to prevent fetal death and to help ensure the best possible fetal outcome. A number of tests can be performed during pregnancy to monitor fetal growth, development, and well-being. Antenatal assessment during the first and second trimesters is directed primarily at the diagnosis of fetal congenital anomalies, whereas the goal of third trimester assessment is to determine the quality of the intrauterine environment for the maturing fetus.

No antepartal testing or antepartal surveillance procedure can guarantee the birth of a perfect child. The woman and her partner must be counseled that prenatal diagnostic tests cannot detect all congenital defects. A baseline risk remains for congenital defects in every pregnancy.

The nurse should remember the woman's right to refuse antepartal testing even though she may have an increased risk for a baby with a birth defect that can be diagnosed with one of these tests. If a screening test suggests an abnormality, the woman may refuse further testing. The nurse and health care team need to respect the woman's personal decisions.

Ultrasonography is the use of high-frequency sound waves to detect differences in tissue density and visualize outlines of structures in the body. The examination can be done abdominally or transvaginally during pregnancy. During the first trimester, ultrasound may be used to confirm the viability and age of a pregnancy, determine the number, size, and location of the gestational sacs, identify uterine abnormalities, rule out an ectopic pregnancy, and locate the presence of an intrauterine contraceptive device. Fetal heart rate can be observed as early as 6 weeks to 7 weeks via real-time echo sonography. In the second and third trimesters, ultrasound is frequently used to confirm fetal viability and gestational age, monitor fetal growth, amniotic fluid volume, placental location and maturity, and assess uterine fibroid tumors and cervical length. Ultrasound is an essential component of the biophysical profile and fetal Doppler studies.

The modified ***biophysical profile (BPP)*** allows conservative treatment of high-risk patients because delivery can be delayed if fetal well-being is jeopardized. It is noninvasive and less costly than some tests because it can be performed on an outpatient basis. The BPP helps identify the presence and severity of hypoxia and anemia because it measures multiple variables.

The individual components of the exam are a combination of acute and chronic markers of fetal well-being. The acute or short-term markers are the fetal heart rate reactivity, fetal breathing movements, gross fetal movements, and fetal muscle tone. The major chronic or long-term marker is the amount of amniotic fluid. A scoring technique is used to interpret the data, with each parameter contributing 0 to 2 points; a score of 10 is a perfect score, and a score of 0 is the worst possible score.

Doppler ultrasound blood flow studies (umbilical velocimetry) is used to study blood flow in the umbilical vessels of the fetus, placental circulation, and maternal uterine circulation. A noninvasive Doppler wave measures the velocity of red blood cell movement through the uterine and fetal vessels. Assessment of the blood flow through the uterine vessels is useful in determining vascular resistance in women at risk for developing placental insufficiency (preeclamptics, postdates, etc). Decreased velocity is associated with poor fetal outcomes.

Chorionic villus sampling (CVS) is an invasive procedure that is performed between 10 weeks and 12 weeks' gestation to diagnose fetal chromosomal, metabolic, or DNA abnormalities. CVS is not used to detect open body wall defects such as spina bifida because an amniotic fluid sample is required. The advantages to using this over amniocentesis are that it can be done earlier in the pregnancy, and the results are obtained sooner. If results are abnormal, and the woman chooses an abortion, she may consider an earlier abortion, which is less physically and emotionally traumatic than one done at a later date.

Alpha fetoprotein (AFP) screening is a maternal blood test offered to women between 16 weeks' and 18 weeks' gestation. AFP is the predominant protein in fetal plasma and is synthesized by the embryonic yolk sac, developing fetal liver, and gastrointestinal tract. It diffuses from fetal plasma into fetal urine and is excreted into the amniotic fluid. A portion of the fluid is ingested by the fetus, and the remainder crosses the placental membranes into maternal circulation (maternal serum alpha fetoprotein [MSAFP] screening). Abnormal concentrations of AFP are associated with serious fetal anomalies.

Multiple marker screening are tests that are added to the AFP, such as human chorionic gonadotropin (hCG) levels and inhibin A, to screen for other abnormalities. Advantages to these tests are that they are done early and allow more time for motor comprehensive diagnostic procedures if abnormal results are found. Multiple marker screening allows patients to examine their options and prepare for the birth of an infant who will need special care.

Amniocentesis is the aspiration of amniotic fluid from the amniotic sac for examination. This procedure traditionally has been performed at 15 weeks' to 20 weeks' gestation. Current techniques allow early amniocentesis at 11 weeks to 14 weeks. The most common purpose for midtrimester amniocentesis is to examine fetal cells in the amniotic fluid to identify chromosome abnormalities. In addition, amniocentesis is performed to evaluate the fetal condition when the woman is sensitized to Rh-positive blood, diagnose intrauterine infections, and investigate amniotic fluid AFP and acetylcholinesterase when the multiple marker test on maternal serum is not normal. It is also used later in pregnancy to detect fetal lung maturity.

Abnormal results are usually known in time to give the woman the choice of pregnancy termination before 20 weeks' gestation. However, this time frame is unacceptable to some women because of the increasing reality of the pregnancy. The risks of amniocentesis include a pregnancy loss rate $< 1\%$. Ultrasound guidance of needle insertion reduces the possibility of the placenta or cord being pierced. Transfer of fetal blood to maternal circulation may occur, resulting in sensitization of the Rh-negative woman carrying an Rh-positive fetus. RhoGAM is administered to prevent sensitization in nonsensitized Rh-negative women after amniocentesis.

Percutaneous umbilical blood sampling (PUBS) involves the aspiration of fetal blood from the umbilical cord for prenatal diagnosis or therapy. Blood is tested for anemia, isoimmunization, metabolic disorders, and infection. The PUBS technique can be used to treat blood diseases and deliver therapeutic drugs that cannot be given to the fetus in any other way. After the procedure, the fetus is monitored for 60 minutes. The Rh-negative woman is given RhoGAM to prevent sensitization by any Rh-positive fetal blood that may have entered her circulation.

The ***NST*** identifies whether an increase in the fetal heart rate occurs when the fetus moves, indicating adequate oxygenation, a healthy neural pathway from the fetal central nervous system to the fetal heart, and the ability of the fetal heart to respond to stimuli. Fetal heart rate accelerations without fetal movement are also considered a reassuring sign of adequate fetal oxygenation. If the fetal heart does not accelerate with movement, however, fetal hypoxemia and acidosis are concerns. A nonreassuring tracing may need to be followed up with a BPP.

The NST takes approximately 40 minutes. The nurse places an external fetal monitor on the patient and a tocotransducer. A tracing (recording of fetal heart rate and contractions on monitor) is considered reactive if there are two fetal heart rate accelerations in a 20-minute period. An acceleration is an increase in fetal heart rate of at least 15 beats above the baseline that remains elevated for at least 15 seconds.

A ***contraction stress test (CST)*** may be done if NST findings are nonreactive, or the test is sometimes the initial test of fetal well-being. Because a BPP often supplements both reassuring and nonreassuring NSTs, the CST is less often performed. The CST records the response of the fetal heart rate to stress induced by uterine contractions, identifying the fetus whose oxygen reserves are insufficient to tolerate the recurrent mild hypoxia of uterine contractions. Variability and accelerations of the fetal heart rate are expected, as in the NST.

The patient is positioned in bed on her side. She is placed on external fetal monitoring devices. The monitor strip is evaluated for the first 10 minutes to see if the patient is having any contractions, then a breast self-stimulation test is performed. The breast self-stimulation test is based on the knowledge that stimulation of the nipples causes release of oxytocin from the posterior pituitary, which causes uterine contractions, The woman brushes her hand over one nipple for 2 minutes, stopping if contractions start. The nipple stimulation is resumed after a 5-minute rest period and continued until an adequate contraction pattern is established.

If the breast self-stimulation test does not effectively stimulate contractions, or if the health care provider prefers to use pitocin (synthetic oxytocin), an IV infusion of pitocin is started. The rate is increased every 20 minutes until the desired contraction frequency is attained. CST results may be interpreted as negative, positive, or equivocal (suspicious). If findings are negative, CST offers > 99% reassurance that the uteroplacental unit is likely to support life for at least 1 more week.

Vibroacoustic stimulation (VAS) can be used to confirm nonreactive NST findings and shorten the time required to obtain high-quality NST data during the third trimester of pregnancy. A vibroacoustic stimulator is applied to the maternal abdomen over the area of the fetal head, and stimulation with vibration and sound is given for up to 3 seconds. VAS can be repeated at 1-minute intervals up to three times. It appears safe for the fetus, although temporary changes in body movements, breathing movements, and heart rate have been described.

Objective L: To Understand Childbirth Education Classes

9.12 Childbirth Education Classes

The goals of perinatal education are to help parents become knowledgeable consumers, take an active role in maintaining health during pregnancy and birth, and learn coping techniques to deal with pregnancy, childbirth, and parenting. Meeting these goals reduces their fear of the unknown and increases parents' abilities to make decisions regarding childbirth and parenting with confidence, satisfaction, and feelings of empowerment.

Perinatal education classes are strongly recommended by the American Academy of Pediatrics and the American Congress of Obstetricians and Gynecologists (formerly the American College of Obstetricians and Gynecologists). A Healthy People 2020 goal is to increase the number of women who attend a series of prepared childbirth classes. Although most perinatal education classes are taught by registered nurses, physical therapists and other health care professionals who have taken special courses may become childbirth educators. Teachers must be versed in adult education theories and techniques and skillful in handling groups of people of diverse backgrounds and ages. Classes may be sponsored by schools, hospitals, medical groups, civic organizations, churches, and health departments. Classes may also be held in less traditional sites, such as workplaces.

People take classes for a variety of reasons. Many have a strong desire to participate actively in all aspects of childbearing. Others are looking for coping strategies to deal with their fears of pain and childbirth. Some women report feeling a greater sense of control during labor and delivery when they have taken childbirth preparation classes. When women feel that they are informed and have some control over what happens to them, they are more likely to expect birth to be satisfying and fulfilling and to experience it as such. Although most people think of perinatal education primarily as preparation for the birth experience, classes are available in all areas of pregnancy, childbirth, and parenting. An added benefit of taking classes is meeting other expectant parents with similar concerns.

Early pregnancy classes focus on the first two trimesters. They cover information on adapting to pregnancy, dealing with early discomforts such as morning sickness and fatigue, and understanding what to expect in the months ahead. Second-trimester classes focus on changes that occur during the second trimester, fetal development, and alterations in roles. Information about body mechanics, work during pregnancy, and what to expect during the third trimester are discussed. Teachers talk about childbirth choices and encourage students to take a class in relaxation techniques to help through labor and delivery. Childbirth preparation classes are offered for the expectant mother and her partner. They learn self-help measures and what to expect during labor and delivery. These "natural childbirth" classes are offered during the third trimester. Women whose last prepared childbirth class was more than a few years ago often take refresher classes for a review of techniques and an update on current practices. Courses usually include a discussion of role changes in the family and sibling adjustment.

Exercise classes help women keep fit and healthy during pregnancy. Some classes also continue into the postpartum period. The instructor teaches low-impact aerobic exercises to prevent injury and overexertion of the pregnant woman.

Planned cesarean birth classes are offered for women who know they will have a cesarean, usually those who have had a cesarean birth previously. These women may remember very little from their first cesarean birth because they were frightened and exhausted. Class discussion makes parents feel that they have some control over events and provides a basis for discussion with caregivers. Vaginal birth after cesarean (VBAC) classes are offered for those parents who wish to have a vaginal birth after having a cesarean (VBAC) or a trial of labor after cesarean (TOLAC). Content includes explanations of the precautions taken, rationale, and coping techniques. Situations that might necessitate another cesarean birth and the emotional aspects of a failed VBAC are also discussed.

Although adolescents may attend regular prenatal classes, those designed to specifically meet the needs of this age group are the most effective. Education for pregnant adolescents is similar to that of adults, but they focus on the teenager's perceptions of childbearing. Clarification of misconceptions in a nonjudgmental manner makes classes more effective. Teenagers feel more comfortable in classes with their peers and will participate more actively when in a peer group situation. Because of their lack of experience and unrealistic expectations of infants, adolescents have a greater need for information about infant care and parenting than do older women. Presentations often include videos, demonstrations, games, and practice with dolls.

Breastfeeding classes are an excellent way to help the pregnant woman build confidence in her ability to breastfeed. These classes are especially useful because the length of stays in birth facilities in the United States have been reduced over recent years, and the opportunity for teaching during the time in the birth facility is minimal. Breastfeeding classes include information on physiology of lactation, feeding routines, feeding techniques, establishing a good milk supply, and solutions to common breastfeeding problems. Partners who attend learn how to provide support to breastfeeding women. Some instructors hold classes postpartum so problems can be addressed as they occur. Lactation specialists often work privately in the community as well, offering private sessions in clients' homes.

Parenting classes offer education on newborn care and cover topics such as preparing the home for a newborn, what to bring to the hospital for the newborn, infant safety, car seat installation and use, general care, and common concerns, such as infant crying, circumcision care, and sibling adjustment. Classes for fathers focus on childbirth from the male perspective. They give men the chance to meet other expectant fathers and ask questions they might not ask in a class with women in it. Classes often involve practicing infant care techniques with dolls.

Classes for other family members are usually held for siblings and grandparents. Sibling classes are usually for children ages 3 years to 12 years. These classes help children learn newborn characteristics and decrease anxiety about the approaching birth. Some younger children may think the new baby will be a playmate and are disappointed when they see the newborn cannot play with them. A tour of the nursery in the birth facility is often helpful, giving siblings the opportunity to see a newborn before the new baby actually comes home. Sibling classes emphasize the fact that children can become helpers and that the new baby can never replace them in their parents' affection. Classes for grandparents provide updates about recent developments in childbearing and parenting practices. Grandparents get the chance to talk with other grandparents and share stories about parenting. Topics include changes in infant care practices, such as putting infants to sleep on their backs, burping, and new feeding guidelines. The art of grandparenting and the importance of grandparents are emphasized.

Objective M: To Understand the Importance of Education for Childbirth

9.13 The Importance of Education for Childbirth

One of the most important goals of childbirth preparation classes is to increase the woman's confidence in her ability to cope with the birth. Most studies agree that couples receiving prenatal preparation for childbirth are more satisfied with their birth experiences and have greater feelings of control, even when unexpected complications occur.

Tension and anxiety during labor cause tightening of the abdominal muscles, impeding contractions and increasing pain by stimulation of nerve endings that heighten awareness of pain. Prolonged muscle tension causes fatigue and increased pain perception. When anxiety and tension are high, uterine contractions become less effective, and the length of labor increases. A woman who can remain relaxed throughout her labor will have the best outcome. Many of the techniques for prepared childbirth are based partially on theories of ***conditioned response,*** in which certain responses to stimuli become automatic through frequent association. Many couples will have difficulty with relaxation and may need to use other methods along with conditioning.

Objective N: To Understand Methods of Childbirth Education

9.14 Methods of Childbirth Education

Although all methods of prepared childbirth use some combination of pain management techniques, each has unique aspects. Many classes take a holistic approach, offering information on a variety of techniques so that couples can choose what works best for them.

Grantly Dick-Read, MD, a British obstetrician, was one of the first to use education and relaxation techniques to help women through childbirth. His theory was that fear in childbirth results in tension and pain. To prevent the fear-tension cycle, he developed a method of slow abdominal breathing in early labor and rapid chest breathing in advanced labor. The ***Dick-Read method*** was the first to be referred to as "natural childbirth."

The ***Bradley method*** was the first to include the father as a coach. Abdominal breathing to increase relaxation and breath control is taught in these classes. The Bradley method also emphasizes avoidance of all medications and other interventions.

The ***Leboyer method*** of childbirth, sometimes called "birth without violence," views birth as a traumatic experience for the newborn. To decrease the trauma of birth, all lights are dimmed, and noise is decreased to help the newborn adapt to extrauterine life. The infant receives a warm bath immediately after birth to promote relaxation. Some mothers deliver in tubs to accomplish this relaxation.

The ***Lamaze method*** is often called "psychoprophylaxis," because it uses the mind to help lessen pain perception. It involves concentration and conditioning to help the woman respond to contractions with relaxation and various techniques to lessen pain perception. Lamaze is the most popular method used today. A variety of techniques are taught, and women are taught that there is more than one way to respond to labor. Lamaze teachers acknowledge that labor is painful and do not promise that these techniques will make it pain-free. Instead, techniques are used to increase the woman's ability to cope with pain by relieving some of the accompanying distress.

The content of specific classes may differ, but most follow a similar pattern. Relaxation techniques, neuromuscular disassociation, touch relaxation, relaxation against pain, cutaneous stimulation (effleurage, sacral pressure, thermal stimulation, massage, and positioning), and mental stimulation (focal point, imagery, and music) are all taught in Lamaze classes. Although controlled breathing techniques were the major focus of these classes, focused or controlled breathing techniques are only one of the coping strategies used today to enhance the woman's ability to work with her labor during birth.

Objective O: To Understand the Role of the Labor Coach

9.15 The Role of the Labor Coach

Almost all methods of childbirth preparation encourage the participation of someone who will remain with the woman throughout labor. This support person shares the experience and helps the woman remain focused and calm.

The person who takes on this role may be the woman's husband, her mother, a friend, or a relative. The role of the support person is an important one and should not be dismissed. The "labor coach" may actively participate in the labor or may be supportive only by his or her presence. Depending on the woman's culture, husbands may not be expected to participate in the labor and delivery; it may only be the women of the family who participate actively. The nurse needs to recognize the woman's cultural practices and be supportive of them.

Objective P: To Understand Preparation for Labor and Birth

9.16 Preparation for Labor and Birth

Aside from attending childbirth education classes and packing a bag for the stay in the birth facility, the woman can prepare her body for the labor and birth by doing certain exercises which help strengthen muscle tone and which promote more rapid restoration of muscle tone after birth.

The ***pelvic tilt,*** or pelvic rocking, helps prevent or reduce back strain and strengthens abdominal muscle tone. To do the pelvic tilt, the woman lies on her back and bends her legs, with her feet flat on the floor. This position helps prevent strain and discomfort. The woman decreases the curvature in her back by pressing her spine toward the floor. With her back pressed against the floor, the woman then tightens her buttocks and abdominal muscles. The pelvic tilt can also be performed on hands and knees. A basic exercise to increase abdominal muscle tone is to tighten the abdominal muscles with each breath. A woman first expands her abdomen by taking a deep breath and as she gradually exhales, pulls in her abdominal muscles until they are fully contracted. She relaxes for a few seconds and then repeats the exercise.

Partial sit-ups strengthen abdominal muscle tone and are done according to individual comfort levels. When doing partial sit-ups, the woman lies on the floor with her knees bent and feet flat. She stretches her arms toward her knees as she slowly pulls her head and shoulders off the surface to a comfortable level. She then slowly returns to the starting position, takes a deep breath, and repeats the exercise. These exercises can be done in a sequence of five and can be repeated several times during the day, if desired.

Kegel exercises, or perineal muscle tightening, strengthens the pubococcygeus muscle and increases its elasticity. This muscle helps support the pelvic organs, including the uterus and bladder. A strong pubococcygeus muscle helps prevent stress incontinence, cystocele, rectocele, and uterine prolapse following childbirth. Kegel exercises involve identifying and contracting the muscle that controls or regulates urination. The woman should be cautioned, however, not to do these exercises while urinating because stopping urination midstream can cause urinary stasis and urinary tract infections. If done properly, the woman does not contract the muscles of the buttocks or thighs. Kegel exercises can be done at almost any time.

During pregnancy, the woman should be encouraged to assume the cross-legged position as much as possible. This "tailor sit" or "Indian style" position stretches the muscles of the inner thighs in preparation for labor and birth.

Review Exercises

True/False

1. ______ Today there are many options for childbirth.
2. ______ A birth plan is a document stating a couple's specific wishes for their childbirth experience.
3. ______ The need for calcium during pregnancy is greatly increased.
4. ______ Travel is contraindicated during pregnancy.
5. ______ Vegetarian diets may not include all the nutrients needed during pregnancy.
6. ______ Culture has a major influence on childbearing practices.
7. ______ Language can be a major barrier to the effective provision of health care.
8. ______ Eye contact is an important aspect of communication for people in the United States.
9. ______ Advance preparation for a baby is avoided in some cultures.
10. ______ Touch by anyone other than the individual's spouse is offensive in some cultures.
11. ______ Culturally competent nursing care requires an awareness of and sensitivity to the cultures of patients.
12. ______ It is important for pregnant women to "eat for two."
13. ______ Sushi is contraindicated in pregnancy.
14. ______ Maternal iron intake must be increased during pregnancy.
15. ______ Fatigue is a common symptom associated with pregnancy.
16. ______ Smoking during pregnancy is associated with low birth weight infants.
17. ______ Many women decide on the method of feeding before their infant's birth.
18. ______ The nurse should discourage women who decide to do combination feeding of infants.
19. ______ Patients should be encouraged to personalize their birth setting.
20. ______ While taking cultural practices of patients into consideration during childbearing, the nurse knows that the safety of the mother and her infant is most important.

Completion

1. ______________ is the ingestion of nonnutritive substances during pregnancy.
2. Vitamin ______________ enhances the absorption of iron.
3. During pregnancy, the recommended daily allowance (RDA) for caloric intake increases slightly, up __________ kcal/day.

4. The ____________________ test involves electronic external fetal monitoring for approximately 40 minutes.

5. Seat belts on a pregnant woman should be placed ______________ and ______________.

6. To be able to call a nonstress test reactive, two ____________________ must take place in a 20-minute period.

7. ______________ is the use of high-frequency sound waves to detect differences in tissue density and visualize outlines of fetal structures during pregnancy.

8. "Morning sickness" is another name for ______________, one of the earliest symptoms of pregnancy.

9. On an airplane, the pregnant woman should be encouraged to ambulate frequently to minimize the risk of ____________________.

10. The three safest exercises for pregnant women are ______________, ____________ and ______________.

11. A danger sign during the first trimester of pregnancy is ______________.

12. A danger sign during the second trimester is ______________.

13. The Family and Medical Leave Act of 1993 guarantees __________ weeks of unpaid maternity leave following the birth or adoption of a child.

14. Amniocentesis can be done early in pregnancy to check for chromosomal abnormalities and later in pregnancy for ______________.

15. Many of the techniques for prepared childbirth are based on theories of ______________ ______________, in which certain responses to stimuli become automatic through frequent association.

Matching Columns

1. Lamaze ____________________ A. "Birth without violence"

2. Biophysical profile (BPP) ______________ B. Test confirms pregnancy

3. Nonstress test ____________________ C. External fetal monitoring to assess fetal environment

4. Chorionic villus sampling (CVS) ________ D. Psychoprophylaxis method of childbirth education

5. Bradley method of childbirth education ____________ E. Test for chromosomal abnormalities

6. Alpha fetoprotein (AFP) ______________ F. Fetal blood test to detect fetal anomalies

7. Human chorionic gonadotropin (hCG) in urine ______________ G. Maternal blood test to determine neural tube defects

8. Maternal serum alpha fetoprotein (MSAFP) ____________________ H. Test assessing five parameters of fetal status

Answers

True/False

1. True
2. True
3. True
4. False. Travel is safe for pregnant women.
5. True
6. True
7. True
8. True
9. True
10. True
11. True
12. False. Pregnant women do not have to "eat for two"; instead, they should increase calories by 300 kcal daily.
13. True
14. True
15. True
16. True
17. True
18. False. Once the patient decides on a feeding method, the nurse should be supportive of her decision.
19. True
20. True

Completion

1. Pica
2. Vitamin C
3. 300 kcal/day
4. Nonstress
5. Above the gravid uterus, across the lap
6. Accelerations
7. Ultrasound
8. Nausea
9. thrombophlebitis
10. swimming, cycling, low-impact aerobics
11. bleeding
12. preterm labor (bleeding, gestational diabetes)
13. 12
14. Fetal lung maturity
15. conditioned response

Matching Columns

1. Lamaze—D
2. BPP—H
3. Nonstress test—C
4. CVS—F
5. Bradley method—A
6. AFP—E
7. hCG—B
8. MSAFP—G

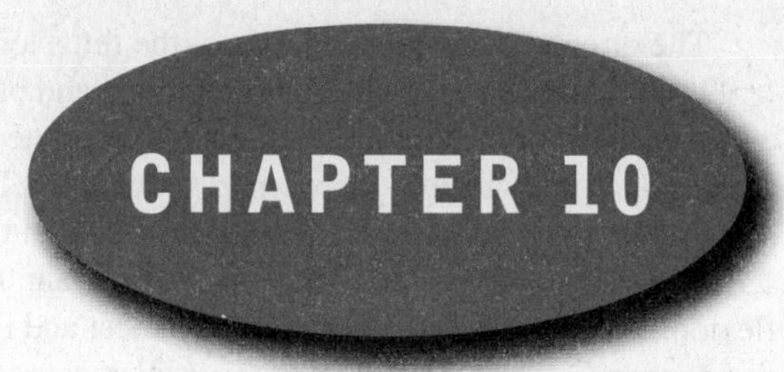

Labor and Birth Process

Objective A: To Understand the Components of the Birth Process

10.1 Components of the Birth Process

Childbirth is both a physical and an emotional experience. It is an irrevocable event that forever changes a woman and a family. The nurse must attend to the physiologic, psychological, and emotional needs of the woman to promote a positive birth experience. The four major factors during normal childbirth are the powers, the passage, the passenger, and the psyche.

The ***powers*** needed for birth are the uterine contractions (UCs) and the maternal pushing efforts. During the first stage of labor, the UCs are the primary force that moves the fetus through the maternal pelvis. During the second stage of labor, UCs continue to propel the fetus through the pelvis, but now the woman feels an urge to push and bear down as the fetus distends her vagina and puts pressure on her rectum. She adds her voluntary pushing efforts to the force of the contractions, making it possible for the baby to be born.

The ***passage*** refers to the maternal pelvis and soft tissue. The bony pelvis is usually more important to the outcome of labor than the soft tissue because the bones and joints do not readily yield to the forces of labor. However, softening of the cartilage linking the pelvic bones occurs at term because of increased levels of the hormone relaxin.

The passenger refers to the fetus, membranes, and placenta. The fetus enters the birth canal in the cephalic (head first) presentation ~97% of the time. The fetal head is composed of bony parts. The skull is composed of three major parts: the face, the base of the skull (cranium), and the vault of the cranium (roof). The bones of the fetal head involved in the birth process are not fused but are connected by sutures composed of flexible fibrous tissue, allowing for molding in order to fit through the birth canal; they also help the clinician identify the position of the fetal head during examination. The five major bones are the two frontal bones on the forehead, the two parietal bones at the crown of the head, and the occipital bone at the back of the head.

The intersection of several cranial sutures forms an irregular space called a ***fontanelle*** that is enclosed by a membrane. The anterior and posterior fontanelles are clinically useful in identifying the position of the fetal head in the pelvis and in assessing the status of the newborn after birth. The anterior fontanelle is diamond-shaped, measures 2 to 3 cm, and is situated at the junction of the sagittal, coronal, and frontal sutures. It permits growing of the brain by remaining unossified for as long as 18 months. The posterior fontanelle is shaped like a small triangle, measures ~1 to 2 cm, and is situated at the intersection of the sagittal and lambdoid sutures. It closes within 8 to 12 weeks after birth.

The orientation of the long axis of the fetus to the long axis of the woman's body is called the ***fetal lie***. In > 99% of pregnancies, the lie is longitudinal and parallel to the long axis of the woman. In the longitudinal lie, either the head or the buttocks of the fetus enter the pelvis first. A transverse lie exists when the long axis of the fetus is at a right angle to the woman's long axis. This occurs in < 1% of all pregnancies. An oblique lie is at some other angle between the longitudinal lie and the transverse lie.

The relation of the fetal body parts to one another is the ***attitude*** of the fetus. The normal attitude is one of flexion, with the head flexed toward the chest and the arms and legs flexed over the thorax. The back is curved in a convex C shape. Flexion remains a characteristic feature of a full-term newborn.

The fetal part that enters the pelvis first is termed the ***presenting part.*** Presentation falls into three categories: cephalic (head first), breech (buttocks first), and shoulder. The ***cephalic presentation*** with the head flexed is the most common and most favorable for vaginal delivery. Because the head is the largest part of the fetal body, once it is delivered, usually the rest of the body is delivered more easily. During labor, the fetal head can mold to fit through the maternal pelvis; because it is smooth, round, and hard, it is effective in dilating the cervix, which is also round.

A ***breech presentation*** is associated with many disadvantages. The buttocks are not smooth and firm like the head and are therefore less effective in dilating the cervix. Also, because the head in the breech presentation is the last part of the fetal body to be born, by the time the fetus is fully delivered, the cord is outside the body, which can cause cord compression.

The breech presentation has three variations, depending on the relationship of the fetal legs to the fetal body. In the most common variation, the ***frank breech*** position, the legs are extended across the abdomen toward the shoulders. The ***full breech*** presentation is a reversal of the cephalic presentation, and the ***footling breech*** occurs when one or both feet are presenting.

Fetal position describes the location of a fixed reference point on the presenting part in relation to a specific quadrant of the maternal pelvis. The fetal position is not fixed but changes as the fetus maneuvers through the maternal pelvis. The presenting part can be right anterior, left anterior, right posterior, or left posterior. The four quadrants designate whether the presenting part is directed toward the front, back, right, or left side of the passageway.

The ***psyche*** is a crucial part of childbirth. Marked anxiety and fear decrease a woman's ability to cope with the pain of labor. Much of nursing care during this time is promoting relaxation and reducing anxiety and fear. The nurse's supportive attitude strengthens positive psychological elements and enhances the process of birth. A negative childbirth experience can have far-reaching implications, which can interfere with bonding and maternal role attainment.

Objective B: To Understand the Onset of Labor

10.2 Onset of Labor

Despite continuing research, the exact mechanism that initiates labor is unknown. The most common hypotheses formed point to decreased levels of progesterone and the release of fetal cortisol, which may stimulate labor and birth.

Objective C: To Understand the Premonitory Signs of Labor

10.3 Premonitory Signs of Labor

Before the onset of labor, a number of physiologic changes occur that signal the readiness of labor and birth. These changes are usually noted by the primigravida woman at about 38 weeks' gestation. In multigravidas, they may not take place until labor begins. These changes are referred to as ***premonitory signs*** of labor. Educating the woman about these signs and giving her guidelines for calling her health care provider can reduce some of the anxiety that surrounds labor and birth.

At about 38 weeks' gestation in primigravidas, the presenting part descends into the pelvic cavity, causing the woman's uterus to move downward as well. This process is called ***lightening*** and marks the beginning of engagement. This drop in the uterus may decrease upward pressure on the diaphragm and result in easier breathing. The downward settling of the uterus can cause maternal symptoms of increased urinary frequency, leg cramps or pains, increased pelvic pressure, edema in the lower legs, and increased vaginal secretions.

As the pregnancy approaches term, most women become aware of irregular sensations called ***Braxton Hicks contractions.*** Because these contractions become stronger and are often uncomfortable, many women think they are in true labor; however, this does not result in dilation or effacement of the uterus and is often called ***false labor,*** or ***prodromal labor.*** It is thought that Braxton Hicks contractions contribute to the preparation of the cervix for true labor.

As full term nears, the cervix softens because of the effects of the hormone relaxin and increased water content. The changes (***ripening***) allow the cervix to yield more easily to the forces of labor contractions. As the fetal head descends with lightening, it puts pressure on the cervix, starting the process of effacement and dilation. Effacement and dilation cause expulsion of the mucous plug that sealed the cervix during pregnancy, rupturing small cervical capillaries in the process. This bleeding, often called ***bloody show,*** is a mixture of thick mucus and pink or dark brown blood. It may begin several days to a few weeks before the onset of labor.

In the weeks before labor starts, some women have a burst of energy and need to get the home ready for the baby's arrival. This behavior, referred to as ***nesting,*** may be related to an increase in the hormone adrenaline, which is needed to support the woman in labor. Women should be cautioned to conserve some of that energy for the childbirth process.

Before the onset of labor, changes in the levels of estrogen and progesterone can lead to electrolyte shifts and may result in a reduction in fluid retention. This increased fluid loss can result in a weight loss of up to 3 lb. Some women experience gastrointestinal disturbances (diarrhea, nausea, vomiting, or indigestion) as a sign of impending labor. The etiology of the gastrointestinal disturbances is generally unknown.

Increased backache and sacroiliac pressure may be experienced by the near-term woman due to the influence of relaxin on the pelvic joints.

About 12% of pregnant women experience spontaneous ***rupture of the amniotic sac*** (ruptured membranes or "broken bag of waters") prior to the onset of labor. Rupture of the membranes is a critical event in pregnancy. After membranes rupture, 80% of women will experience spontaneous labor within 24 hours. If membranes rupture and labor does not begin spontaneously within 24 hours, labor may be induced to avoid infection (once the membranes have ruptured, there is an open pathway into the uterine cavity). It is important that the woman be taught to note the color, amount, and odor of the amniotic fluid and to call her health care provider immediately to let him or her know that the membranes have ruptured. The amniotic fluid should be clear and odorless. A yellow-green tinged amniotic fluid may indicate infection or fetal passage of meconium; this finding always signals the need for further assessment and electronic fetal heart rate (FHR) monitoring. Confirmation of amniotic fluid can be done by a nitrazine test or by a ferning test. The nitrizine pH paper will turn blue-green if amniotic fluid is placed on paper. In the ferning test, a slide is prepared placing amniotic fluid on the slide. Under a microscope, the amniotic fluid on the slide looks like fern.

Objective D: To Understand How to Distinguish True Labor from False Labor

10.4 True Labor and False Labor

True labor contractions lead to progressive dilation and effacement of the cervix. They occur with regularity and increase in intensity, frequency, and duration. The pain in true labor starts in the woman's back and radiates to the abdomen. It often intensifies with activity, such as walking. In contrast, the contractions of false labor are irregular and do not increase in intensity, frequency, or duration. False labor does not lead to dilation and effacement. The sensations associated with false labor are mostly felt in the groin and abdomen and are often considered annoying rather than truly painful. False labor pain is often relieved with comfort measures, such as positioning and warm showers.

For many couples, this can be a disappointing and frustrating experience. The nurse needs to provide reassurance and review the signs and symptoms of true labor in a sensitive manner and instruct the woman when to return to the birth facility.

Objective E: To Understand the Maternal Physiologic Response to Labor

10.5 Maternal Physiologic Response to Labor

The labor process affects nearly every major body system. Each system adapts to these changes through various compensation mechanisms. The most obvious changes occur in the reproductive system. Normal labor contractions are coordinated, involuntary, and intermittent. They are rhythmic in nature.

Each contraction consists of three phases. The ***increment,*** or "building up" phase, occurs as the contraction begins in the fundus and spreads throughout the uterus. The ***peak,*** or acme, is the period during which the contraction is most intense. The ***decrement*** is the period of decreasing intensity as the uterus relaxes. Between contractions is a period of relaxation. This period of relaxation, or ***resting tone,*** allows uterine muscles to rest and provides respite for the laboring patient. It also restores uteroplacental circulation and adequate circulation in the uterine blood vessels.

Contractions are often described in terms of their frequency, intensity, and duration. The ***frequency*** of a contraction is measured from the beginning of one contraction to the beginning of the next. The ***duration*** of a contraction is measured from the beginning of a contraction to the end of that same contraction. The ***intensity*** of a contraction is most frequently measured by uterine palpation and is described as mild, moderate, or strong.

Contractions bring about changes in uterine musculature. The upper portion of the uterus, or fundus, becomes thicker and more active. The lower uterine segment becomes thin-walled and passive. With each contraction the uterus elongates. Elongation causes a straightening of the fetal body so that the upper body is pressed against the fundus, and the lower, presenting part is pushed toward the lower uterine segment and the cervix. As the uterus elongates, the longitudinal muscle fibers are stretched upward over the presenting part. This force, along with the hydrostatic pressure of the fetal membranes, causes the cervix to open (dilate).

Contractions are usually measured via electronic monitoring. Monitoring may be external or internal and can provide a continuous assessment of uterine activity. With external contraction monitoring, the pressure that is exerted against the device as the uterus contracts is measured and recorded on graph paper. External monitoring may be continuous or intermittent. It provides information about the frequency and duration of contractions, but it does not give accurate data about their strength. Contraction intensity is best assessed by palpation.

Effacement and dilation are the major cervical changes during labor. They occur simultaneously during labor but at different rates. Before labor the cervix is a cylindric structure ~2 cm long at the lower end of the uterus. Labor contractions push the fetus downward against the cervix while pulling the cervix upward. The cervix becomes shorter and thinner as it is drawn over the fetus and amniotic sac. A fully thinned cervix is 100% effaced. As the cervix is pulled upward and the fetus is pushed downward, the cervix dilates. Dilation is expressed in centimeters. Full dilation is 10 cm, sufficient to allow delivery of a full-term fetus.

The woman's cardiovascular system is stressed by both the UCs and the pain, anxiety, and apprehension the woman experiences. In pregnancy, the resting pulse rate increases 10 to 18 beats per minute (bpm). During labor there is a significant increase in cardiac output. Each strong contraction gently decreases or stops the blood flow to the placenta and a redistribution of blood into the peripheral circulation. The result is an increase in the systolic and diastolic blood pressure, a slowing of the pulse rate, and an increase in cardiac output. It is therefore very important for the nurse to take the woman's vital signs between contractions.

Perfuse perspiration (diaphoresis) occurs during labor. Hyperventilation also occurs, altering electrolyte and fluid balance from insensible fluid loss. The muscle activity elevates the body temperature, which increases sweating and evaporation from the skin. In some instances, parenteral intravenous (IV) fluids are administered.

The depth and rate of respirations increase, especially if the woman is anxious or in pain. A patient who breathes rapidly and deeply may experience symptoms of hyperventilation if respiratory alkalosis occurs. She may feel dizzy or experience tingling of her hands and feet or numbness. The nurse or labor partner needs to encourage the woman to slow her breathing to alleviate these symptoms.

Polyuria is common during labor. This results from the increase in cardiac output, which causes an increase in the glomerular filtration rate and renal plasma flow. Slight proteinuria occurs in one third to one half of laboring women.

During labor there is an increase in maternal rennin, plasma rennin activity, and angiotensinogen. This elevation is thought to be important in the control of uteroplacental blood flow during birth and the early postpartal period.

Gastric motility is reduced in labor to various degrees, which can result in nausea and vomiting. Most women are not hungry but very thirsty while in labor, and ice chips are usually permitted. Solid food is usually withheld to prevent vomiting and aspiration of undigested food in the event that general anesthesia is needed.

The fluid requirements for women in labor have not been clearly established. In some instances, oral hydration is the primary goal. In other situations a saline lock may be inserted so that IV access is available if needed. If IV fluids are used, caution should be taken with glucose solutions, as there is an increase in maternal blood glucose that can lead to fetal hyperglycemia and hyperinsulinemia in the newborn.

The white blood cell (WBC) count of a woman in labor increases to 25,000 to 30,000/mm^3 during labor and early postpartum. The change is probably due to a physiologic response to stress. The increased WBC count makes it difficult to identify the presence of infection.

Maternal blood glucose levels decrease in labor because glucose is used as an energy source during UCs. The decreased blood glucose levels lead to a decrease in insulin requirements. Glucose levels can drop significantly during a prolonged or difficult labor.

Most authorities recognize 500 mL as the maximum normal blood loss during a vaginal birth. Women usually tolerate this well because of the increased blood volumes amassed during pregnancy of 1 to 2 L. A woman who is anemic at the beginning of labor has less reserve for normal blood loss and a poor tolerance for excess bleeding. Normal blood loss during a cesarean birth is 1,000 mL.

Levels of several clotting factors, especially fibrinogen, are elevated during pregnancy and continue to be higher during labor and after delivery. The greater number of clotting factors provides protection from hemorrhage but also increases the woman's risk for a venous thrombosis during pregnancy and after birth.

Objective F: To Understand Fetal Responses to Labor

10.6 Fetal Responses to Labor

When the fetus is normal, the mechanical and hemodynamic changes of normal labor have no adverse effects. The exchange of oxygen, nutrients, and waste products between the woman and fetus occurs in the intervillous spaces without the mixing of maternal and fetal blood. During strong labor contractions, the maternal blood supply to the placenta decreases and eventually stops temporarily as the spiral arteries supplying the intervillous spaces are compressed by the uterine muscle. The placental circulation usually has enough reserve compared with fetal basal needs to tolerate the periodic interruption of blood flow. The fetus might not tolerate labor contractions well in conditions associated with reduced placental function, such as maternal diabetes and hypertension.

The fetal cardiovascular system reacts quickly to events during labor. Alterations in the rate and rhythm of the fetal heart may result from normal labor effects or suggest fetal intolerance to the labor. The FHR ranges from 110 to 160 bpm.

The fetal lungs produce fluid (surfactant) to allow normal development of the airways. Lung fluid must be cleared to allow normal breathing after birth. As term nears, production of fetal fluid decreases to ~65% of its normal production. Labor speeds up the absorption of lung fluid, and some fluid is expelled as the thorax is compressed during passage through the birth canal. A small amount is absorbed into the baby's interstitial spaces and then into the circulatory system, and some is cleared by the lymphatic system. Infants born by cesarean birth are more likely to have transient breathing difficulty.

Catecholamines are produced as a response to the stress of labor and aid in the newborn's response to extrauterine life. They stimulate cardiac contraction and breathing, quicken the lung absorption, and aid in temperature regulation.

Objective G: To Understand the Mechanisms of Labor

10.7 Mechanisms of Labor

The mechanisms (cardinal movements) of labor occur as the fetus is moved through the pelvis during birth. The fetus undergoes several positional changes to adapt to the size and shape of the mother's pelvis at different levels. In a vertex presentation, the mechanisms include

- ***Descent*** of the fetal head
- ***Engagement*** of the fetal head as its widest diameter reaches the level of the ischial spine of the mother's pelvis
- ***Flexion*** of the fetal head downward onto the chest, allowing the smallest head diameter to align with the smaller diameter of the midpelvis as it descends
- ***Internal rotation*** to allow the largest fetal head diameter to align with the largest maternal pelvic diameter
- ***Extension*** of the fetal head as it passes under the symphysis pubis
- ***External rotation*** of the fetal head, aligning the head with the shoulders during expulsion. Through expulsive efforts of the laboring woman and after the external rotation, the anterior shoulder meets the undersurface of the symphysis pubis and slips under it. As lateral flexion of the shoulder and head occur, the anterior shoulder is born before the posterior shoulder, with the body following quickly.

Objective H: To Understand the Stages and Phases of Labor

10.8 Stages and Phases of Labor

Labor is divided into four stages. Each stage has its unique qualities. These represent therapeutic separations in the process. A laboring woman usually will not experience distinct differences from one to the other. The time for a normal labor will depend on whether the woman is a nullipara or a multipara.

1. The first stage begins with the start of true labor and ends when the cervix is completely dilated.
2. The second stage begins with complete dilation and ends with the birth of the baby.
3. The third stage begins with the birth of the baby and ends with the expulsion of the placenta.
4. Some clinicians identify a fourth stage of labor, or recovery stage, which lasts 1 to 4 hours after expulsion of the placenta. During this stage the uterus effectively contracts to control bleeding at the placental site.

The ***first stage*** of labor is divided into the latent, active, and transition phases. Each phase of labor is characterized by physical and psychological changes. The ***latent phase*** begins with the onset of regular contractions. As the cervix begins to dilate, it also effaces, although little or no descent is evident. In this early phase, the contractions are usually mild, lasting 20 to 40 seconds, with a frequency of 3 to 30 minutes. The woman feels able to deal with her discomfort. She may be relieved that labor has finally started. The woman is often very talkative and smiling and is eager to talk about herself and answer questions. Although she may be anxious, she is able to recognize and express those feelings of anxiety. Excitement is high, and her partner or support person is often as elevated as she is. For a woman in her first labor (nullipara), the latent phase averages 8.6 hours but should not exceed 20 hours. The latent phase in multiparas averages 5.3 hours but should not exceed 14 hours.

When the woman enters the early ***active phase,*** her anxiety tends to increase as she senses the intensification of contractions and pain. She begins to fear a loss of control and may use a variety of coping mechanisms. Some women exhibit a decrease in coping ability and feel a sense of helplessness. Women who have support persons and family available experience greater satisfaction and less anxiety than those without support. During this phase the cervix dilates from 4 to 7 cm. Fetal decent is progressive. The cervical dilation should be at least 1.2 cm per hour in nulliparas and 1.5 cm in multiparas. This is the ideal time to give pain medications, if the patient desires. Pain medications given too early in labor can slow the labor. Giving medications after this time increases the risk that the newborn will be born with respiratory depression.

The ***transition phase*** is the last part of the first stage. When the woman enters the transition phase, she may demonstrate significant anxiety. She becomes acutely aware of the increasing intensity of the contractions. She may fear being left alone. Cervical dilation slows as it progresses from 8 to 10 cm, and the rate of fetal head descent increases. During transition, contractions have a frequency of 1.5 to 2 minutes and a duration of 60 to 90 seconds. As dilation approaches 10 cm, there may be increased rectal pressure and an uncontrollable urge to bear down, an increase in bloody show, and rupture of the membranes. The woman may also feel that she will be "torn apart" by the force of the contractions. The transition phase should not be longer than 3 hours for nulliparas and 1 hour for multiparas. The total duration of the first stage may be increased by approximately 1 hour if epidural anesthesia is used.

The ***second stage*** of labor begins when the cervix is completely dilated (10 cm) and ends with the birth of the infant. Contractions continue with a frequency of 1.5 to 2 minutes, a duration of 60 to 90 minutes, and strong intensity. The woman has the urge to push because of pressure on the rectum and pelvic floor causing an involuntary pushing response in the mother. She may say she has the need to "have a bowel movement" or say "the baby's coming." As the fetal head continues its descent, the perineum begins to bulge, flatten, and move anteriorly. With succeeding contractions and maternal pushing efforts, the fetal head descends further and starts to crown. Crowning occurs when the fetal head is encircled by the external opening of the vagina and means birth is imminent. Some women report feeling a "burning" sensation as the perineum distends. The woman may state again that she feels "she is going to rip apart," but the nurse has to instruct her to push through the pain and the burning. The duration of the second stage of labor averages 30 minutes to 3 hours in nulliparas and 5 to 30 minutes in parous women.

Usually, a childbirth-prepared woman is relieved to be able to push and recognizes that the end of labor is near. Others, particularly those without childbirth preparation, may become frightened. The woman may feel that she has lost control and become embarrassed and apologetic, or, she may demonstrate extreme irritability toward the staff and her support person. Such behavior is often frightening and disconcerting to her support person. The nurse needs to provide reassurance to the support person that this is a common reaction. The woman feels tremendous relief and excitement as the second stage ends.

The ***third stage*** of labor begins with the birth of the baby and ends with the expulsion of the placenta. This stage is the shortest, lasting up to 30 minutes, and averaging 5 to 10 minutes. There is no difference in duration between nulliparas and parous women. Massaging the perineum helps relax the muscles to allow for delivery. Sometimes an episiotomy has to be cut to make more room to allow the fetal head to be delivered or if delivery needs to be hastened.

An ***episiotomy*** is a surgical incision of the perineal body. The procedure is performed with a sharp scissors that has rounded points, just before birth, when ~3 to 4 cm of the fetal head is visible during a contraction. There are two types of episiotomies: midline and mediolateral. A ***midline episiotomy*** is performed extending down from the vaginal orifice to the fibers of the rectal sphincter. This type of episiotomy avoids muscle fibers and major blood vessels because it entails less blood loss, is easy to repair, and heals with less discomfort to the mother. The major disadvantage is that a tear of the midline incision may extend through the anal sphincter and rectum.

In the presence of a short perineum, macrosomia, and instrument-assisted birth (use of forceps or vacuum extractor), a ***mediolateral episiotomy*** provides more room and decreases the possibility of a traumatic extension into the rectum. The mediolateral episiotomy begins in the midline of the posterior fourchette and extends at a 45-degree angle downward to the right or to the left. It may be complicated by greater blood loss, a longer healing period, and more postpartal discomfort. The episiotomy is usually performed with regional or local anesthesia but may be performed without anesthesia in emergency situations. Adequate anesthesia must be given for the repair. Repair of the episiotomy and any laceration is usually performed after the expulsion of the placenta in case a manual removal of the placenta or a uterine exploration is indicated.

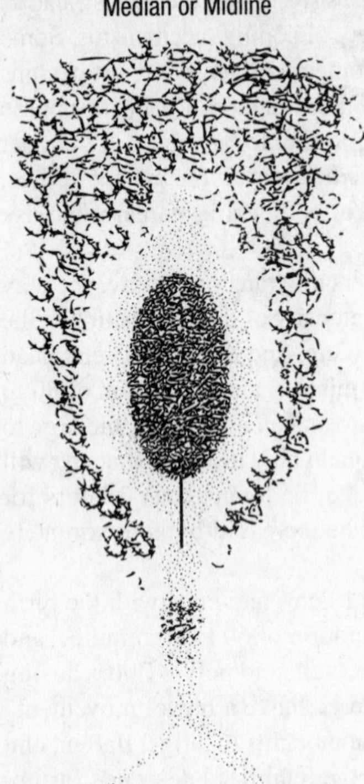

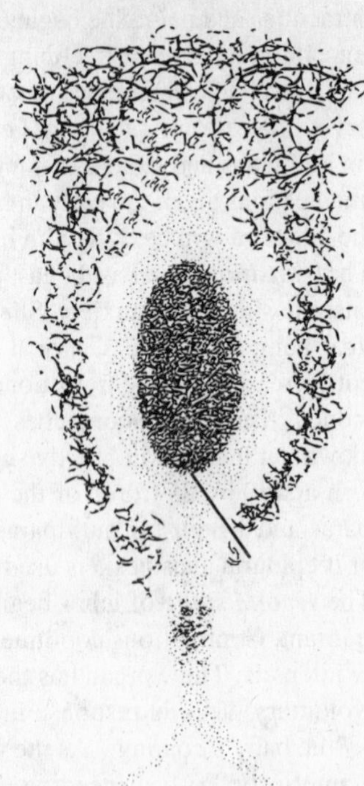

Median or Midline: *ADVANTAGES*	Median or Midline: *DISADVANTAGES*	Mediolateral: *ADVANTAGES*	Mediolateral: *DISADVANTAGES*
Minimal blood loss Neat healing with little scarring Less postpartum pain than the mediolateral episiotomy	An added laceration may extend the median episiotomy into the anal sphincter Limited enlargement of the vaginal opening because perineal length is limited by the anal sphincter	More enlargement of the vaginal opening Little risk that the episiotomy will extend into the anus	More blood loss Increased postpartum pain More scarring and irregularity in the healed scar Prolonged dyspareunia (painful intercourse)

Figure 10.1 Types of episiotomies.

Pain relief measures may begin immediately after birth with application of an ice pack to the perineum. For optimal effect, the ice pack should be applied for 20 to 30 minutes and removed for at least 20 minutes before being reapplied. If the ice pack is left in place longer than 30 minutes, vasodilation and subsequent edema may ensue.

Indications for the ***use of forceps*** include the presence of any condition that threatens the woman or fetus and that can be relieved by birth. Conditions that put the mother at risk include heart disease, acute pulmonary edema or pulmonary compromise, certain neurologic conditions, intrapartal infection, prolonged second stage, and exhaustion. Fetal conditions include premature placental separation, prolapsed umbilical cord, and nonreassuring fetal status. Forceps may be used electively to shorten the second stage of labor and spare the woman's pushing effort or when regional anesthesia has affected the woman's motor innervations and she cannot push effectively. If a good application cannot be obtained or if no descent occurs with the application, a vacuum technique can be attempted. If this yields no descent, then a cesarean birth is the method of choice.

Maternal risks of forceps-assisted delivery include trauma such as lacerations of the birth canal, periurethral lacerations, and extensions of a median episiotomy into the anus, resulting in increased bleeding, bruising, hematomas, and pelvic floor injuries. In addition, an increase in postpartum infections, cervical lacerations, and urinary and rectal incontinence may occur.

Risks to the newborn from a forceps-assisted delivery include small areas of ecchymosis or edema, or both, along the sides of the face as a result of forceps application. Transient facial paralysis, as well as cephalohematoma or caput succedaneum, may occur. Other reported complications include low Apgar scores, retinal hemorrhage, corneal abrasions, ocular trauma, elevated neonatal bilirubin levels, and prolonged hospital stay.

Vacuum extraction is an obstetric procedure used to assist the birth of the fetus by applying suction. A vacuum extractor is composed of a soft suction cup attached to a suction bottle (pump) by tubing. The suction cup is placed against the occiput of the fetal head, and negative pressure of 50 to 60 mm Hg is created while the clinician applies traction in coordination with contractions. The fetal head should descend with each contraction until it emerges from the vagina. The American Congress of Obstetricians and Gynecologists (ACOG) advises a 30-minute limit on the duration of use. In addition, if more than three "pop-offs" occur (the suction cup pops off the fetal head), the procedure should be discontinued. A birth by cesarean section may be indicated after a failed forceps/vacuum extraction attempt.

Maternal complications include perineal trauma, edema, third- and fourth-degree lacerations, postpartum pain, and infection. Neonatal complications include scalp lacerations, bruising, subgaleal hematomas, cephalohematomas, subconjunctival hemorrhages, neonatal jaundice, fractured clavicle, Erb palsy, damage to the sixth and seventh cranial nerves, retinal hemorrhage, and fetal death. Women who give birth with the aid of a vacuum extractor report more sexual difficulties in the postpartum period.

Cesarean birth is the birth of an infant through an abdominal uterine incision. It is one of the oldest surgical procedures known. As malpractice rates have skyrocketed in the United States and as more women are waiting later to have children, the prevalence of cesarean birth has grown. Also, some women would like to choose the type of delivery they are having, sometimes called "designer births." This raises a lot of ethical issues that will not be discussed at this time. The majority of cesarean sections performed in the United States today are done because of a previous cesarean birth or dystocia. Cesarean birth requires both skin and uterine incisions, which are not necessarily the same type of incision. The skin incision is either transverse (Pfannenstiel) or vertical and is not indicative of the type of incision made on the uterus. The type of skin incision is determined by time factor, client preference, cosmetic reasons, and physician preference.

The ***transverse incision*** is made across the lowest and narrowest part of the abdomen. Because the incision is made just below the pubic hair line, it is almost invisible when healed. Other advantages of this type are less bleeding, less uterine rupture, and better healing. The limitations of this incision are that it cannot be extended if needed and that it may develop more scar tissue if subsequent surgeries are needed. The ***vertical incision*** is made between the navel and the symphysis pubis. This incision is quicker and is preferred in cases of nonreassuring fetal status when rapid birth is indicated, with preterm or macrosomic infants, or when the woman is obese.

The type of uterine incision depends on the need for the cesarean. The choice of incision affects the woman's opportunity for a subsequent vaginal birth and her risks of a ruptured uterine scar with a subsequent pregnancy. The most common uterine incision is the transverse. It is less likely to rupture in subsequent pregnancies, it requires only moderate dissection of the bladder from the underlying myometrium, and it is easier to repair. The disadvantages include the fact that it takes longer to make a transverse incision, it is limited in size because of the presence of major blood vessels on either side of the uterus, and it has a greater tendency to extend laterally into the uterine vessels. The lower uterine segment vertical incision is preferred for multiple gestation, abnormal presentation, if the woman has had no labor, and for preterm and microsomic fetuses.

One other incision, the ***classical incision,*** is rarely used today. The vertical incision is made in the upper uterine segment. There is a greater blood loss in this part of the uterus, and it is more difficult to repair. Most importantly, it carries a greater risk of uterine rupture with subsequent pregnancy, labor, and delivery because the upper uterine segment is the most contractile portion of the uterus.

There is no preferred method of anesthesia for cesarean birth. Each has its advantages and disadvantages, possible risks, and side effects. The anesthesia chosen often has to do with the scenario related to the reason for the cesarean birth. In a planned cesarean, a woman usually has more options as opposed to an emergency, when general anesthesia is usually warranted.

When the infant is born, the uterine cavity becomes much smaller. The reduced size decreases the size of the placenta site, causing it to separate from the uterine wall. Four signs suggest placenta separation: the uterus having a spherical shape, the uterus rising upward in the abdomen as the placenta descends into the vagina and pushes the fundus upward, the cord descending farther from the vagina, and a gush of blood that appears as blood trapped behind the placenta is released. The placenta may be expelled in one of two ways. In the more common Schultze mechanism, the placenta is delivered with the shiny fetal side presenting first ("shiny Schultze"). In the Duncan mechanism, the rough maternal part is presenting ("dirty Duncan").

The placenta should be examined by the clinician after birth. It should be checked to see if all lobules are intact so that the patient will not have retained placenta, and the cord should be examined for three vessels, two arteries, and one vein. The umbilical artery is the largest vessel, and the arteries are smaller vessels. The presence of only one artery is associated with genitourinary abnormalities in the newborn. The number of vessels is recorded on the birth and newborn records. Blood from the cord is drawn up by the clinician and sent to the lab to determine the infant's blood type, Coombs test, and Venereal Disease Research Laboratories (VDRL) test.

The ***fourth stage*** of labor is the stage of physical recovery for the mother and infant. It lasts from the delivery of the placenta through the first 1 to 4 hours after birth. It is during this time that the woman could have an early postpartum hemorrhage, so it is crucial that the nurse assess the new mother regularly to avoid this complication. The woman also becomes acquainted with her newborn at this time. If she is breastfeeding, the woman should be encouraged to put the baby to breast during this time, as the infant is born awake and alert, in order to promote a positive breastfeeding experience.

Objective I: To Understand Evaluation of Labor Progress

10.9 Evaluation of Labor Progress

Intrapartal nursing care requires competent assessment and clinical skills and a comprehensive knowledge of maternal-fetal anatomy and the physiology of the labor process. An ongoing accurate assessment of both the woman and fetus and their response to labor is necessary to provide the data required to make sound clinical judgments and provide appropriate care. Assessment of the fetus during labor and birth is a fundamental component of caring for a woman in labor. Intrapartal assessment of the fetus should be included in the maternal assessment at admission and remain ongoing throughout the intrapartal period. Fetal assessments include identification of fetal position and presentation, as well as auscultation.

Approximately 85% of all labors are monitored electronically, making ***electronic fetal monitoring (EFM)*** the most prevalent assessment procedure in maternal-fetal health care. Since its introduction into clinical practice in the late 1960s, EFM has continuously been researched and evaluated in regard to its ability to improve fetal outcomes and reduce morbidity and mortality. It was thought that continuous EFM could identify nonreassuring fetal status earlier, facilitate earlier interventions, and prevent fetal morbidity and mortality. However, that has not been proven over intermittent auscultation. Professional organizations and individual health care institutions generally set the guidelines for the level of intrapartum monitoring. The frequency of the maternal-fetal assessment and documentation depends on the stage of labor and the presence of risk factors.

Assessment of the fetus during labor and birth is a fundamental component of caring for a woman in labor. Intrapartal assessment of the fetus should be included in the maternal assessment at admission and remain ongoing throughout the intrapartal period. Fetal assessments include identification of fetal position and presentation, as well as auscultation. Generally speaking, for low-risk pregnancies, FHR tracings can be reviewed every 30 minutes in first-stage labor and every 15 minutes in second-stage labor. The FHR tracings for high-risk pregnancies need to be reviewed more frequently—every 15 minutes in first-stage labor and every 5 minutes in second-stage labor. Periodic documentation should accompany each review of the FHR tracing.

To assess ***fetal position,*** there are four methods; some are more accurate than others. The nurse may attempt to identify fetal position in the following ways:

1. Abdominal palpation (Leopold maneuvers)
2. Location of the point of auscultation of FHR
3. Vaginal exam
4. Ultrasound

Leopold maneuvers are a systematic way of palpating the maternal abdomen to assess the fetal position. Performing Leopold maneuvers takes practice and is not always accurate in identifying fetal position. The first maneuver is done with the nurse facing upward toward the fundus and placing the hands on the upper uterus to determine what fetal part is in the upper uterus. The second maneuver is trying to locate the fetal back. The nurse palpates the maternal abdomen with her palms. The right hand should be steady, while the left hand explores the right side of the uterus. The nurse then repeats the maneuver, probing with the right hand and steadying the uterus with the left. Next, the nurse should determine what fetal part is lying above the inlet by gently grasping the lower portion of the abdomen just above the symphysis pubis with the thumb and fingers of the right hand. This maneuver yields the opposite information from what was found in the fundus and validates the presenting part. If the head is not engaged, it may be gently pushed back and forth. The fourth maneuver is done from the opposite direction, with the nurse facing the woman's feet and taking the fingers of both hands, pressing gently down on both sides of the uterus toward the pubis. The cephalic prominence (brow) is located on the side where there is greatest resistance to the descent of the fingers toward the pubis. It is located on the opposite side from the fetal back if the head is well flexed.

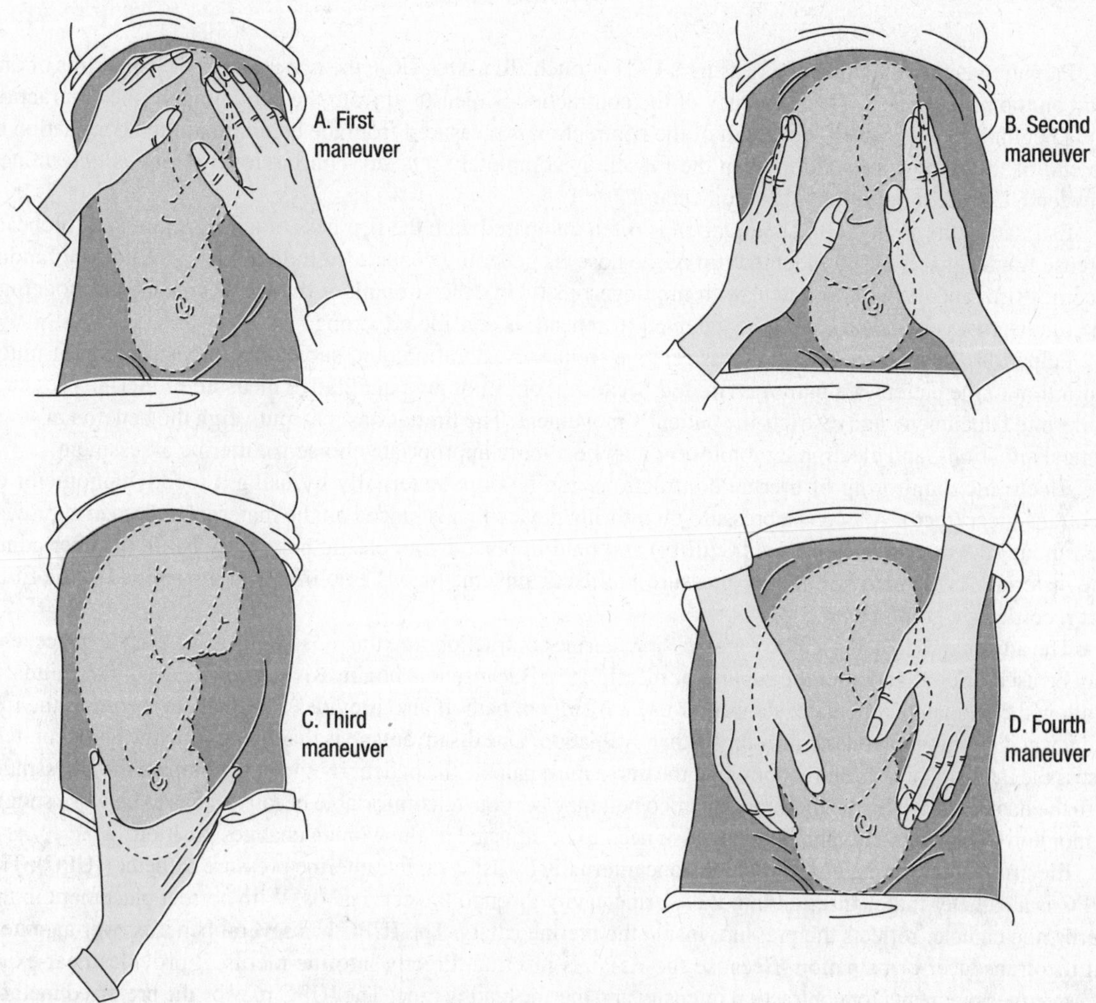

Figure 10.2 Leopold's maneuvers for determining fetal head position, presentation, and lie.

Another method of assessing the fetal position is by vaginal exam. The examiner may be able to palpate the fontanelles or cranial suture to identify that the fetus is in the cephalic position. Ultrasound may be used when the practitioner is unable to identify the position by abdominal palpation or when it is necessary to determine the fetal position with the most accuracy.

Monitoring ***uterine activity*** throughout labor is essential and provides data regarding the labor progress and fetal well-being. Numerous internal and external factors affect the maternal and fetal well-being. UCs interrupt the flow of blood to the placenta and reduce the amount of oxygen immediately available to the fetus. Decreased oxygen and blood flow directly affect the FHR. The pattern and intensity of contractions have a direct effect on the duration and progress of labor and the ability of the fetus to adapt to the intrapartal process. It is impossible to interpret the FHR without considering its relationship to the uterine activity.

UCs occur in wavelike patterns. The contraction begins in the fundus and progresses downward through the lower segments of the uterus and is then followed by a similar wave of relaxation. By monitoring the changes in the fundus, the nurse can determine the timing and intensity of the UCs and the resting tone of the uterus between contractions. There are three methods currently used for monitoring UCs:

1. Palpation
2. External monitoring with a tocodynamometer
3. Internal electronic monitoring with an intrauterine pressure catheter

Palpation is the technique of assessing a UC by touch. To assess UCs, the nurse places the fingertips of one hand on top of the uterus. The frequency of the contraction is measured from the beginning of one contraction to the beginning of the next. The length of the contraction is measured from the beginning of the contraction to the end of the same contraction, when the muscle is completely relaxed. Uterine resting tone is determined between UCs, when optimum relaxation occurs.

Estimating the strength of a contraction is often compared with the firmness of a nose, chin, and forehead. A tense fundus that is easily indented (tip of the nose) is generally considered mild intensity. When the fundus becomes firm and difficult to indent with the fingertips (chin), the strength of the UC is considered moderate. The fundus that is hard and cannot be indented (forehead) is considered strong.

Palpation allows the nurse to assess relative frequency, duration, and subjective intensity without much restriction to the patient. Palpation is limited because it does not give qualitative measure of uterine pressure, or a printed document, and restricts the patient's movement. The limitations may outweigh the benefits in some clinical situations, and electronic monitoring may be a more appropriate choice for uterine assessment.

Electronic monitoring of uterine contractions can be done externally by using a tocodynamometer or tocotransducer (toco). A toco is a pressure monitoring device that is placed on the maternal abdomen at or near the fundus (the area of greatest contractility) and held in place by an elastic belt, belly band, or other adhesive material. As the uterus contracts, pressure exerted against the toco is amplified and transmitted to the EFM and recorded on graph paper.

The advantages to using a toco for assessing uterine contractions are that it is noninvasive, easy to place, and may be used prior to and after the rupture of membranes. Because it is noninvasive, it can be used intermittently to allow the woman to ambulate, shower, or use a whirlpool bath. It also provides a permanent record of the frequency and duration of contractions for further evaluation. One disadvantage is that it does not always accurately assess the intensity of the contractions, and the nurse must palpate the patient routinely to compare the assessment with the data recorded by the monitor. The toco belt may become uncomfortable because it has to be worn snugly to monitor UCs accurately. The belt may also need to be adjusted as the woman changes position.

Electronic monitoring of UCs can be done internally by using an intrauterine pressure catheter (IUPC). The IUPC is a catheter that is inserted into the uterine cavity through the cervical os. With correct placement in the uterus, the catheter reflects the pressure inside the uterine cavity. The IUPC has several benefits over an external tocotransducer or palpation. Because the IUPC is inserted directly into the uterus, it provides near-exact pressure measurements for contraction intensity and uterine resting tone. The IUPC may be the preferred method of monitoring when it is particularly important to avoid hyperstimulation and possible uterine rupture in a woman with a previous history of cesarean birth who is attempting a vaginal birth (VBAC) and is receiving pitocin. If a woman's labor is prolonged, internal monitoring can be used to assess the frequency and strength of contractions. If a nonreassuring FHR tracing is present, internal monitoring with an IUPC and fetal scalp electrode may be essential to correlate UC timing and FHR pattern response.

However, with all of its benefits, the IUPC has its limitations and risks. Use of the IUPC is limited by the clinical situation. Membranes must be ruptured, and adequate cervical dilation must be achieved for insertion. The procedure is invasive and increases the risk of uterine infection or uterine perforation or trauma. Insertion of an IUPC with a low-lying placenta can result in placenta puncture, which can cause hemorrhage and nonreassuring fetal status.

Objective J: To Understand Fetal Surveillance During Labor

10.10 Fetal Surveillance During Labor

EFM may be done on an intermittent or continuous basis. In a large number of American and Canadian hospitals, women are routinely monitored on admission for a short period of time to assess fetal well-being and then monitoring is conducted periodically throughout labor. This practice is referred to as intermittent fetal monitoring. Situations in which EFM is recommended continuously for assessing fetal well-being include the presence of a high-risk pregnancy, induction of labor with pitocin, or when monitoring identifies a nonreassuring tracing. EFM can be done externally as well as internally.

The external EFM is involves a process that is very similar to the nonstress test (NST). The external monitor is composed of a Doppler ultrasound transducer and tocodynamometer that is applied to the external abdomen to monitor and display the FHR and contractions. Most hospitals have central monitoring systems where all tracings (recordings) from all the patients on the unit can be viewed in a central location, usually the nurse's station.

The internal fetal monitor features a spiral electrode that must be inserted into the fetal scalp during a vaginal examination. The cardiac signal is transmitted through the spiral electrode, and a fetal electrocardiogram tracing is produced. The internal method of FHR monitoring is more accurate than fetal monitoring.

The interpretation of the FHR pattern requires a thorough assessment of the maternal risk factors, uterine activity, baseline FHR, FHR patterns, variability and presence of accelerations, and identification of any decelerations. Nurses who work in labor and delivery units often have specialized training regarding fetal monitoring to aid in accurate interpretation.

In 1997 the National Institute of Child Health and Human Development (NICHD) published a proposed nomenclature system for EFM interpretation. Standardized definitions for FHR monitoring were proposed and later adopted by ACOG and the Association of Women's Health, Obstetric, and Neonatal Nurses.

The ***baseline FHR*** is the average FHR observed between contractions over a 10-minute period, rounded to increments of 5 bpm. The recorded baseline excludes periodic FHR changes that are evidenced by increased variability or accelerations. The normal baseline heart rate at term is 110 to 160 bpm. There are two abnormal variations of the baseline: tachycardia (baseline > 160 bpm) and bradycardia (baseline < 110 bpm).

Fetal tachycardia is a sustained baseline fetal heart rate > 160 bpm for a duration of 10 minutes or longer. The causes of tachycardia may be idiopathic, maternal, fetal, or a combination of maternal and fetal. Some of the most common causes are maternal fever, dehydration, anxiety, maternal hyperthyroidism, maternal drugs (beta-sympathetic and parasympathetic), early fetal hypoxia, fetal anemia, prematurity, and prolonged fetal stimulation. Fetal tachycardia is considered a nonreassuring sign if it is accompanied by other FHR patterns, such as decelerations or absent variability. Intervention for tachycardia usually requires treatment of the underlying cause. Fetal arrhythmia or dysrhythmia needs to be ruled out. The neonatologist should be notified, because tachycardia may cause heart failure in the newborn.

Fetal bradycardia is defined as a sustained baseline FHR < 110 to 120 bpm over more than 10 minutes. It may be associated with late hypoxia, medications (beta-adrenergic blocking drugs), maternal hypotension (supine hypotension, epidural anesthesia), prolonged umbilical cord compression, fetal dysrhythmia, and accidental monitoring of maternal pulse. When bradycardia is accompanied by decreased variability or late decelerations, or both, it is considered ominous and a sign of advanced fetal compromise.

Baseline ***variability*** is a reliable indicator of fetal cardiac and neurologic function and well-being. Variability of the FHR is manifested by fluctuations in the baseline FHR observed on the fetal monitor. The pattern denotes an irregular, changing FHR rather than a straight line that indicates few changes in the rate. Variability can further be classified as short- or long term. ***Short-term variability*** is the beat-to-beat changes in the FHR and is most accurately assessed with an internal electrode. ***Long-term variability*** refers to the changes in FHR over a longer period of time, such as 1 minute. The absence of variability is considered nonreassuring.

The absence of variability may indicate normal variations, such as fetal sleep (the sleep state should not last longer than 30 minutes); a response to certain drugs that depress the central nervous system (CNS), such as analgesics and barbiturates; and general anesthesia or a pathologic condition, such as hypoxia, a CNS abnormality, or acidemia. In addition to the changes in the average FHR baseline range, the FHR may exhibit intermittent or transient deviations or changes from the baseline that are commonly referred to as accelerations and decelerations.

An ***acceleration*** is defined as an increase of 15 bpm above the FHR baseline that lasts for at least 15 to 30 seconds. Accelerations are considered a sign of fetal well-being when they accompany fetal movement. At gestational ages of 32 weeks or less, an acceleration of 10 beats above baseline by 10 seconds is acceptable. A prolonged acceleration is any acceleration that lasts longer than 2 minutes. Prolonged accelerations that last longer than 10 minutes are considered a change in baseline. FHR accelerations are associated with fetal movement, vaginal exams, application of a fetal scalp electrode, occiput posterior presentation and UCs, fundal pressure, abdominal palpation, vibroacoustic stimulation (VAS), scalp stimulation, and other environmental stimulation.

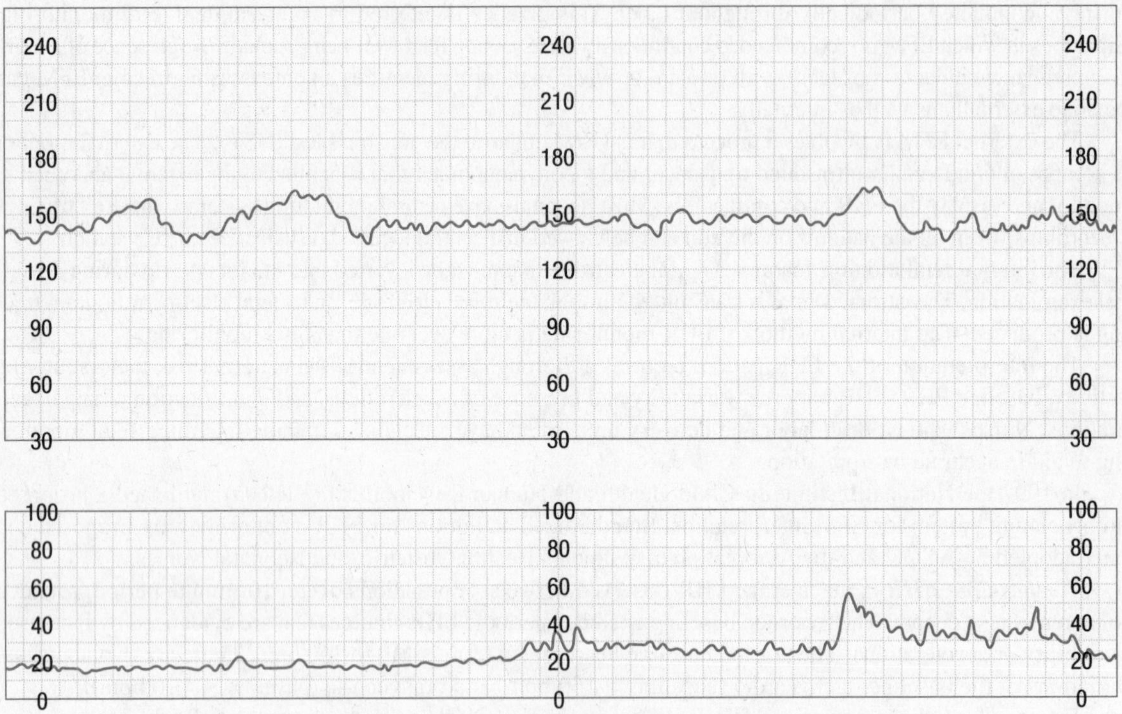

Figure 10.3 *Top.* Fetal heart rate accelerations. *Bottom.* Uterine contractions.

Decelerations, often referred to as "decels," are defined as any decrease in FHR below the baseline. Each type of deceleration has its own characteristics, etiology, and significance. Decelerations are further defined according to their onset and are characterized as early, variable, or late.

Early decelerations are characterized by a deceleration in the FHR that resembles a mirror image of the contraction. The onset of the decelerations begins near the onset of the contraction, and the lowest part of the deceleration occurs at the peak of the contraction, with the FHR returning to baseline by the end of the contraction. The deceleration is rarely more than 30 to 40 bpm. Early decelerations are a result of vagal nerve stimulation caused by fetal head compression that occurs during UCs. They occur most frequently during the active phase of labor (between 4 and 7 cm dilated) and are considered benign. They are also considered reassuring unless they are seen with a lack of descent of the fetal head into the pelvis.

Early decelerations are considered benign, and no nursing intervention is needed. However, it is important to document precisely what is occurring so they can be differentiated from late or variable decelerations. When documenting the findings, terms associated with EFM such as marked variability and variable decelerations should be avoided because they reflect visual descriptions of the patterns produced on the monitor tracing. Terms that are numerically defined (ie, bradycardia and tachycardia) may be used. When auscultated, FHR must be described as a baseline number or range and as having a regular or irregular rhythm. The presence or absence of accelerations or decelerations that occur during and after contractions should be noted.

Variable decelerations, as the name implies, are decelerations that are variable in terms of their onset, frequency, duration, and intensity. The decrease in FHR below the baseline is 15 bpm or more, lasts at least 15 seconds, and returns to the baseline in less than 2 minutes from the time of onset. The deceleration is unrelated to the presence of UCs. Variable decelerations are thought to be a result of umbilical cord compression. Occasional decelerations are often considered benign but repetitive, worsening variable decelerations are cause for concern.

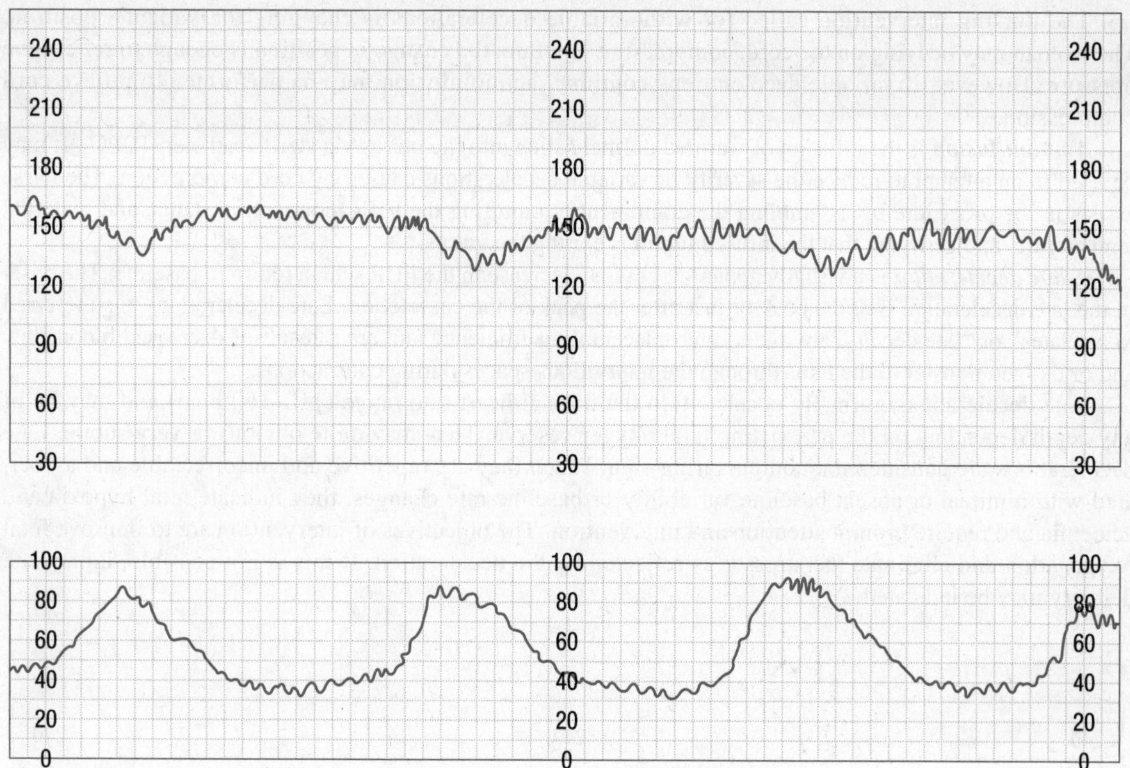

Figure 10.4 *Top.* Early decelerations. *Bottom.* Uterine contractions.

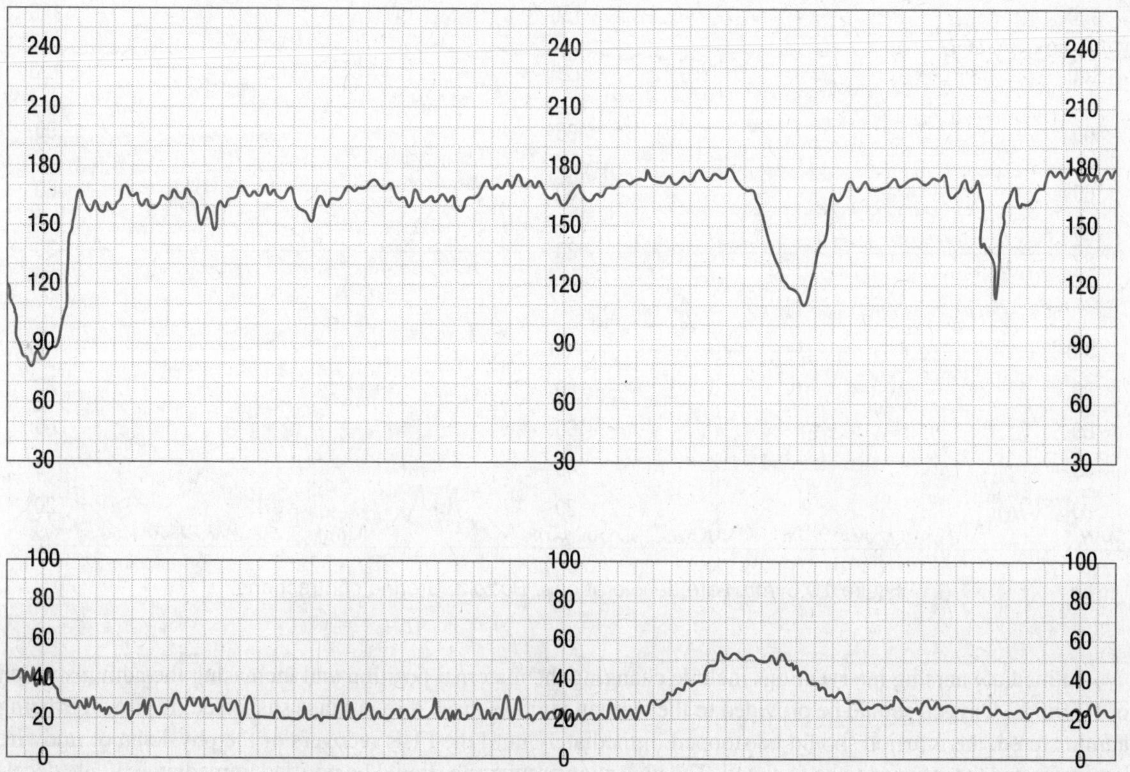

Figure 10.5 *Top.* Variable decelerations. *Bottom.* Uterine contractions.

The nursing intervention called for with variable decelerations is changing the patient's position. The woman may be lying on the cord, compressing it. Often, the change in position is enough to relieve the pressure. However, if variable decelerations continue, amnioinfusion may be performed to relieve cord compression.

Amnioinfusion is the infusion of warmed normal saline into the uterus via sterile catheter (IUPC). It may be used in an attempt to reduce the severity of variable decelerations caused by cord compression. The nurse assists in the procedure by assembling the equipment, monitoring the FHR, contraction status, and maternal temperature, and verifying that the infused liquid is exiting the uterus.

A ***late deceleration*** is a visually apparent, gradual decrease in the FHR with a return to baseline. The onset of the late deceleration is at the peak or just after the peak of the contraction. Late decelerations, also referred to as "lates" or "late decels," are due to uteroplacental insufficiency and are a result of decreased blood flow and/or oxygen transfer to the fetus through the intervillous spaces during contractions.

Late decelerations normally occur within the normal heart rate range (110–160 bpm) and may be of any depth depending on the preexisting fetal oxygen reserve. They may quite obvious or very subtle. Late decelerations are considered a nonreassuring sign. When they are repetitive and uncorrectable and associated with minimal or absent baseline variability or baseline rate changes, they indicate fetal hypoxia and acidemia and require prompt attention and intervention. The objectives of intervention are to improve fetal oxygenation and eliminate the stressor as reflected by the deceleration. If this is not possible, immediate delivery may be indicated.

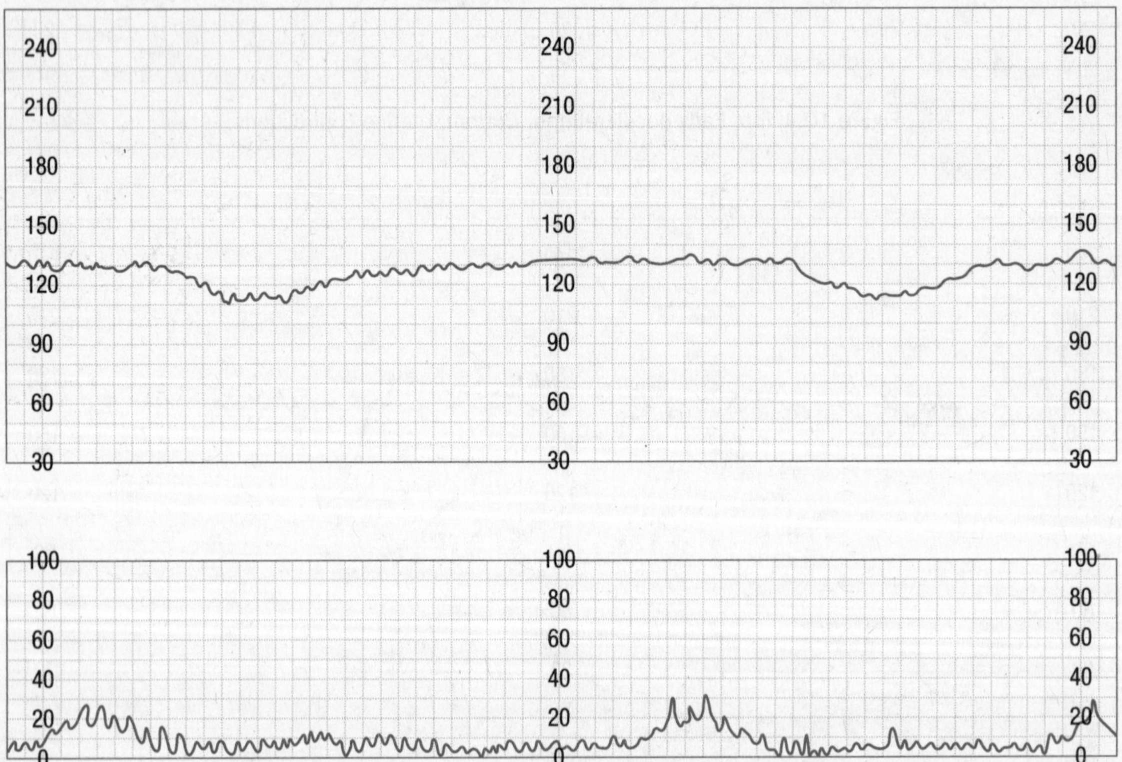

Figure 10.6 *Top.* Late decelerations. *Bottom.* Uterine contractions.

Immediate nursing interventions include changing the maternal position and increasing the administration of IV fluids. Oxygen should be provided to the woman via face mask if hypoxia is suspected. If pitocin is being administered, the infusion should be stopped immediately until the FHR recovers or the physician or midwife has instructed the infusion to be resumed. The physician or midwife should be notified immediately if late decelerations occur.

Objective K: To Understand Comfort Promotion and Pain Management During Labor and Delivery

10.11 Comfort Promotion and Pain Management

Pain is a complex, multidimensional experience. There are many definitions of pain. One such definition states pain is whatever the person who is experiencing it says it is. Another definition says pain includes not only the perception of an uncomfortable sensation but also the response to it. The International Association for the Study of Pain defines it as an unpleasant sensory and emotional experience arising from actual or potential tissue damage or described as such damage.

The pain experienced during childbirth is an unpleasant sensation that is localized to the back and abdomen. For most, the pain associated with childbirth intensifies an already highly emotional experience for both the laboring woman and her support person. How well the woman is able to cope with her pain significantly affects the overall birth experience. The experience of pain is shaped by many factors, including the patient's age, educational background, state of wellness, degree of family and social support, and mastery of coping mechanisms. The expression of pain is also influenced by a number of psychosocial and cultural factors.

During assessment, the nurse may identify physiologic and psychological changes that are indicative of maternal pain. These may include an increased pulse and blood pressure, changes in mood, increased anxiety and stress, marked agitation, changes in mood, confusion, decreased urine output, decreased intestinal motility, and guarding of the target area of discomfort. Despite the presence or absence of physiologic indicators of pain, only the patient can validate with certainty her present level of discomfort.

When a woman experiences discomfort during labor and birth, the nurse can help her to have a positive birth experience by providing effective comfort measures. Nursing interventions directed toward pain relief begin with nonpharmacologic measures. For other women, the progression of labor brings increasing levels of pain that interfere with their ability to cope effectively. For these women, pharmacologic agents may be used to decrease discomfort, increase relaxation, and reestablish the ability to participate more actively in the labor and birth experience.

Nurses need to recognize that the decision to have an unmedicated or medicated birth involves many factors and reflects a great deal of thought and planning for most women and their families. For the woman who has advised the nursing staff that she wants no pharmacologic remedies, the nurse should offer alternative comfort measures. All nurses in the intrapartum setting should be familiar with various nonpharmacologic techniques available to help women cope with the pain they may experience. The nurse should avoid offering these women pain medications unless they specifically ask for them or for information about pharmacologic options. The woman who signs a birth plan and states she does not want pain medication "under any circumstances" can change her mind at any time, and the nurse needs to be aware of this. The support person may restate the woman's former wishes regarding pain medication, but ultimately it is the woman who, at any time, can request medication.

The nurse also needs to know that feelings of inadequacy and guilt may accompany such decisions for pain medication. The nurse plays an important role in assisting the woman and her support person to explore options for pain relief realistically. The nurse should reassure the woman and her support person that accepting medication for pain is not a failure. The emphasis should be on the goal of a healthy, satisfying outcome for the family.

10.12 Types of Pain

The pain experienced in labor and during birth has both visceral and somatic origins. UCs during the first stage of labor bring about cervical dilation and effacement. During each contraction, arteries that supply the myometrium are compressed, causing uterine ischemia.

During the first stage of labor, pain impulses are transmitted via the T11 and T12 spinal nerve segments and accessory lower thoracic and upper lumbar sympathetic nerves. These nerves originate in the uterus.

Visceral pain describes the predominant discomfort experienced during the first stage of labor. It is related to changes in the cervix, distention of the lower uterine segment, and uterine ischemia. It is a slow, deep, poorly localized pain that occurs over the lower abdomen, the lumbosacral area of the back, the iliac crests, the gluteus maximus, and down the thighs.

Somatic pain is a faster, sharper, burning, tingling, localized intense pain that occurs during the second stage of labor. Somatic pain is associated with stretching and distention of the perineal body to allow for birth. During the second stage of labor, pain impulses are transmitted via the pudendal nerve through S2 to S4 spinal nerve segments and the parasympathetic system.

10.13 Psychological Factors of Pain

A number of psychological factors influence a woman's response to pain, such as anxiety, fear, previous experiences, support systems, and childbirth preparation. Maternal anxiety during labor triggers the release of catecholamines, which increase the amount of pelvic pain stimuli sent to the brain, resulting in an intensified perception of pain. As muscle tension increases, the effectiveness of the UCs decreases, and maternal discomfort and pain increase. The woman's confidence in her ability to cope with the pain erodes, and therapeutic interventions to help reduce pain and discomfort become less effective.

Prepared childbirth classes provide the patient and her partner with an understanding of what to expect during childbirth and empower them to become knowledgeable consumers of health care. These classes generally focus on educating the woman and her support person about strategies to achieve comfort and relief of pain during labor. Methods of distraction are learned and practiced in prepared childbirth, such as breathing patterns, massage, and use of focal points and imagery, to reduce or completely block the capacity of the nerve pathways to transmit pain. According to the ***gate control theory*** of pain, it is believed that these distractions "shut the gate" in the spinal cord so that pain signals are unable to reach the brain.

10.14 Nonpharmacologic Pain Measures

One of the best ways the nurse can assist the laboring woman is to help her find comfortable positions. Movement and changes in ***maternal position*** not only help with the patient's comfort level but also facilitate descent of the fetus. The woman may feel more comfortable ambulating in early labor or "slow dancing" with her support person, whom she can lean on during a contraction. The woman may want to assume a squatting position, which helps open the pelvic inlet, facilitating the fetus's downward movement.

A ***birthing ball*** may be used to promote comfort during labor. The birthing ball is a physical therapy ball that provides support for the laboring woman. She sits carefully on the ball and rhythmically rocks back and forth or moves the ball in a circular motion. Assuming a squatting position on the birthing ball opens the pelvis to allow fetal descent in preparation for birth. Warm compresses can be applied to the patient's back to enhance relaxation. The birthing ball should be big enough to allow the woman to sit comfortably on it with her knees bent at a 90-degree angle with her feet flat on the floor and ~2 feet apart.

During childbirth education classes, the pregnant woman and her support person learn about ***conscious breathing patterns*** that involve slowed respirations to enhance relaxation. Specific breathing methods are also taught as attention-focusing and distraction techniques to help relieve discomfort and pain during labor. The woman is instructed to take a slow, deep cleansing breath through the nose and out through the mouth at the beginning of every contraction. Slow breaths are encouraged. As the labor progresses and the contractions increase in intensity, the patient may need to change to modified paced breathing. This breathing technique is shallower and approximately twice the rate of the woman's normal breathing (32–40 breaths per minute).

During the transition period, when contractions are the most intense, patients usually find it hard to concentrate on breathing techniques. At this time, the pattern-paced breathing technique is often used. In this technique, following a cleansing breath, the woman begins with a 3:1 pattern: breathe in, breathe out; breathe in, breathe out; breathe in, then blow (as if blowing out a candle). As with other breathing patterns, a cleansing breath is taken at the end of the contraction. The patient can use and modify any of the breathing techniques that work best for her at any stage of her labor.

If a woman starts pushing before her cervix is completely dilated, she risks injury to her cervix and the fetal head. Blowing prevents closure of the glottis and breath holding, helping to overcome the urge to push strongly. The patient should be encouraged to blow repeatedly using short puffs when the urge to push is strong and she is not completely dilated. Some women vary the blowing by taking one short breath and then blowing. The patient's support person may learn to blow along with her to help her concentrate.

Hyperventilation may occur when a woman breathes very rapidly over a prolonged period of time. It is the result of an imbalance of oxygen and carbon dioxide. The signs and symptoms of hyperventilation are numbness or tingling of the fingers, lips, nose, or toes; dizziness; spots before the eyes; or spasms of the hands or feet. If hyperventilation occurs, the nurse needs to encourage the woman to slow her breathing rate and to take shallow breaths. If the signs or symptoms persist or become more severe, having the woman breathe into a mask or into her hands will help. The nurse should remain with the patient to reassure her.

Massage and ***touch*** are techniques that have long been used to facilitate comfort and relaxation during labor. Massage increases circulation and reduces muscle tension. In self-massage, the woman may rub her abdomen, legs, or back during labor to counteract discomfort. Some women find relief from palm or sole stimulation and may rub their palms vigorously during a contraction. In massage by others, the support person can rub the patient's back, shoulders, legs, or any area where she finds massage helpful. The nurse should be aware that some women find touch and massage irritating, especially over the abdomen. The nurse needs to explain this to the support person who may have gone to childbirth education classes with the woman and who now may feel rejected when the woman refuses to let this person touch her.

Counterpressure is sacral pressure that is most helpful when the woman has back pain, usually most intense when the fetus is in the occiput posterior position. Sacral pressure may be applied using the palm of the hand, the fist, or a firm object, such as a tennis ball.

Thermal stimulation is warmth applied to the back, abdomen, or perineum during labor. Warmth increases local blood flow, relaxes muscles, and raises the pain threshold. Massage is often more comfortable to a tense woman after her skin is warmed. Cool, damp washcloths provide comforting coolness if the laboring woman complains of feeling hot. Ice chips cool the mouth and also can provide hydration.

Hydrotherapy provides thermal stimulation, and studies have shown benefits of water therapy during labor, including immersion in a tub or whirlpool. Sitting in the shower during labor is very comforting for many women, and many rooms on the labor and delivery unit are equipped with seats in the shower area for this purpose.

In ***guided imagery,*** the laboring woman can imagine herself in a pleasant and relaxing place during contractions. Imagery can help the woman dissociate herself from the painful aspects of labor. Some hospitals have screens printed with peaceful images that patients can look at in order to distract themselves.

Some childbirth education classes encourage the use of a ***focal point***. A woman may bring a picture of a relaxing scene or an object to use as a focal point, or she may choose an object in the labor room to focus on during a contraction. This may divert her attention away from the pain of the contraction.

10.15 Pharmacologic Pain Measures

Pharmacologic methods for pain relief include systemic drugs, regional pain management techniques, and general anesthesia. Decisions for any method must be made as part of a risk-benefit process, as any drug taken by the woman is likely to affect her fetus. Any drugs that the pregnant woman ingests, whether it be therapeutic or abused, including herbal preparations, may also affect the fetus. Fetal effects may be direct or indirect, and their durations of action may be more pronounced than in the pregnant woman.

Pharmacologic pain relief should be given, for the most part, only during the active phase of labor (4–7 cm dilated). If given too early, pain medications can slow labor. If given too late, the chances that the infant will be respiratory depressed at birth are greater.

Systemic drugs have effects on multiple systems because they are distributed throughout the body. ***Opioid analgesics*** are the most common parenteral medications given to reduce the perception of pain without loss of consciousness. Analgesics commonly used for labor include meperidine (Demerol), butorphanol (Stadol), nalbuphine (Nubain), and fentanyl (Sublimaze). They are given in small, frequent doses by the IV route during labor to provide a rapid onset of analgesia and a predictable duration of action.

The primary side effect of opioids is respiratory depression, which is more likely to affect the newborn. Naloxone (Narcan) reverses opioid-induced respiratory depression, and although not used in obstetrics, it should be on hand to be given to the infant if born respiratory depressed. The neonatal resuscitation dose is 0.1 mg/kg by IV or intratracheal route for most reliable absorption.

Adjunctive drugs during the intrapartum period include those with antiemetic and tranquilizing effects, as well as sedatives. Promethazine (Phergan) relieves nausea and vomiting, which may occur when opioid drugs are given. It is given either intramuscularly (IM) or by the IV route, usually in conjunction with the opioid. Hydroxyzine (Vistaril) is an antihistamine with antiemetic effects that can be given IM.

Sedatives are not routinely given in labor; however, a small dose of a short-acting barbiturate may be given to promote rest if a woman is fatigued from false labor or is prodroming (prolonged latent phase).

Regional pain control methods may be used for intrapartum analgesia, surgical anesthesia, or both. These methods provide pain relief without loss of consciousness. The major advantage of regional pain methods is that the woman can participate in the birth yet have good pain control. Disadvantages depend on the specific technique. The effects on the fetus depend on how the woman responds rather than direct drug effects on the fetus.

The lumbar ***epidural block*** is the most popular regional pain method. It is used for both vaginal and cesarean births. Epidural blocks are started and maintained by an anesthesiologist or nurse anesthetist. It is not recommended for those with coagulation disorders, a low platelet count, uncorrected hypovolemia, an infection or reaction in the area of insertion, allergy, or condition in which immediate delivery of the fetus is warranted. Women who have had spinal surgery are evaluated on a case-by-case basis.

The epidural block is performed by injecting a local anesthetic agent, often combined with an opioid, into the epidural space. The epidural space is entered at L3–L4, and a catheter is passed through the needle into the epidural space. The catheter allows for continuous infusion or intermittent injection of medication to maintain pain relief during labor and vaginal or cesarean birth. Epidural block can have several side effects. Maternal hypotension can occur due to vasodilation, with possible reduction in placental perfusion. It is most likely to occur in the first 15 minutes of an epidural's initiation or injection of an intermittent bolus dose to maintain pain relief.

The nurse should take the patient's blood pressure every 5 minutes for 1 hour after the administration of an epidural. Rapid infusion of a warmed, nondextrose IV solution before the initiation of the block fills the vascular system to offset vasodilation. If hypotension occurs, IV ephedrine promotes vasoconstriction to raise the blood pressure. Additional nondextrose IV fluid is given rapidly, accompanied by oxygen administration and uterine displacement as needed.

The woman's bladder will fill up rapidly because of the large quantity of IV fluid being given during an epidural. Because the woman has reduced sensation, it is important for the nurse to assess the woman's bladder frequently. Intermittent or indwelling catheterization is common. After epidural placement, catheter migration may occur. The anesthesiologist should be notified immediately if there is a question about catheter placement.

For reasons that are not readily clear, fever after epidural analgesia during labor is common. This fever may be due to the reduced hyperventilation and decreased heat dissipation that occur when a woman's pain is relieved. Because fever is also a marker for infection, other indications for infection should be monitored.

Epidural or spinal headaches are another adverse reaction. If the dura is accidentally punctured with the needle used to introduce the epidural catheter, leakage of cerebrospinal fluid can occur, which may result in a headache. A spinal headache is postural and may feel worse when a woman is upright and may disappear when she is lying flat. Bed rest and IV hydration help relieve the headache. Caffeine may be helpful in some cases. A blood patch may provide definitive relief. The blood patch involves injection of 10 to 15 mL of the woman's blood into the epidural space. The blood clots and forms a plug in the hole in the dura, stopping the spinal leakage. The blood patch can be repeated if needed.

Late maternal respiratory depression may occur up to 24 hours after the administration of an epidural opioid, depending on the duration of action of the drug used. Adverse effects associated with opioids may result, including nausea and vomiting, pruritis, and delayed maternal respiratory depression.

Intrathecal injection of an opioid provides another option for pain management. The subarachnoid space is entered with a spinal needle, and an opioid is injected. The drug chosen usually depends on the anticipated duration of labor. Drugs used for this route are often fentanyl, sufentanyl, and morphine. As with epidural opioids, nausea, vomiting, and pruritis may occur. Delayed maternal respiratory depression may occur, depending on the drug used.

Subarachnoid (spinal) block is a simpler procedure than the epidural block and may be performed when a quick cesarean birth is necessary and an epidural catheter is not in place. It also can be performed just prior to a vaginal birth. Contraindications and side effects are similar to those with epidural block.

Vaginal birth anesthesia includes local infiltration and pudendal block. Infiltration of the perineum with a ***local anesthetic*** is done by the physician or nurse midwife just before he or she performs an episiotomy or sutures a laceration. Local infiltration does not alter pain from UCs or distention of the vagina. The local agent provides anesthesia in the immediate area of the episiotomy or laceration. Local infiltration rarely has adverse effects on the woman or the fetus.

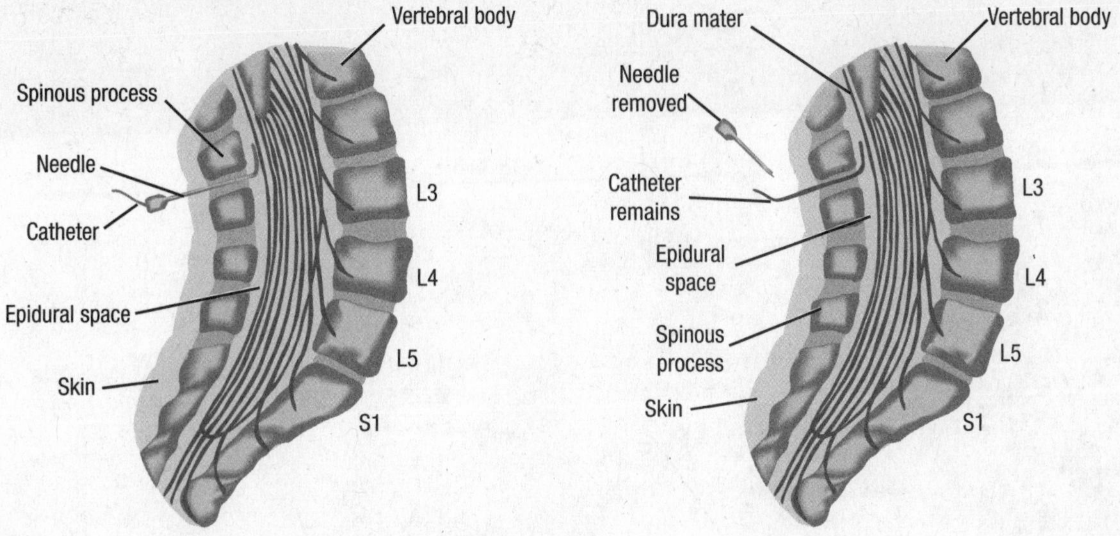

Figure 10.7 Technique for epidural block.

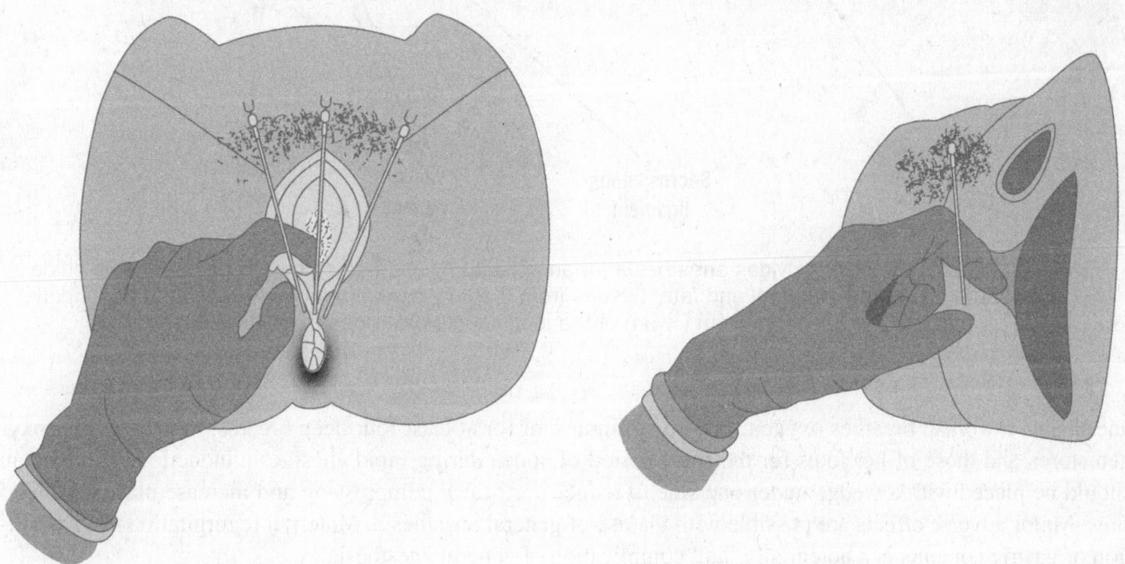

Figure 10.8 Local infiltration anesthesia numbs the perineum just before birth for an episiotomy or after birth for suturing of a laceration. The birth attendant protects the fetal head by placing a finger inside the vagina while injecting the perineum in a fanlike pattern or as needed.

A ***pudendal block*** anesthetizes the lower vagina and part of the perineum to provide anesthesia for an episiotomy and a vaginal birth, with low forceps if needed. A pudendal block does not block pain from UCs, and the woman feels pressure. An injection is given in each pudendal nerve near the ischial spine with a local anesthetic. The perineum is infiltrated with local anesthetic because the pudendal block does not fully anesthetize this area. Possible maternal complications include a toxic reaction to the anesthetic, rectal puncture, hematoma, and sciatic nerve block. If maternal toxicity is avoided, the fetus is usually not affected.

General anesthesia is a systemic pain control method that involves loss of consciousness. It is not used for vaginal births but is usually used for cesarean births in an emergency situation. Occasionally, a planned epidural or subarachnoid block proves to be inadequate, and general anesthesia is warranted. Before the induction of

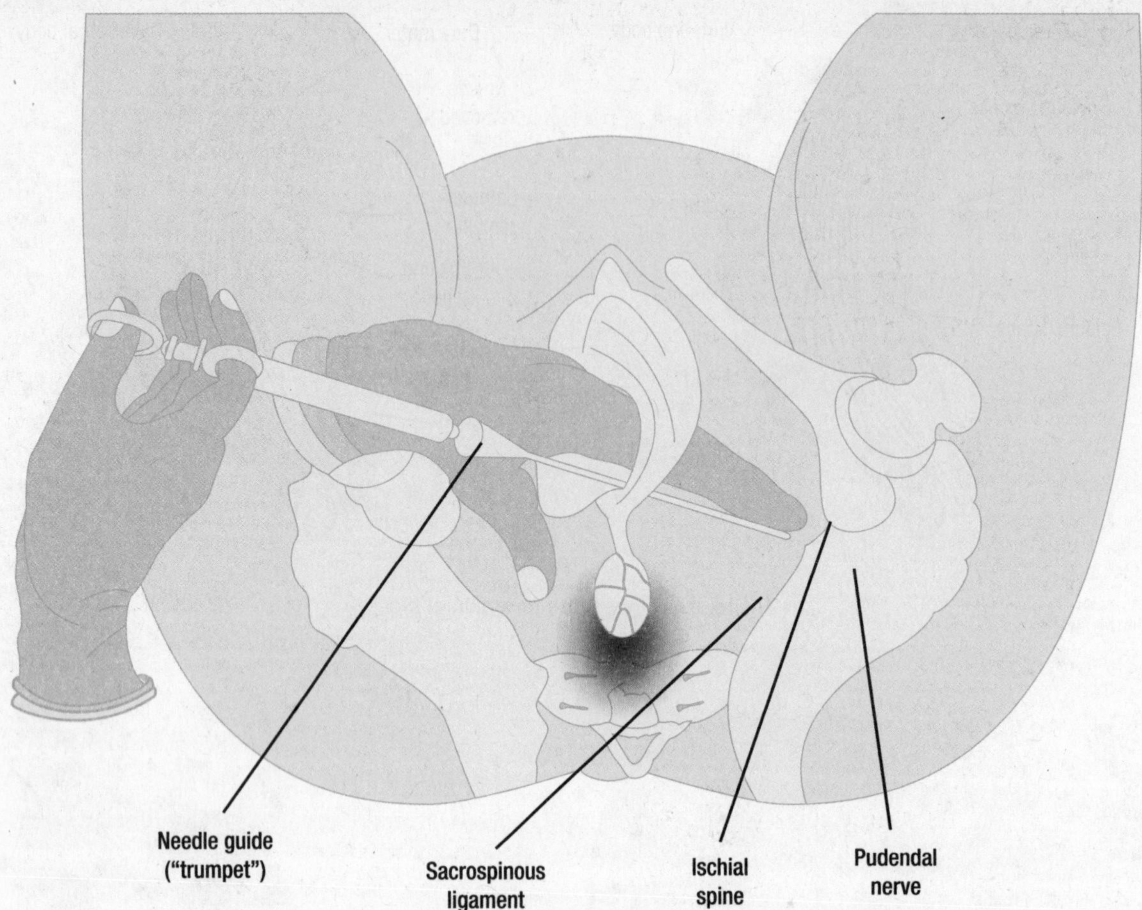

Figure 10.9 Pudendal block provides anesthesia for an episiotomy and use of low forceps. A needle guide ("trumpet") protects the maternal and fetal tissues from the long needle needed to reach the pudendal nerve. Only about 1.25 cm ($^1/_2$ in) of the long needle protrudes from the guide.

anesthesia, a woman breathes oxygen for 3 to 5 minutes, or for at least four deep breaths, to increase her oxygen stores and those of her fetus for the short period of apnea during rapid anesthesia induction. The woman should be placed with a wedge under one side to reduce aortocaval compression and increase placental blood flow. Major adverse effects are possible with the use of general anesthesia. Maternal regurgitation with aspiration of gastric contents is a potentially fatal complication of general anesthesia.

Respiratory depression may occur in the mother or the infant but is more likely in the baby. This is more likely if the interval between induction of anesthesia and cord clamping is long. Some inhalational anesthetics can cause uterine relaxation, and postpartum hemorrhage may occur.

Safety is a major consideration for the patient who has used pharmacologic methods of pain relief. Because the woman will have altered sensations, it is up to the nurse to anticipate the woman's needs and provide the care necessary to prevent injury.

Review Questions

True/False

1. ______ Childbirth is both a physical and an emotional experience.
2. ______ The component of childbirth called the passage refers to the maternal pelvis and soft tissue.

3. _______ The fetal lie refers to the orientation of the long axis of the fetus to the long axis of the pregnant woman's body.

4. _______ The relation of the fetal body parts to one another is the attitude of the fetus.

5. _______ Flexion is characteristic of a preterm infant.

6. _______ A breech presentation is associated with many disadvantages.

7. _______ The psyche is a crucial part of childbirth.

8. _______ Most of the nursing care during childbirth involves promoting relaxation and reducing anxiety and fear.

9. _______ Despite continuing research, the exact mechanism that initiates labor is unknown.

10. _______ Braxton Hicks contractions help dilate the cervix.

11. _______ Pushing before a woman is fully dilated can cause injury to the cervix and the fetal head.

12. _______ Focal points help the woman focus on something other than her contractions while in labor.

13. _______ Showering during labor helps promote relaxation.

14. _______ A precipitous delivery is a birth that ensues very quickly.

15. _______ The support person plays an important role in labor.

16. _______ Most laboring patients in the United States are placed on external fetal monitors for periodic fetal assessment of well-being.

17. _______ Uterine resting tone is the period of uterine relaxation between contractions.

18. _______ The patient with an epidural in place during labor may have to be catheterized.

19. _______ Uterine contractions interrupt the flow of blood to the placenta and reduce the amount of oxygen immediately available to the fetus.

20. _______ Amnioinfusion can be done to relieve cord compression during labor.

Completion

1. The four major factors that affect childbirth are _____________, _____________, _____________, and _____________.

2. The _____________ presentation with the head flexed is the most favorable for a vaginal delivery.

3. Labor initiation is hypothesized to be caused by decreased levels of _____________ and release of _____________.

4. Premonitory signs of labor in primigravidas are usually experienced at _____________ weeks' gestation.

5. In primigravidas, the presenting part descends into the pelvic cavity in a process known as _____________.

6. As full term nears, the cervix softens because of the hormone _____________.

7. _____________ describes the burst of energy and activities seen as the expectant mother prepares the home for the arrival of the newborn.

8. ____________________ is a mixture of mucus and blood that a woman sees several days to a few weeks before delivery.

9. With rupture of membranes, the amniotic fluid should be ______________ and ______________.

10. Confirmation of the rupture of membranes is done by a ____________ test or a ____________ test.

11. Contractions are described in terms of their ______________, ______________, and ______________.

12. ______________ and ______________ are the major cervical changes during labor.

13. Full dilation is ________________________, sufficient to allow delivery of a full-term fetus.

14. The exchange of oxygen, nutrients, and waste products between the woman and the fetus takes place in the ____________________________.

15. Infants born by ________________ are more likely to have transient breathing difficulty.

16. The mechanisms of labor that occur as the fetus is moved through the pelvis during birth are also known as ______________________________.

17. Labor is divided into ___ stages.

18. The shortest stage of labor is the ______________ stage.

19. The placenta is delivered in the ________________ stage.

20. For low-risk pregnancies, fetal heart rate tracings can be reviewed every ____________ minutes in the first stage of labor and every ____________ minutes in the second stage of labor.

21. ______________ ______________ are a systematic way of palpating the maternal abdomen to assess fetal position.

22. Uterine contractions occur in ______________ patterns.

23. Cervical dilation and effacement are evaluated by ______________________.

24. Fetal tachycardia is sustained baseline fetal heart rate > ____________ beats per minute.

25. ______________ decelerations are characterized by a deceleration in the fetal heart rate that resembles a mirror image of the contraction.

26. ______________ pain is the predominant discomfort experienced during the first stage of labor.

27. ______________ may occur when a woman breathes very rapidly over a prolonged period of time.

28. ______________ is sacral pressure that is most helpful when the laboring woman has back pain.

29. ____________ are those that have effects on multiple systems because they are distributed throughout the body.

30. The primary side effect of opioids for pain relief is ______________________.

31. The epidural block is a ______________________ type of pain relief method.

32. The epidural block is not recommended for those with ______________________.

33. In an epidural block, the epidural space is entered at the ______________.

34. Maternal hypotension after epidural placement is most likely to occur in ______________.

35. Spinal headaches are caused by puncture in the ______________.

36. Late maternal respiratory depression may occur up to ______________ of administration of an epidural opioid.

37. ______________ anesthesia involves loss of consciousness.

38. After general anesthesia for a cesarean section, the ______________ is more likely to have respiratory depression.

39. ______________ is a major concern for patients using pharmacologic pain relief methods.

40. The drug ______________ should be on hand when a pregnant woman receives opioids for the relief of pain during her labor and delivery in the event the newborn is born respiratory depressed.

41. Correct placement in the uterus of an ______________ provides near-exact measurements for contraction intensity and resting tone.

42. Late decelerations indicate______________________.

43. The ______________ uterine incision for cesarean sections is the most likely result in a ruptured uterus in subsequent pregnancies.

44. The most commonly made incision for cesarean sections is the ______________ incision.

45. The umbilical cord should contain three vessels: ______________, ______________, and ______________.

46. The major advantage of using a tocotransducer for fetal heart rate assessment in labor is that it is ______________________.

47. Two abnormal variations of the baseline fetal rate are ______________ and ______________.

48. A sustained decrease in the fetal heart rate is known as a ______________.

49. An ______________________ is a surgical incision of the perineum to allow more room for the fetus to deliver or to help prevent the mother from pushing too strenuously.

50. The most common complication of an epidural block is ______________________.

Answers

True/False

1. True
2. True
3. True
4. True
5. False. Flexion is characteristic of a full-term infant.
6. True
7. True
8. True
9. True
10. False. Braxton Hicks contractions do not help dilate the cervix; only true contractions help.
11. False. Only 12% of women rupture their membranes before labor starts.
12. True
13. True
14. True
15. True
16. False. Maternal blood pressure increases with contractions, so blood pressure should be monitored between contractions.
17. True
18. False. A white blood cell count of 30,000 is normal for a laboring woman and not a sign of infection.
19. True
20. True

Completion

1. the powers, the psyche, the passage, and the passenger
2. cephalic
3. progesterone, fetal cortisol
4. 38
5. Lightening
6. Relaxin
7. Nesting
8. Bloody show
9. clear, odorless
10. Nitrazine tape test, ferning test
11. frequency, intensity, duration
12. Effacement, dilation
13. 10 cm
14. intervillous spaces
15. cesarean
16. cardinal movements
17. four
18. third
19. third
20. 30 minutes, 15 minutes
21. Leopold maneuvers
22. Wavelike
23. Vaginal
24. 160
25. Early
26. Visceral

27. Hyperventilation
28. Counterpressure
29. Systemic
30. Respiratory depression
31. Regional
32. coagulation disorders (or low platelet count)
33. L3–L4
34. first 15 minutes
35. Dura
36. 24
37. General
38. Infant
39. Safety
40. Narcan
41. Intrauterine pressure catheter
42. Uteroplacental insufficiency
43. Transverse
44. Classical
45. two arteries, one vein
46. Noninvasive
47. Tachycardia, bradycardia
48. Bradycardia
49. Episiotomy
50. Maternal hypotension

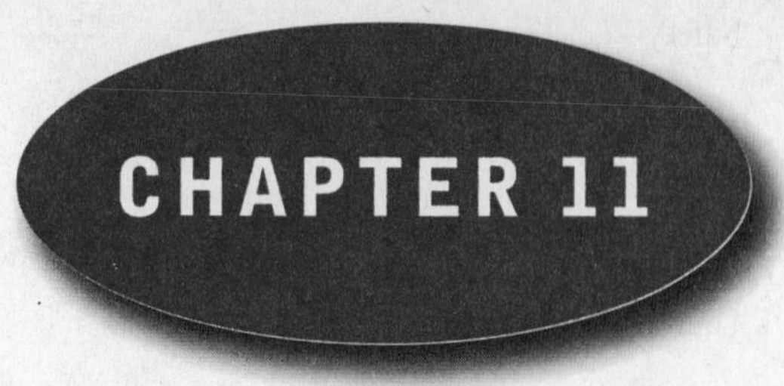

Postpartum

Objective A: To Understand What the Postpartum Period Entails

11.1 The Postpartum Period

The first 6 weeks after the birth of an infant is known as the ***postpartum period,*** or ***puerperium***. During this period, a woman goes through many psychological and physiologic changes. There is probably no other time in a family's history that requires such rapid change in roles, relationships, and structure than the birth of a baby. Both the mother and father begin the process of attachment with the newborn, and siblings must adapt to a new standing in the family structure and cope with feelings of jealousy and rivalry that may occur with the birth. Because of these changes, the first 12 weeks (3 months) after the birth of the baby is often called the ***"fourth trimester,"*** when the family adjusts to the addition of a new family member.

The responsibility of the maternity nurse includes the care not only of the mother–infant dyad but of the whole family. With the changing health care system in the United States, it may be particularly difficult to provide this care. Although postpartum mothers typically remain only a short time in the hospital (48 hours for a vaginal delivery and 96 hours for a cesarean birth), their need for care extends beyond this period. Added to the limitations of time is the potential matter of language barrier and cultural influences that affect the childbearing family in a multicultural society.

Objective B: To Understand the Psychological Needs in the First Postpartum Hour

11.2 Psychological Needs in the First Postpartum Hour

Immediately after the birth, the woman feels a sense of relief, because labor is over and because she can now meet her baby for the first time. The health care provider may place the infant on the patient's chest if the baby is pink and crying at birth, to allow for bonding. If the health care provider brings the infant over to the infant warmer, the nurse should dry the infant off, place a hat on the baby's head, do a quick assessment, and swaddle the infant for presentation to the mother.

Current research points to the importance of this time for bonding and for the initiation of breastfeeding. The first period of reactivity in the infant begins at birth. Infants are active at this time and are awake, alert, and interested in their surroundings. They move their arms and legs energetically, root, and appear hungry.

This is the best time to initiate breastfeeding if the mother has chosen this method of feeding. Prophylactic erythromycin administration should be delayed so mother and infant can gaze into each other's eyes.

The term ***bonding*** refers to the rapid initial attraction felt by parents soon after childbirth. It is unidirectional, from parent to child, and is enhanced when parents and infants are allowed to touch and gaze at each other. This time, called the ***sensitive period,*** extends through the first 30 to 60 minutes after birth. It is believed that infants can see clearly up to 12 inches as a newborn, so parents should be encouraged to hold the infant close and maintain eye contact. ***Attachment*** is the process by which the enduring bond between parent and child is developed through pleasurable, mutual interaction. The process of attachment begins in pregnancy and extends for many months after childbirth.

Maternal behavior, especially touch, changes rapidly as the mother progresses through a discovery phase with her infant. Initially, she may not reach for her infant, but wait for the nurse to present the child to her. If the infant is placed in her arms, she holds the infant in an en face position, in which she looks at the infant in the same vertical plane as the baby's. The mother will run her fingertips over the infant in an exploratory fashion initially. She then begins what is called "claiming" behavior, in which she relates physical features of the baby to family members (eg, "She has her father's eyes").

Verbal behavior is an important indicator of maternal attachment. Some women will refer to the infant by name after seeing it on ultrasound; others may call the infant "it," "the baby," or "he or she" but should progress to using the given name prior to discharge. In some cultures, a baby-naming ceremony may take place after discharge, and the mother may not call the baby by its given name until that time. The nurse needs to be aware of the patient's cultural practices when assessing the woman's psychological relationship with the infant. He or she must observe interactions between the mother and infant and, if necessary, teach and model behaviors that foster early attachment.

Objective C: To Understand the Process of Maternal Adaptation

11.3 Maternal Adaptation

There are several phases a woman goes through to attain comfort in the role of mother. Knowing these phases can help the nurse anticipate maternal needs and intervene to meet those needs in order to support this process.

During the ***"taking in" phase,*** the woman is trying to recover from the delivery. She is focused primarily on her own needs—food, pain reduction, sleep, and so on. The major task of this phase is to integrate her birth experience into reality. This process helps the woman realize that her pregnancy is over and that the newborn is now a separate individual. This process can be delayed in the case of an unplanned cesarean section or in women who may have negative feelings about their birth experience. The nurse needs to keep this in mind and provide sensitive nursing care.

During the ***"taking hold" phase,*** the woman becomes more independent. She assumes responsibility for her own care and shifts her attention from herself to the baby.

This period is often referred to as "the reachable, teachable moment," and the nurse needs to use this time to teach the mother about infant care and allow her to perform as many of the duties as possible. The father should also be encouraged at this time to participate in the infant's care. Some men lack the confidence or experience they feel they need and may view their role as only to support the mother. The nurse can assist both the mother and father in promoting confidence by giving praise for infant care activities and support of decisions made for the infant. Classes offered through the maternity unit, as well as other instructional mediums, should address both maternal and paternal needs.

The ***"letting go" phase*** is a time of relinquishment for the mother and father. If this is their first child, they must give up their previous role as a childless couple and acknowledge the loss of their previous lifestyle. At this time, the couple must give up their idealized expectations of the birth experience and what they thought the baby would look like and accept the real infant. This may provoke feelings of subtle grief. The nurse needs to encourage them to talk about these feelings and the expectations they had and let them know that these feelings are common in all new parents.

Objective D: To Understand the Process of Maternal Role Attainment

11.4 Maternal Role Attainment

Role attainment is a process by which the woman achieves confidence in her ability to care for the infant and becomes comfortable with her new identity as a mother. The process begins during pregnancy and continues for several months after childbirth. The transition to the maternal role has four stages: the anticipatory, formal, informal, and personal.

The ***anticipatory stage*** begins during pregnancy when a woman chooses a health care provider and a location for the birth. During this stage, women seek out role models to help them learn the role of a mother.

The ***formal stage*** begins with the birth of the infant and continues for 4 to 6 weeks. During this stage, behavior is largely guided by others (pediatrician, family, etc). A major task during this time is for the woman to become acquainted with the infant and try to familiarize herself with cues from her child.

The ***informal stage*** follows. It begins once the woman has learned appropriate responses to her infant's cues and signals. She responds to her infant's unique needs and personality and develops the maternal role that suits her as opposed to what she has read or been told.

The ***personal stage*** is attained when the woman feels a sense of harmony, enjoys the infant, and has internalized the maternal role. She accepts the role of parent and is comfortable in it.

Objective E: To Understand Paternal Role Attainment

11.5 Paternal Role Attainment

The transition to fatherhood is influenced by many factors, including participation in childbirth, relationships with significant others, competence in child care, the family role organization, the father's cultural background, and the method of infant feeding. The father's developing bond to his infant is a process called ***engrossment***. Similar to what mothers experience, fathers go through a predictable three-stage process during the first 3 weeks. The three stages are expectations, reality, and transition to mastery.

During the ***expectations stage,*** the man thinks about what his preconceived life will be like when the infant arrives.

During the ***reality stage,*** he begins to realize that his preconceptions are not realistic. His feelings change from elation to ambivalence, then frustration. He often does not feel confident that he will be able to care for an infant.

During the ***transition to mastery stage,*** the new father makes a conscious decision to take control and be part of his child's life despite how unprepared he may feel. The nurse needs to encourage him to become involved in the infant's care and develop a bond with the newborn. Reinforcement of engrossing behavior can help the father develop a lifelong bond with his child.

Objective F: To Understand Redefined Roles after the Birth of an Infant

11.6 Redefined Roles

Although nurses are not actively involved in redefining the roles of members of the family, they can use their communication skills to encourage family members to express their feelings and concerns so that all members are aware of each other's needs and concerns.

Respect for different cultural practices and family structure is important for the nurse to be aware of because, although patients are educated in certain practices, they may be held to cultural practices of their families of origin.

As long as the practices are not unsafe, some deviation may be acceptable and may be therapeutic for the healing mother. One such practice is that of support of the woman during labor and birth. Although it is expected in the United States that the father/partner is the main source of support for the laboring woman, in certain cultures it is the other women of the family who support the mother through labor and delivery, and the man is not involved at all. Provision of care for the mother and new baby by female relatives is actually a common thread among cultures. Cultural beliefs and practices provide a sense of security for new mothers. Tact and sensitivity are necessary to determine what care is appropriate for each woman and to find a compromise, if necessary.

Siblings' responses to the birth of a new brother or sister depend on their age and developmental level. It can be very overwhelming to have another family member introduced into their small, stable world where they feel safe and secure. They may view the new baby as competition or a replacement for their parents' love and affection. All siblings need reassurance that they are loved and important and will not lose that from their parents. Parents often need to be reassured that sibling rivalry is normal, even in a young child.

Negative behavior such as bedwetting, thumb sucking, and regression to more infantile behavior is a sign of stress in the older child. Parents need to emphasize the advantages of being an older sibling and should allow children to participate in age-appropriate aspects of infant care. Parents need to spend time alone with older children so they still feel special. Sibling classes, available through many agencies, may help older children in transitioning into their new place in the family. Siblings are encouraged to visit their mother and the new baby at the birth facility.

The involvement of grandparents depends on many factors, including their proximity to the newborn and nuclear family, their willingness to become involved, and the cultural expectations of their role. Grandparents can be a source of support and comfort to the new family if effective communication skills are used and roles defined. Nurses can assist in the grandparents' role transition by assessing the communication skills and role expectations. Although first-time parents lack parenting skills, they often seek their own parents' support, although they do not want criticism. Grandparents should recognize their adult children's need for autonomy, respect their wishes, and remain resource people for them when requested. Grandparent classes, offered through many agencies, may ease the transition to "grandparenthood." These classes can help them to understand new parenting concepts and bring them up to date on child-rearing practices of today.

Objective G: To Understand Major Maternal Concerns

11.7 Major Maternal Concerns

Nurses need to be aware that as a new mother becomes more confident in her ability to care for her infant and her discomfort level decreases, her concerns related to the self become more evident. Concerns about body image, the experience of postpartum blues, and resuming sexual intercourse are particularly important in the early postpartum period.

Women are very concerned with regaining their normal figures after delivery. Some have unrealistic expectations about the amount of weight they will lose and how long it will take to regain their pre-pregnant figures. Approximately 4.5 to 5.5 kg (10–12 lb) are lost during childbirth, which includes the weight of the fetus, the placenta, amniotic fluid, and blood. An additional 2.3 to 3.6 kg (5–8 lb) is lost as a result of diuresis during the early postpartum days. Nurses must emphasize that weight loss should be gradual and can take as long as 1 year. A strict weight loss diet should be avoided to prevent depleted energy levels and decreased immunity. Nurses need to address the diets of postpartum mothers because increased calories, high protein, and appropriate amounts of fluids are needed not only for tissue repair, but also for breastfeeding. Muscle tone is also diminished and it may take several months of exercise before an improvement in their figure results.

Mild depression, also known as ***"postpartum blues,"*** is a frequently expressed concern of new mothers. It is a mild, transient condition that affects ~70% of women in the United States who have given birth. The condition typically begins 3 to 4 days after birth and resolves itself by 10 days to 2 weeks postpartum. It is characterized by anxiety, irritability, insomnia, crying, loss of appetite, and sadness. Throughout the state of mild depression, the woman maintains contact with reality consistently, and the condition does not interfere with the woman's ability to care for herself or her infant. The nurse needs to encourage the new mother to talk about her feelings and concerns, and should demonstrate patience and understanding with her and her family. Providing phone numbers to support people and organizations (lactation consultant, pediatrician, hospital, nursery, La Leche League, etc) may also be helpful.

Depression that lasts for more than two weeks is a more severe form of depression and the woman needs to be referred for therapy and possibly medication. Family members should be instructed to observe for signs of postpartum depression in the new mother prior to discharge from the hospital, and know that they need to assist her in getting medical treatment for this condition.

Sexuality is an important and integral part of every woman's life and is a vital component of physical and emotional well-being for women and men in every society. However, it is probably the most superficially discussed topic during a woman's postpartum experience. Despite the importance of sexuality in their lives, many women are reluctant to ask their health care providers questions or express their concerns. It is up to the nurse working with the postpartum patient to assume anticipatory guidance, reassurance, counseling, or referral when addressing the woman's concerns regarding sexuality.

During postpartum, many women experience fatigue, weakness, perineal discomfort, vaginal bleeding, hemorrhoids, sore breasts, decreased vaginal lubrication from decreased estrogen levels, and dyspareunia. They may be hesitant to resume sexual intercourse for a variety of reasons. A patient may be fearful that she will tear the episiotomy or have intense pain or that her partner may feel differently toward her. The issues of fatigue and the woman's increased investment in the mothering role can make her partner feel secondary and can pose some problems for the couple's relationship.

When counseling the couple about sexuality, the nurse should determine what concerns the couple has about their sexual relationship and should inform them about what to expect when resuming sexual intercourse. To prevent any discomfort, the nurse can suggest the use of water-based lubricants and instruct the mother about pelvic floor exercises that may be helpful. Typically, sexual intercourse can be resumed when bright red bleeding has stopped and the perineum has healed from an episiotomy or laceration. This is usually between the third and sixth week postpartum.

Instruction on contraceptive options should be given at this time. Most couples, though, are not ready for a lengthy discussion of contraceptives in the early postpartum period, as they are overwhelmed by the amount of information given to them in the short hospital stay. A discussion of contraception should include effectiveness, acceptability, and safety. Presenting a short review of the various options, along with written literature for referral, may be appropriate. If culturally and religiously appropriate for the couple, suggesting a barrier method of contraception may be helpful, especially if the woman's postpartum checkup will not occur until 6 weeks after childbirth. A condom and spermicidal foam or gel should be used until a permanent method is decided upon, as many couples resume sexual intercourse before the postpartum checkup.

The woman's choice and use of postpartum contraception are often dictated by the infant feeding method. Also, discussing the couple's needs and preferences is important when selecting a contraceptive method. This approach allows for sharing of responsibility and provides an opportunity to review the advantages and disadvantages of methods, clarify misconceptions, and discuss preventing sexually transmitted infections (STIs).

Objective H: To Understand the Physiologic Changes that Occur During the Postpartum Period

11.8 Physiologic Changes During the Postpartum Period

Most of the changes that occur are regressive, meaning that the changes that occurred during pregnancy reverse. One progressive change that occurs is that of lactation.

Reproductive System

The changes that occur in the uterus are termed ***involution***. Involution starts immediately after delivery of the placenta. Uterine muscle fibers contract firmly around the maternal blood vessels where the placenta was attached to the uterus. These contractions control bleeding and help the uterus shrink to its pre-pregnant state.

Immediately after birth, the uterine fundus can be palpated midway between the umbilicus and symphysis pubis. During the first 12 hours after birth, the muscles relax slightly, and the fundus returns to the level of the umbilicus. Beginning on postpartum day 1 or 2, the progression of uterine descent into the pelvis is 1 cm daily (or one fingerbreadth). By day 10, the fundus of the uterus usually cannot be palpated because it has descended into the true pelvis. Descent is documented in relation to the umbilicus. For example, U ↓ 1 indicates that the fundus is palpable 1 cm (one fingerbreadth) below the umbilicus. The location of the uterine fundus helps determine whether involution is progressing normally.

The uterus, which usually weighs ~1000 g (2.2 lb) soon after birth, weighs ~500 g (1 lb) at 1 week after birth and ~60 g (2 oz) at 6 weeks (the prepregnant weight). The uterus of a multipara remains slightly heavier. If retrogressive changes do not occur as a result of infection or retained placental fragments, ***subinvolution*** occurs.

Factors that would inhibit involution include prolonged labor and birth, incomplete expulsion of the amniotic membranes and placenta, uterine infection, overdistention of the uterine muscles (as a result of a large infant, multiple gestation, or hydramnios), a full bladder (which displaces the uterus and makes it boggy), anesthesia (which relaxes the uterine muscles), and close childbirth spacing (frequent and repeated distention decreases tone and causes muscular relaxation). Intermittent uterine contractions, known as ***afterpains,*** are experienced by all women after childbirth. The discomfort, which usually can be relieved by analgesics, is more acute for multiparas because of repeated stretching of the uterus leading to loss of muscle tone. Afterpains can be particularly severe when breastfeeding. Oxytocin, released from the posterior pituitary to stimulate the milk-ejection reflex, also stimulates contractions of uterine muscles.

Exfoliation, the process of placental site healing, occurs over the first 6 weeks after birth and is necrotic sloughing of the superficial tissues. A reparative process follows in which the endometrium regenerates from the margins and base of the site where the placenta was attached to the uterus.

Lochia is the uterine discharge that occurs after birth. Changes in the amount and color of the lochia also provide information about whether involution is progressing normally. For the first 3 days after birth, the lochia is bright red to brownish red and is called ***lochia rubra***. It consists almost entirely of blood, decidua, and mucus and is equated to the menstrual period. Lochia flow is the greatest immediately after delivery and gradually decreases. It is less after a cesarean birth because the uterine cavity is suctioned after delivery of the placenta. The amount of bleeding decreases by the fourth day, when leukocytes invade the area. The lochia then changes from red to pink or brown-tinged and is called ***lochia serosa***. Lochia serosa is composed of serous exudate, erythrocytes, leukocytes, and cervical mucus. By approximately the 10th day, the lochia changes to ***lochia alba***. Lochia alba is white or cream-colored and contains leukocytes, decidual cells, epithelial cells, fat, cervical mucus, and bacteria. It can last up to the sixth week postpartum.

When documenting the lochia, the nurse needs to note the amount as well as the color. The most common method for documenting the amount of lochia in a 1-hour timeframe is as follows: heavy = pad saturated, moderate = 4 to 6 inch stain (10–15 cm), and scant = 1 inch stain (< 2.5 cm). It is important to determine how long the peripad has been in place when making the assessment of lochia amount.

Lochia flow will be very heavy when the new mother gets up for the first time after delivery, and when the postpartum mother gets up after sleeping, as the blood pools in the vagina and will flow freely in an upright position. Immediately after childbirth the cervix is formless and open wide enough to allow a hand to enter. This allows for manual extraction of the placenta and examination of the uterus when necessary. Although the cervix may remain edematous for several months, rapid healing takes place, and by the end of the first week, the cervix feels firm. The internal os closes to what it was previously, but the external os remains slightly open and appears slitlike rather than round as in the nulliparous woman.

The vagina and introitus are stretched greatly during birth to allow delivery of the fetus. After childbirth, the walls of the vagina are edematous and may have small tears. Few rugae are present. The voluntary muscles and supports of the pelvic floor gradually regain tone during the first 6 weeks postpartum. Nurses should encourage women to restore vaginal tone by performing perineal tightening exercises (Kegel exercises). Not maintaining and restoring perineal muscle tone can lead to urinary incontinence later in life for many women.

The return of menses and ovulation varies between women. The first menstrual period after childbirth usually returns within 7 to 9 weeks postpartum in nonnursing women. Menstruation in nursing patients varies widely and usually returns between 2 and 18 months, depending on estrogen levels.

Estrogen and progesterone levels drop dramatically after the placental delivery, and there is minimal gonadotropin activity. As hormone levels return to normal, ovulation returns approximately 7 to 9 weeks after birth in nonnursing women and 17 weeks in women who are breastfeeding. The delay in the resumption of menses in breastfeeding women may be due in part to elevated prolactin levels.

Cardiovascular System

The cardiovascular system undergoes dramatic changes after childbirth. The heart, which was displaced and lifted during pregnancy, reverses. Cardiac output remains high for the first few days postpartum but gradually declines to nonpregnant values within 2 to 4 weeks. The decrease in cardiac output is reflected in bradycardia (50–70 bpm) for the first 2 weeks postpartum. Tachycardia (≥ 100 bpm) in the postpartum woman warrants further investigation. It may indicate hypovolemia, dehydration, or hemorrhage.

Blood volume, which increased substantially during pregnancy, drops rapidly after birth and returns to normal within 4 weeks postpartum. The decrease in cardiac output and blood volume allows for the normal childbirth loss of 500 cc during a vaginal birth and 1000 cc loss during a cesarean birth. Despite the decrease in blood volume after birth, there should not be a decrease in hematocrit. A decrease of 10% lower than admission hematocrit may indicate hemorrhage.

Clotting factors in the blood that are increased during pregnancy remain elevated for the first 2 to 3 weeks during the postpartum period. This hypercoagulable state, along with vessel damage during birth and immobility, places the woman at great risk for thromboembolism (blood clots) in the lower extremities. Nurses need to encourage early ambulation after childbirth. Postpartum women should also refrain from wearing tight clothing, crossing their legs/ankles, massaging legs, and sitting with their legs dependent for great lengths of time during this period.

Respiratory System

Respirations remain within the normal adult range of 16 to 24 breaths per minute after childbirth. As the abdominal organs resume their nonpregnant position, the diaphragm returns to its normal position. Tidal volume, minute volume, vital capacity, and functional residual capacity return to pre-pregnant values 1 to 3 weeks postpartum.

Metabolic System

The basal metabolic rate remains elevated for 7 to 14 days after birth (it is elevated up to 25% during pregnancy because of fetal metabolic activity).

The decreases in progesterone and estrogen stimulate the anterior pituitary to produce prolactin. For those who breastfeed, prolactin levels increase with every nursing episode. In formula-feeding women, the prolactin level returns to normal between the third and fourth week postpartum.

Thyroid function returns to normal within 4 to 6 weeks postpartum. There is a slightly increased risk of hyperthyroidism postpartum.

Low levels of estrogen, lactogen, cortisol, growth hormone, placental enzyme, and insulinase reduce their anti-insulin effect in the early postpartum period. This results in lower glucose levels and a reduction in insulin requirements for insulin-dependent diabetic women. Women with gestational diabetes often have normal glucose levels immediately postpartum. Breastfeeding may precipitate hypoglycemic episodes in women with insulin-dependent diabetes, and patients need to be aware of this and make sure their nutritional needs are being met.

In the first 2 hours postpartum, plasma rennin and angiotensin II levels (blood pressure maintenance) fall to normal, nonpregnant levels, then rise again and remain elevated for up to 14 days. Blood pressure should remain stable postpartum, but women may become hypotensive due to the lowered vascular resistance in the pelvis. Postpartum women need to be cautioned to rise from bed slowly and sit at the edge of the bed for a few minutes before standing. An increase in blood pressure postpartum (30 mm Hg systolic and 15 mm Hg diastolic), especially if accompanied by a headache, may indicate preeclampsia and warrants further evaluation.

Neurologic System

In the early period after childbirth, the woman may have temporary neurologic changes, such as a lack of feeling in the legs, no urge to urinate, or lightheadedness from analgesia or anesthesia. Safety is a priority.

Carpal tunnel syndrome that resulted from compression of the median nerve by the edema of pregnancy is relieved by postpartum diuresis.

Headaches may result from fluid shifts in the first week after birth, leakage of cerebrospinal fluid into the extradural space during spinal anesthesia, fluid and electrolyte imbalance, preeclampsia, or stress. Careful assessment of the headache and vital signs are necessary, as postpartum eclampsia is often preceded by severe headache or visual disturbances.

Urinary System

The glomerular filtration rate and renal plasma flow that increased significantly during pregnancy begins to slow down and are both normalized by 6 weeks after birth. Pregnancy-induced hypotonia and dilation of the ureters and renal pelvis return to normal by 8 weeks postpartum.

Labor may result in displacement of the urinary bladder, stretching of the urethra, and a decrease in sensation when the bladder is full. An inability to void leads to bladder overfilling and distention. The uterus may become displaced and may be unable to contract effectively, causing uterine atony, placing the woman at great risk for hemorrhage. Spontaneous voiding should resume by 6 to 8 hours after birth, and bladder tone usually returns to normal levels 5 to 7 days later. If catheterization is necessary, rapid emptying of the bladder should be avoided, and no more than 800 mL of urine should be removed at one time. This measure will avoid a precipitous drop in intra-abdominal pressure, which can result in splenetic engorgement and hypotension. Urinary stasis can also result in urinary tract infections. Women should be encouraged to void every 2 hours, whether they have the sensation to or not, to prevent bladder overfilling.

Many women complain of stress incontinence during the first 6 weeks postpartum. Impairment of muscle function in and around the urethra is an underlying cause of stress incontinence. Persistent stress incontinence due to obstetrical factors diminishes over 3 months. Muscle-strengthening exercises (Kegel exercises) and prompt emptying of the bladder help to improve muscle tone.

Postpartum diuresis occurs within 12 hours after childbirth and continues throughout the first week postpartum. Women may complain of profuse sweating but should be reassured that this is a normal finding. Changes of clothing or showering frequently may help the woman feel more comfortable.

Gastrointestinal System

The gastrointestinal system quickly returns to normal after childbirth. The gravid uterus is no longer encompassing the abdominal cavity and producing pressure on the abdominal organs.

Constipation is often a common problem postpartum. Bowel tone and gastric motility, which were diminished during pregnancy as a result of progesterone, remain sluggish for several days. The first bowel movement usually occurs within 2 to 3 days postpartum, with normal patterns of bowel elimination resuming between 1 to 2 weeks postpartum.

Women with episiotomies, lacerations, or hemorrhoids may be fearful of pain or damage to the perineum with their first bowel movement and may attempt to delay it. Stool softeners and laxatives are frequently prescribed for all women on the postpartum unit to prevent or treat constipation.

Most women are thirsty and hungry after childbirth because of the energy expended during labor and the restrictions placed upon them during labor. The nurse should anticipate each mother's needs and provide fluids and food soon after childbirth.

Musculoskeletal System

In the first few days after birth, many women experience muscle fatigue and aches due to the effort exerted during labor and delivery. These muscle aches are often felt in the arms, shoulders, neck, and thighs and may be relieved with warmth to the affected areas and analgesics.

Also in the first few days after birth, the ligaments and cartilage of the pelvis begin to return to their pre-pregnant positions as the levels of the hormone relaxin subside. This sometimes causes hip and joint pain, but the new mother should be reassured that this is normal and that the condition should resolve itself shortly. Proper body mechanics and good posture are important to prevent any permanent injury.

Separation of the rectus abdominus muscles, also known as ***diastasis recti,*** may occur during pregnancy but usually reapproximates by the late postpartum period. Mild stretching and flexing of the abdominal muscles may help restore muscle tone and can be initiated 1 to 2 weeks postpartum.

In rare cases, a condition known as ***separated symphysis pubis (SSP)***, also known as pelvic girdle relaxation, is seen. SSP is a condition that results in separation of the symphysis pubis bone in late pregnancy or during delivery. It occurs in otherwise healthy pregnancies as a result of hormonal and/or biomechanical factors. Most cases of SSP result during normal spontaneous deliveries without evidence of forceful expulsion. Diagnosis is made from complaints offered by the patient, palpation, and by x-rays.

Symptoms of SSP range from mild discomfort to total debilitation. Symptom severity and duration vary among individuals. Mild cases often go undiagnosed but commonly present as mild pain over the symphysis pubis itself, pain with palpation, and mild discomfort with ambulation. Milder cases typically resolve in 2 days to 2 weeks. In more severe cases, patients complain of severe symphysis pubis pain and difficulty walking. In severe cases, the symptoms can interfere with activities of daily living, infant care, and normal postpartum adaptation. It may take up to 6 months for the condition to resolve itself in severe cases.

Priorities of nursing care for these patients include relieving discomfort, providing emotional support, and education. Analgesics should be ordered on an as-needed basis. A walker or crutches should be used if the extent of the separation is severe. Women should be instructed to shuffle instead of picking up their feet during ambulation. Stairs should be avoided until the problem has been resolved.

Patients typically need a support person to assist them in the early postpartum period on an around-the-clock basis to assist them in activities of daily living and infant care. Nurses should make referrals as needed to an orthopedic surgeon, physical therapist, and home health nursing service, as well as a social worker for help in dealing with the physical and psychosocial implications of SSP. Support for the family is also important, as they may have to shift their roles in order to accommodate the postpartum patient with SSP.

The postpartum woman's joints may not stabilize after delivery until 6 to 8 weeks postpartum, and vigorous exercise should be avoided.

Endocrine System

After expulsion of the placenta, there is a rapid decline in placental hormones. The pituitary hormone prolactin returns to pre-pregnant levels in approximately 2 weeks if the woman is not breastfeeding. The average time for nonbreastfeeding mothers to resume menstruation is 7 to 9 weeks after childbirth, although it varies among individuals. In lactating mothers, menses may resume as early as 12 weeks or as late as 18 months. In general, breastfeeding delays the return of both ovulation and menstruation. However, their return depends on several factors, such as the frequency of feedings, supplementation, and duration of lactation. In industrialized nations, it is not recommended that women use breastfeeding as a method of contraception. Therefore, contraceptive needs need to be addressed before sexual relations are resumed.

Integumentary System

Many of the skin changes that occurred during pregnancy revert to their pre-pregnancy states. Linea negra and chloasma fade and eventually disappear within a few months. Striae gravidarum (stretch marks) will fade to a silvery gray color but will not disappear completely. Hair loss peaks between 3 and 5 months after birth, but regrowth generally occurs by 9 months.

Immune System

An Rh-negative women who delivers an Rh-positive baby needs to be given 300 μg (micrograms) of anti-D immune globulin vaccine (RhoGAM). It is most effective if given within 72 hours after the delivery to prevent the development of maternal antibodies that would affect subsequent pregnancies.

The woman's rubella status (German measles) should be noted after birth. A woman who is nonimmune should be immunized against rubella, even if she is breastfeeding. The patient should be advised that she may experience a low-grade fever and joint aches. She should be encouraged not to become pregnant for 4 weeks after immunization, as the live virus can be harmful to a developing fetus during that period.

Women who are currently being treated for human immunodeficiency virus/acquired immunodeficiency syndrome (HIV/AIDS) with antiretroviral regimens such as zidovudine (ZDV) should continue their treatment regimen and follow-up during the postpartum period. HIV-infected mothers and their newborns can be cared for on postpartum units, and the infant can stay in the mother's room with her with the use of standard (universal) precautions. Gloves should be worn among personnel whenever contact with mucous membranes, blood, or body fluid is anticipated. Safety glasses should be worn when there is a chance blood or body fluids may spray.

Objective I: To Understand Focused Assessment After Vaginal Delivery

11.9 Assessment After Vaginal Delivery

Immediate postpartum assessment needs to be done once the woman has been bathed and assisted into a comfortable position for her recovery period, which is typically 1 to 4 hours on the labor and delivery unit. Frequency of assessment varies, depending on the facility's protocol. Generally, a full assessment is done every 15 minutes for 1 hour. Depending on the specifics of her delivery, including whether or not she received anesthesia, she may then be assessed every half hour for 1 hour, or every 4 hours for 24 hours. There are no data from prospective clinical trials to determine how often maternal status should be assessed during the postpartum period to promote optimal outcomes and safety. Generally, a focused assessment of a woman who delivered vaginally will include examination of vital signs, fundus, lochia, perineum, bladder elimination, breasts, lower extremities, and psychosocial status.

Vital Signs

Temperature. A temperature of up to 100.4°F (38°C) is a common finding during the first 24 hours after delivery, usually caused by postpartum dehydration. If an elevated temperature persists more than 24 hours or is higher than 100.4°F (38°C), the nurse should suspect an infection and report the finding to the health care provider.

Blood pressure. The postpartum blood pressure should be compared with the blood pressure of the predelivery period so that deviations can be quickly identified. Blood pressure should remain within the normal predelivery range for that patient. Lower blood pressure can indicate dehydration or hypovolemia resulting from blood loss. An increase in blood pressure can signify preeclampsia. It is important to monitor the woman at risk for orthostatic hypotension after delivery. Blood pressure should be taken in the same arm with the woman in the same position, and safety should be a priority concern when helping the woman out of bed. A patient with hypotension may feel dizzy or faint when getting out of bed.

Pulse/respirations. Transient cardiac output and pulse rate increases during the first 1 to 2 hours postpartum may occur when uteroplacental circulation returns to maternal circulation. After that, bradycardia with pulse rates between 40 and 50 bpm may occur during the immediate postpartum period. Tachycardia during this period may be a sign of infection, sign of hypovolemia due to hemorrhage or infection, or an effect of pain or anxiety. Tachycardia plus tachypnea may occur before a drop in blood pressure and may be an early sign of hemorrhage or impending shock.

Pain. Pain during the postpartum period may be caused by many factors. It is important for the nurse to assess the patient because unrelieved pain may interfere with the woman's ability to care for herself and her newborn. Uterine assessment, episiotomy or laceration pain, trauma, uterine incisions, after birth contractions, hemorrhoids, and nipple tenderness can all be sources of pain for the postpartum patient. Nursing interventions should be directed toward elimination of pain or reducing the sensation of pain to a tolerable level. Alternative methods of pain relief and analgesics may be employed for the relief of pain in the immediate postpartum period.

The acronym BUBBLE-HE is often used to guide the postpartum exam. It is a systematic way of doing a postpartum exam in the cephalocaudal fashion. The letters stand for breasts, uterus, bladder, bowel, lochia, episiotomy, Homan's sign, and emotional state.

Breasts. Breasts should be assessed for fullness, tenderness, nipple intactness, fissures, and bleeding. Breastfeeding should be initiated within 1 hour of birth. Successful latch-on and suckling at this time greatly reduce sucking disorganization or dysfunction later on and contribute to increased breastfeeding duration.

Analgesics given during labor have the potential to interfere with breastfeeding. The perinatal nurse may be able to offset this by encouraging early breastfeeding, keeping the newborn and mother together, and teaching the mother to put the newborn to the breast when he or she demonstrates hunger cues, such as sucking sounds and sucking on a fist.

Fundus. Under normal circumstances in term singleton pregnancy, immediately after birth, the fundus of the uterus should be firm and palpable halfway between the umbilicus and symphysis pubis. By 1 hour postpartum, the fundus typically is even with or slightly below the level of the umbilicus.

The presence of a boggy or soft fundus and inability to palpate the fundus are primary signs of uterine atony. The uterus should be massaged until it has contracted and is firm. However, continuing to massage after firmness is achieved or overaggressive massaging puts the woman at an increased risk of or exacerbates uterine atony.

To check the fundus, two hands should be used. The nurse should place one hand over the suprapubic area to support the lower uterine segment and to prevent uterine prolapse or inversion, while using the other hand to palpate the fundus (or top of the uterus).

A variety of medications can be given to stimulate uterine tone, such as pitocin and prostaglandin preparations. It is common for pitocin to be added to an existing intravenous (IV, 10–20 mu) dosage after delivery, or an intramuscular IM, 10 mu) injection of pitocin can be given after delivery to stimulate uterine tone.

Bladder. The bladder is often assessed in conjunction with the fundus. Upon inspection of the abdomen, a full bladder will often be observed. In other cases, the uterus may be displaced up and to the left by a full bladder. The patient may not feel the urge to urinate because of the trauma from the delivery or may have had epidural anesthesia. She will need to be helped onto a bedpan or up and out of bed for the first few times to urinate in the bathroom. The ability to ambulate and an assessment of potential hypotension are factors the nurse must keep in mind. Measurement of the first void or first few voids is often done to ensure output is adequate.

Bowel. Some patients pass stool when they are pushing and/or delivering vaginally. Patients need to be reminded that it may be several days before they are able to pass stool because of this, as well as because most patients are not allowed to eat during labor. Many patients are concerned about passing stool because they believe it will be painful or because they are fearful that their episiotomy may tear. They need to be reassured that this most often is not the case. Most postpartum units have standing orders for stool softeners to help make the passage of stool easier for postpartum women.

For women who deliver by cesarean section, early ambulation will aid in the passing of flatus due to not eating and surgery. Most patients who have had cesarean sections are given clear fluids after surgery but are not given food until they pass flatus. Each birth facility has its own policy on the advancement of diets for postoperative patients.

Lochia. Lochia flow is heaviest immediately after delivery. The nurse needs to assess the amount of lochia on the perineal pad and under the buttocks. If more than one pad is saturated within 15 minutes, bleeding is considered excessive, and the health care provider should be notified.

Perineum. The nurse needs to assess the condition of the perineum. The perineum may be swollen or have sustained lacerations, or an incision (episiotomy) may have been made.

Perineal lacerations are classified by the extent and severity in relation to how deep they extend into the perineal tissue. A first-degree laceration is limited to the perineal skin and vaginal mucous membranes. A second-degree laceration includes the fascia and perineal muscles. A third-degree laceration extends into the anal sphincter muscle. A fourth-degree laceration extends through the anterior rectal mucosa, exposing the rectal lumen. Superficial lacerations may not need repair, as they may approximate and heal spontaneously, whereas deeper lacerations need surgical repair.

An ***episiotomy*** is an incision made into the perineum during the second stage of labor. This is often done to allow more room for the fetal head to pass and to shorten the second stage, when forceful pushing is contraindicated, as in cardiac patients, in women who are exhausted and are pushing ineffectively, or when immediate delivery is warranted.

A midline episiotomy extends straight toward the rectum. A mediolateral episiotomy is an incision made diagonal to the midline. The mediolateral episiotomy is often used to prevent the extension into the rectum with forceful pushing.

In assessing the condition of the episiotomy, a woman is helped onto her side in bed with her upper leg flexed at the knee. By separating her labia and with the use of a flashlight, the episiotomy is assessed for redness, edema, bruising, hematomas, and bleeding. The acronym REEDA (redness, ecchymosis, edema, discharge, and approximation) is often used to guide assessment of episiotomies and other surgical incisions.

Hematomas typically appear as bulging, purplish masses on the perineum. A hematoma is an accumulation of blood in pelvic tissue caused by damage to a vessel wall without laceration of the tissue. Small hematomas usually resolve without treatment. Some hematomas may be deep within the vagina and may not be noticeable. Complaints of unrelenting perineal pain often point to hematoma formation, and closer examination of the perineum is called for. Excision and draining of the hematoma are warranted in cases of large hematomas.

Among the most critical postpartum complications are pulmonary emboli, which occur when all or part of a blood clot detaches from a vessel wall and becomes lodged in a pulmonary vein. Embolism is one of the leading causes of maternal mortality in the United States.

Thrombus, or clot formation, can lead to thrombophlebitis or thromboembolism, and vigilance by both the patient and the nurse is important. A superficial vein thrombus appears as a painful, often hard, unusually red vein. Deep vein thrombosis (DVT) carries the potential for clot fragmentation. Thrombophlebitis is the inflammation of the lining of a blood vessel due to the formation of blood clots. Sites are superficial, red, and painful to touch. They are often found in the veins of the leg, pelvis, and thigh. Onset is often rapid with severe pain and swelling.

Homan sign is assessed by dorsiflexion of the foot. A positive Homan sign is detected when there is pain in the calf with dorsiflexion. Further assessment is needed when there is a positive Homan sign, as it is not definitive of DVT. Later in the postpartum period the patient needs to be taught the signs and symptoms of thrombophlebitis and thromboembolism, along with measures to prevent clot formation.

Emotional. Assessment of the woman's interaction with her infant is important. The patient's fatigue level, for example, can interfere with attachment behavior. Noting whether the mother looks directly at the infant and maintains eye contact (en face) and whether she holds the infant close, touches, and speaks to the infant are all important clues to the mother's emotional readiness to parent. The nurse needs to provide an early opportunity for the mother to hold the infant and keep the infant with her as much as possible during the postpartum stay in the hospital.

Objective J: To Understand Cesarean Birth Assessments of the Postpartum Patient

11.10 Assessment After Cesarean Birth

After a cesarean birth, the patient should be closely monitored until she is bleeding minimally, passing at least 30 mL of urine hourly, and has a blood pressure reading within normal limits.

Assessment following cesarean birth includes the vital signs and fundal and lochia assessment similar to that for a woman who has had a vaginal birth and according to hospital policy; monitoring of the patient's level of consciousness according to the type of anesthesia or analgesia used, according to hospital policy; monitoring of the IV flow rate, the condition of the insertion site, and the IV connection; auscultation of bowel sounds in all four quadrants at intervals of approximately 4 hours; monitoring of the condition of any surgical dressings; evaluation of incisions based on the REEDA scale elements; assessment of the amount, color, and character of urine; monitoring of the side effects from anesthesia; assessment of pain and pain relief measures; and assessment of the patient's interaction with her infant.

11.11 Ongoing Assessment of the Postpartum Patient

The nurse caring for a postpartum patient must take into consideration that any time spent is a "reachable, teachable moment." While doing an assessment, the nurse can encourage the woman to participate in self- and infant care activities. This is especially important because the stay for new mothers in the hospital is typically very short.

The nurse needs to constantly reinforce what other nurses have taught the patient and should ask for return demonstration. Although patients from certain cultures, as well as their infants, will be taken care of by family members, the new mother is ultimately responsible for herself and her infant, so she must show basic proficiency in self- and infant care activities before she can be discharged home with the infant. It is important for the nurse to observe this and document it appropriately on the patient's chart. Discharge teaching begins the minute the patient walks into the hospital to deliver her baby.

During each shift (or more often if necessary or as hospital policy dictates), the nurse needs to do a full assessment of the postpartum patient. The nurse should become familiar with the patient's chart before seeing the patient, being aware of the patient's history and what specific areas of assessment and teaching may be necessary, in order to prioritize care.

An assessment begins the minute the nurse walks into the patient's room. First, the nurse should observe the general tone set by the patient. Is the patient awake and smiling? Is the room dark, with the patient crying on the edge of her bed? Much can be learned about the patient's psychosocial status through such observations. The nurse needs to explain to the patient all that will be done during the assessment. The nurse must respect the patient's privacy and ask the patient, for example, if it is acceptable to do the assessment with the patient's husband or partner present. Because of cultural practices, the patient may not be comfortable exposing more than one body part at a time.

Doing vital signs first allows time to establish a therapeutic relationship with the patient. Also, providing pain relief for the patient is important before doing a hands-on physical examination. Once that is taken care of, the nurse can move on to doing the actual exam. Physical assessment is an essential component of comprehensive nursing care during the postpartum period. Before beginning the exam, it is helpful to ask the patient to void. A full bladder can alter the true findings of a postpartum exam. It is at this time that the nurse can reinforce proper perineal cleansing and care with the patient.

The patient should be encouraged to use a peribottle, or squeeze bottle, to wash the perineum after voiding. The peribottle is filled with warm water, without additives, and sprayed on the perineum after voiding to cleanse the area. It is important to cleanse the area of blood, as any blood will serve as a medium for the growth of bacteria. An episiotomy or laceration can become infected if the perineum is not cleansed properly. In the case of women who have had a cesarean section, they can develop an ascending infection in the uterus from not cleansing the perineal area properly.

The patient should then be instructed to wipe the area, from front to back, to dry the perineum and prevent germs from entering the anus over the episiotomy/laceration or urethra, which can cause an infection. The postpartum patient should be encouraged to try to urinate every 2 hours. Because of the loss of sensation, she may not feel the urge to void until the bladder is so overdistended that she may have an accident on the way to the bathroom. Also, a full bladder may cause the uterus to become boggy, which puts the woman at risk for a postpartum hemorrhage. If the patient is unable to void or the output is < 150 cc, she may have residual urine and may have to be straight-cathed. Up to 800 cc can be released at a time before an indwelling catheter should be inserted.

The postpartum patient needs to be encouraged to change her peripad every 2 hours after she voids and does pericare. Blood on the pads creates a medium for the growth of bacteria and should be changed often. Lochia has a fleshy, musty odor; patients should report a foul odor if it should occur. This may indicate an infection. The patient can save the pad to show the nurse in order to assess how much bleeding has occurred since the last peripad change.

After voiding, the nurse can follow the BUBBLE-HE acronym in the postpartum assessment of the patient. The nurse starts by observing the woman's breasts. The nurse is checking for symmetry, dimpling, cracked nipples, fissures, nipple abnormalities (ie, inverted nipples), and bleeding. If the patient is breastfeeding, the nurse should inquire how it is going. It is important to reassure women about their ability to breastfeed their infants. Many feel they have an insufficient milk supply and may want to supplement with formula. However, only a small percentage of women have an insufficient milk supply. It is not acceptable to question a patient on why she has decided not to breastfeed or pressure her to do so. It is the patient's decision, and the nursing staff has to respect her wishes.

The nurse should ask for permission before she palpates the patient's breasts. This is a good time to inquire whether or not the patient does a monthly self-exam. The nurse can ask the patient to show her how she does the self-exam and can reinforce or teach the exam to the patient at this time. If the patient states she believes she does not have enough milk for the baby or that she has not seen anything from her breasts, she should be instructed on how to express some colostrum. Patients become more confident when they are able to see the colostrum.

The postpartum patient should be encouraged to wear a bra. If the woman is not breastfeeding, a tight sports bra should be worn 24 hours a day, and stimulation to the breasts should be avoided. The patient needs to know that the breasts will become engorged, but that the feeling should pass and that milk will dry up on its own within 1 week. For women who are breastfeeding, a breastfeeding support bra with convenient flaps should be worn to support the breasts and to make breastfeeding easier. The breastfeeding mother will also become engorged between days 3 and 5 when the milk comes in, and she should be encouraged to breastfeed more often to relieve her discomfort from the engorged breasts. This feeling will also pass within 1 week.

The patient should be asked about latch and sucking by the infant. The nurse needs to observe both and document on the patient's and infant's charts that the infant latched properly and sucked well, and that the nurse heard the infant swallow. Successful breastfeeding needs to be documented before a newborn can be discharged home with his or her mother to prevent adverse outcomes later on.

Women may complain of sore, cracked, or bleeding nipples. They can apply lanolin, Lansinoh, tea bags, cabbage leaves, or warm compresses to relieve the soreness. Patients need to be encouraged to continue to breastfeed even if they are experiencing these conditions; skipping feedings can lead to premature discontinuation of milk production and resulting formula supplementation.

The next area for assessment is the uterus. The nurse should ask the patient if she is having after pains. The nurse must next check for placement and firmness of the uterus. The uterus should be midline in the body. To palpate the uterus, the nurse needs to place one hand in the suprapubic area to support the uterus, and with the other hand, palpate the abdomen starting at the umbilicus as the reference point until the fundus is found. The fundus should be firm and centered in the abdominal cavity. The height of the fundus depends on the timing since the delivery. The fundus should descend into the pelvis by one fingerbreadth each day (1 cm ↓ U) until approximately the 10th day, when it should be contracted and so deep in the pelvis it cannot be palpated. In multiparous women, the descent may be slightly slower.

Assessment of the bladder follows. If a woman has a full bladder, the nurse may be able to see it before she palpates the uterus. The patient should be instructed to void before proceeding with the exam. A full bladder can push up the uterus and displace it toward the woman's right side. It also can cause the uterus to become boggy and puts the patient at an increased risk for hemorrhage. The nurse needs to ask the patient how often she is voiding. The nurse should ask about any problems the patient may be experiencing (burning, incontinence, etc). This is a good time to reinforce pericare techniques and reassure the patient if she complains of frequency of urination due to diuresis.

Bowel status is the next assessment to be done by the nurse. Patients on the postpartum unit are often anxious about having their first bowel movement. For those with episiotomies, they often state they are afraid it will tear the episiotomy open, and those patients who have had a cesarean section fear the bowel movement will tear open the abdominal incision. Patients can be reassured that this will not occur. Often stool softeners will be prescribed for all patients on the postpartum unit to ease the transition to having regular bowel movements again. Nurses need to encourage the patient to maintain a well-balanced diet and drink plenty of fluids. For those patients who had cesarean births, early and frequent ambulation helps relieve gas and promotes emptying of the bowel.

Lochia is assessed for amount, color, and odor. The presence of clots should be monitored by the nurse. Expression of clots is important, as they may cause the uterus to become boggy and put the patient at a greater risk for hemorrhage. This is also a good time for the nurse to reinforce pericare techniques.

Episiotomies, lacerations, and abdominal incisions should be assessed. Using the REEDA acronym, the nurse will look for redness, ecchymosis, edema, discharge, and approximation. Episiotomy discomfort can be addressed with ice, topical ointments, witch hazel pads, and analgesics. Patients should be instructed to sit straight on their buttocks in chair; sitting sideways in hopes of relieving pressure on the episiotomy actually puts more (uneven) pressure on the episiotomy and will cause more discomfort. Also, perineal strengthening exercises, or Kegel exercises, should be encouraged. The patient should tighten her perineal/buttock muscles, hold for 10 seconds, and release. A set of 10 repetitions is appropriate at one time.

Homan's sign should be evaluated next. The nurse needs to check the legs for varicosities, warmth, redness, heat, knots, or calf pain. It is not unusual for patients who have pushed for a long period during delivery to have calf aches. This is usually accompanied by shoulder or arm aches, also from the force of pushing. To assess Homan's sign, the patient should be supine in bed with knees bent slightly, and the nurse should dorsiflex a foot.

The pain of a positive Homan's sign has been equated with the pain of hitting the elbow ("funny bone" pain), a sharp, shooting pain up the leg. The nurse should remember that a positive Homan sign is not a positive indicator of a DVT, and further evaluation is needed.

If the woman has varicosities, she should be encouraged to continue wearing compression stockings. If she does not have compression stockings, the nurse should obtain an order and measure the patient for them. The woman should also be encouraged not to sit with her legs dependent for long periods, cross her legs or ankles, or sit cross-legged. She should also be discouraged from wearing a tight girdle in the early postpartum period. Any site where there is a restriction of blood flow can encourage clot formation. The patient should also refrain from having her legs massaged. If there is a clot, it can be dislodged by massage.

Finally, emotional status needs to be assessed. How is the patient responding to the nurse? Is she excited and talking about her experience and her baby, or is she sad, complaining, and stating the she does not know how she is going to manage? Is she participating in self- and infant care activities? Is she exhibiting attachment behavior with her infant? Does she have a support system in place? All of these issues are important and demonstrate the patient's healthy or unhealthy adaptation to her experience and to becoming a parent. They are important to assess and to document as the nurse prepares the patient for discharge home with her infant.

11.12 Lengths of Stay and Discharge Preparation

The length of stay in hospitals for postpartum women and their newborns in the United States has improved since the passage of the Newborns' and Mothers' Health Protection Act of 1996. This law requires that health insurance plans cover at least a 48-hour hospital stay following childbirth (96 hours following a cesarean section). These lengths of stay are more appropriate for accommodating the physical and psychosocial needs of women and their families than the shorter mandates that insurance companies were making previously in order to cut costs.

Although lengths of stay have improved, they are still relatively short periods of time for a new mother to get acquainted with her newborn and feel confident in self- and infant care techniques.

The inpatient perinatal nurse influences the patient's successful transition from hospital to home by assessing individual learning needs, giving accurate information, encouraging independence in self- and newborn care, and promoting confidence in the mothering role. A positive experience during childbirth and in the immediate postpartum period sets the stage for continued adaptation to parenthood at home.

Primary responsibility for patient and family education varies with the institution. Patient education may be coordinated by a clinical nurse specialist, perinatal educator, case manager, or lactation specialist; ultimately, however, it is the responsibility of the bedside nurse to ensure that women and their families have the information and skills necessary for appropriate maternal and infant care. Critical concepts and essential information that families need should be reviewed with the postpartum woman and her family. They should be presented to the family regardless of the family's past experience or self-assessment.

Maternal care includes the following concepts: activity and rest; pain relief and comfort measures; care of the perineum, including lacerations/episiotomies; breast care for breastfeeding women and lactation suppression for women who are formula feeding; postoperative cesarean birth instructions; expected emotional adaptations; and signs of postpartum complications to report to their health care provider. Women also need to be reminded to see their health care provider for a 6-week postpartum checkup. Those who have had cesarean births are usually seen 2 weeks after discharge.

Strict hand washing should be encouraged by the postpartum woman to prevent infecting herself and the newborn. Patients need to wash their hands with soap and water for at least 20 seconds before touching the baby, breastfeeding, before and after pericare, when changing the baby's diaper, or giving care to the baby.

Activity and rest. Extreme fatigue is normal after childbirth. Rest and sleep are emotionally and physically restorative, and the new mother should be encouraged to rest as much as possible. In the early weeks after birth, she should be encouraged to nap when the infant sleeps.

Although the woman is encouraged to ambulate as soon as possible, she needs to be encouraged to slowly increase her activity postpartum. Ambulation is considered exercise that is safe for the postpartum patient. Kegel exercises can also be done early on to help strengthen the perineal muscles. Strenuous exercise at a gym should be avoided until after the postpartum checkup at 6 weeks. If the woman notices an increase in bleeding or bleeding that reverts to bright red, she is doing too much activity and needs to rest. If the bleeding does not subside within a couple of hours, she should contact her health care provider.

Pain relief and comfort measures. Patients may be given prescriptions for analgesics upon discharge. Over-the-counter medications such as nonsteroidal anti-inflammatory agents are helpful for relief of cramping. For episiotomy pain, acetaminophen is often very helpful. Narcotics may be given to women who have had cesarean sections. Topical anesthetic ointments, ice packs, or witch hazel pads may provide relief for laceration/episiotomy/hemorrhoidal pain. For breast tenderness, more frequent feedings are suggested.

Patients can use extra pillows for comfort and to aid in breastfeeding. Keeping legs elevated when sitting may ease leg pain due to swelling.

Postpartum patients should not lift anything heavier than the weight of the newborn. Heavy lifting is contraindicated and can cause fatigue and an increase in bleeding.

Perineal care. The patient needs to be instructed to continue using the peribottle to wash the perineum after voiding until the bleeding stops. Because the uterus takes a full 6 weeks to heal, nothing should be placed in the vagina until the woman goes for her 6-week postpartum checkup. The nurse should discourage the use of tampons, douching, tub baths, and swimming for 6 weeks to prevent infection.

Foul-smelling lochia is usually an indication of infection and should be reported to the health care provider. Large clots also should be reported.

Patients who may have used a diaphragm previous to the birth for birth control need to be refitted by their health care provider at the 6-week postpartum checkup. Having condoms available in the home until the woman can be refitted for a diaphragm or for emergency protection is recommended.

Breast care. Care of the breasts needs to be reinforced, and the postpartum patient should be encouraged to wear a supportive bra. If she is formula feeding, she should be instructed to wear a sports bra and avoid stimulation to the breasts. Breasts do not need to be washed before each breastfeeding session; daily bathing is sufficient. Lanolin or Lansinoh may be applied to the nipples after feedings to keep them from cracking and bleeding.

The nurse should educate the patient on the signs of mastitis: one red, shiny, inflamed breast with chills and high fever present. If mastitis is suspected, the woman needs to see her health care provider and obtain antibiotic treatment. Ice may be applied for short periods for comfort measures. Analgesics may also be helpful. Other treatments used for comfort, such as cabbage leaves and tea bags, will not heal the infection of mastitis. The woman needs antibiotic therapy and must finish the whole course of treatment, as with other antibiotics, even if she feels better after a few days. Women who are breastfeeding are often told to pump the affected breast and discard milk. It is important for the nurse to reinforce the fact that the patient needs to continue to stimulate her breast by pumping (although she will be discarding the milk), in order for milk to be produced. If the affected breast is not stimulated during the course of antibiotic treatment, the woman's milk supply to that breast may dry up.

Those who decide to pump some of their milk, to allow someone else to feed the baby, to go out, or because they are returning to work, should be given information about the type of pumps available and local outlets from which to obtain a pump. They should be encouraged to pump after each feeding to ensure the infant gets what he or she needs at each feeding.

Women need to be given information about storing their milk. Breast milk should be stored in clean glass or plastic containers with tight lids. It can be stored in the refrigerator for up to 48 hours, frozen for 3 months, or kept in a deep freezer at −20°C (−4°F) for 6 months. It is important to label the containers with the date and time so the oldest milk is used for each feeding. Only amounts needed for each feeding should be stored in each container. Any milk left over from a feeding should be discarded. Breast milk should be heated by putting the bottle in a pan of warm water and should never be put in a microwave to be warmed. Microwaving causes uneven heating, and the infant may be burned by milk that contains hot spots.

Some women may be able to get breast pumps as a benefit from their health insurance company or may be able to obtain one from a community agency. Electric pumps can also be rented at many local pharmacies or from some hospitals that offer maternity care. The nurse needs to convey this information to the postpartum woman so that she can inquire from the appropriate sources.

Postoperative cesarean section instructions. Postoperative postpartum women take longer to heal. Cesarean sections are considered major abdominal surgery. Women need to progress slowly with activities of daily living, avoid heavy lifting, and maintain a well-balanced nutritional diet to aid in tissue repair. They need to observe their suture line for redness, drainage, or inflammation, which would indicate infection, and report it to their physician. Frequent ambulation will help the patient pass flatus and encourage emptying of the bowel. Frequent rest periods should also be encouraged.

Expected emotional adaptations. The postpartum woman and her family need to know that "postpartum blues," or mild depression, is a common phenomenon that occurs in many women starting during the first week after birth. New mothers may experience sadness and tearfulness and often cannot say why they feel "blue." This is generally a transient condition that is self-limiting and does not last longer than 2 weeks. It is characterized by fatigue, insomnia, tearfulness, mood instability, anorexia, and anxiety. The woman often questions her ability to care for the infant and is often worried about her attractiveness. Family members need to be supportive during this period.

Although the direct cause of postpartum blues/depression is unknown, it is thought to be the result of a combination of factors, including the drop in hormones with the placenta delivery, the emotional letdown after the delivery, fatigue, and discomfort.

Nurses need to teach the family to call the health care provider if the postpartum woman is depressed for more than 2 weeks after the birth or if she is unable cope with daily self- and infant care.

New fathers may also become depressed in the months surrounding childbirth. It is estimated that up to 30% of new fathers suffer from postpartum depression, most often when the baby is between 3 and 6 months. The rate is higher if the mother is also depressed. This finding dispels the theory that postpartum depression in women is only due to hormones and supports the need for extended family support.

The postpartum woman should be instructed to report any of the following signs and symptoms of physical or psychological complications to her health care provider as soon as they are identified:

- Fever > 100.4°F (38°C)
- Reappearance of bright red lochia that has turned brownish
- Vaginal discharge that has a foul odor or is accompanied by irritation
- Excessive lochia flow or large clots in lochia
- Swelling of the legs, especially if they are red, painful, or warm to the touch
- Swelling or pain of the breasts
- Burning or painful sensation upon urination, frequent urination, or inability to urinate
- Pain in the pelvic or perineal area
- Severe headaches, blurred vision
- Swelling in the face or around the eyes
- Persistent or severe mood swings
- Thoughts of harming herself or her baby

Prior to discharge, knowledge and skills for self- and newborn care need to be validated. Validation can be accomplished by discussion and by return demonstration. Written materials should also be given to the woman and family to reinforce what was taught.

Some institutions have "warm lines" with designated staff to triage calls from new mothers or provide the numbers to the postpartum unit or newborn nursery. Other institutions have discontinued this service because of liability issues. However, the new mother needs to know where or who she can call if she has questions or concerns after discharge. If there is an obvious emergency, the woman should be encouraged to visit the emergency room rather than wait for a call back from a health care provider.

The discharging nurse should evaluate the patient's support system. The patient may report friends or others as her support system and not necessarily family. Patients can be given names of support groups and community agencies that may offer support to new mothers or new parents. If there is some question that the postpartum woman may be having difficulty adjusting to her role as a new parent for any reason, a postpartum home visit may need to be scheduled. Most health insurance plans will pay for one maternal postpartum home visit and one newborn home visit. The nurse and social worker can initiate these visits before the patient is discharged home. The discharging nurse needs to document the discharge circumstances well, including topics covered, skills demonstrated, verbal understanding expressed by the woman and family, and method of exit from hospital, and should note who accompanies the patient from the hospital. The patient should be escorted to the front door of the birth facility and should be relieved of carrying anything.

Review Exercises

True/False

1. _______ A woman experiences many psychological and physiologic changes during the postpartum period.

2. _______ Women should be encouraged to breastfeed during the first hour after birth to promote successful breastfeeding and prevent breastfeeding dysfunction later on.

3. _______ An episiotomy is performed for every vaginal delivery.

4. _______ The uterine bleeding that occurs after childbirth is called lochia.

5. _______ REEDA is an acronym used to guide the assessment of the perineal area and incisions after childbirth.

6. _______ Uncontrolled pain in the postpartum woman can interfere with attachment behavior.

7. _______ Immediately after a vaginal birth, the nurse would expect to palpate the fundus halfway between the symphysis pubis and umbilicus.

8. _______ Two days postpartum, the nurse would expect to palpate the fundus four fingerbreadths below the umbilicus.

9. _______ Early ambulation after a cesarean birth should be encouraged for the prevention of thrombus formation.

10. _______ Hypotension is a risk for postpartum women after receiving analgesia/anesthesia for delivery; therefore patients should rise slowly from a sitting position and when getting out of bed.

11. _______ Cultural practices should be taken into consideration when caring for a postpartum patient.

12. _______ Improper latch is the most common cause of sore nipples in the postpartum woman.

13. _______ It is important to monitor bowel sounds in the postop cesarean section patient.

14. _______ Postpartum patients should be given discharge instructions only on the day of discharge.

15. _______ A boggy uterus should first be treated with an intramuscular injection of pitocin.

16. _______ A full bladder can cause the uterus to become boggy, displace the uterus, and put the woman at risk for hemorrhage.

17. _______ A positive Homan's sign is a positive indicator of a deep vein thrombosis (DVT).

18. _______ Diuresis in the postpartum woman is a normal process that begins within 12 hours after delivery and lasts up to 5 days.

19. _______ Fatigue is a common complaint of postpartum patients.

20. _______ Afterpains or painful uterine contractions are common in the first few days after birth.

21. _______ Heart rate increases normally during the immediate postpartum period.

22. _______ The first menstrual period postpartum usually occurs within 7 to 9 weeks in the nonnursing woman.

23. _______ The first menstrual period postpartum in nursing women varies.

24. _______ Sexual intercourse may be resumed between 3 and 4 weeks postpartum.

25. _______ Uterine palpation for assessment postpartum should be done with two hands.

Completion

1. The process of uterine contraction after birth is called ________________.
2. __________ exercises can be done to strengthen perineal muscles after a vaginal delivery.
3. ______________ is the acronym for the systematic assessment of the postpartum patient.
4. A woman loses an average of ___________ pounds during childbirth.
5. Bowel movements typically resume ______________ days after birth.
6. ______________ is a transient mood disturbance that occurs in many women a few days after birth (3 to 6 days) and is self-limiting.
7. ______________ is responsible for stimulating and sustaining lactation.
8. Urine output in the immediate postpartum period may be ____________ mL or more each day.
9. Spontaneous voiding should resume by ___________ hours after delivery.
10. Blood loss during an uncomplicated vaginal delivery is ___________ mL.

Multiple Choice

1. The red uterine discharge that occurs immediately after birth and the next few days in the postpartum woman is called

   A. Lochia rubra

   B. Lochia serosa

   C. Lochia alba

   D. Lochia accreta

2. Signs and symptoms of thrombophlebitis would include

   A. Pain, swelling, and redness

   B. Decreased lochia flow

C. Increased lochia flow

D. Varicose veins

3. Pain relief for the postpartum patient may include all of the following (choose all that apply):

A. Analgesics

B. Alternative therapies

C. Ambulation

D. Carbonated beverages

4. When assessing a patient for performance of self-care activities, the best indication that the patient understands instructions and is participating in self-care activities would be

A. Patient gives a return demonstration.

B. Patient states she is changing her peripad twice daily.

C. Patient asks why she needs to use a peribottle, as she had a cesarean section.

D. Patient states that she "wants to rest and will walk when she gets home."

5. A patient says she wants to breastfeed; however, in her culture, mothers wait 2 weeks to start breastfeeding. What response by the nurse is the most appropriate?

A. Tell the patient that her cultural practices are the best for the infant.

B. Tell the patient that this is unacceptable behavior.

C. Call the social worker to do a psychosocial assessment of the patient.

D. Instruct the patient on how beneficial colostrum is to the infant, and that early action promotes successful breastfeeding.

6. When providing family-centered care, it is important for the nurse to be aware that

A. The patient cannot have more than one significant other at the bedside at any one time.

B. The only person allowed at the patient's bedside is her husband.

C. The patient's family is whomever she designates as family.

D. Call the social worker if the patient is not married.

7. A patient who is 1 day postpartum wants to be discharged early. What anticipatory guidance should the nurse initiate?

A. A consultation with the social worker

B. A postpartum/well-baby home visit

C. A family support meeting

D. A consult with a psychiatrist

8. Which symptom would be reportable by the postpartum mother to her health care provider after being home 1 week after childbirth?

A. Temperature of 100°F

B. Foul-smelling lochia

C. Small clots expelled when urinating

D. Headache

9. The Rh-negative mother who delivers an Rh-positive infant will be given RhoGAM

A. At her 6-week postpartum checkup

B. Before the delivery of the placenta

C. Within 72 hours of the delivery

D. One week after childbirth

10. The postpartum patient who receives the rubella vaccine postpartum should be instructed

A. Not to breastfeed

B. That her urine may turn orange

C. She should not get pregnant for at least 4 weeks after administration of the vaccine

D. She may experience a high fever after administration of the vaccine

11. A postpartum mother who is HIV positive should be

A. Put on isolation

B. Transferred to the intensive care unit

C. Taken care of on the postpartum unit

D. Sent home from the labor and delivery unit after childbirth

12. Breastfeeding with mastitis should be

A. Discouraged

B. Encouraged, although milk from the affected breast should be discarded

C. Encouraged

D. Discouraged while on antibiotics and resumed after a course of treatment

13. All of the following are signs/symptoms of postpartum blues except

A. Insomnia

B. Tearfulness

C. Anxiety

D. Overeating

14. The postpartum patient needs to be encouraged to void

A. Every 2 hours

B. Every 4 hours

C. Once a shift

D. When she has the urge to void

15. The use of tampons by postpartum women

A. Should be discouraged for 6 weeks

B. Should be used by all postpartum patients

C. Cannot be used once a woman gives birth

D. Should only be used during the night

Answers

True/False

1. True
2. True
3. False. Episiotomies are only performed when necessary to allow more room for the head to be born.
4. True
5. True
6. True
7. True
8. False. The nurse would expect to palpate the fundus in a 2-day postpartum woman two finger breadths below the umbilicus (↓2).
9. True
10. True
11. True
12. True
13. True
14. False. Discharge planning should begin on the day of admission.
15. False. A boggy uterus should be gently massaged until it gets firm; in the case of a full bladder, the woman should void and be reassessed by the nurse.
16. True
17. False. A positive Homan's sign is not a positive indicator of a deep vein thrombosis but requires further evaluation.
18. True
19. True
20. True
21. False. Heart rate decreases slightly immediately postpartum.
22. True
23. True
24. True
25. True

Completion

1. Involution
2. Kegel
3. BUBBLE-HE
4. 12
5. 3 to 5
6. postpartum blues
7. Prolactin
8. 3000
9. 8 hours
10. 500 mL

Multiple Choice

1. A
2. A
3. A, B, C, D
4. A
5. D
6. C
7. B
8. B
9. C
10. C
11. C
12. B
13. D
14. A
15. A

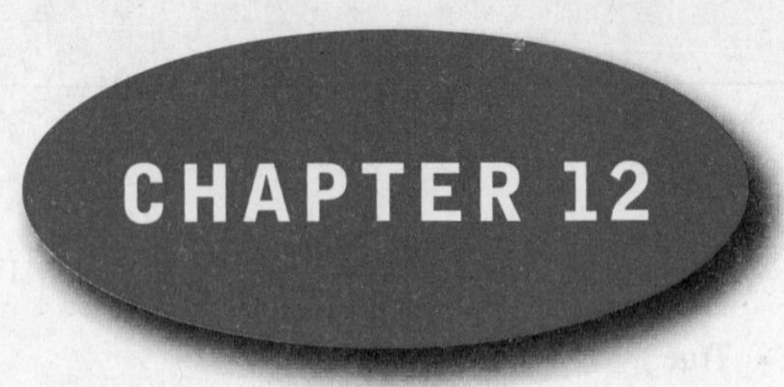

The Newborn

Objective A: To Understand the Physiologic Adaptations of the Newborn

12.1 Physiologic Adaptations of the Newborn

The transition from fetal to newborn life is a critical period. The infant must make profound physiologic changes to adapt to extrauterine life and meet his or her own respiratory, digestive, and regulatory needs. Critical to adaptation to extrauterine life is the establishment of respiration as the lungs become the organ of gas exchange after separation from maternal uteroplacental circulation. Initiation of breathing is a complex process that depends on chemical and sensory stimulation of the respiratory center in the brain and mechanical stimulation of the lungs.

At birth, the infant's first breath must force fetal lung fluid into the interstitial spaces around the alveoli so that air can enter the respiratory tract.

Chemoreceptors in the carotid arteries and aorta respond to changes in blood chemistry brought about by the hypoxia that occur with a normal birth. A decrease in the blood oxygen level (PO_2) and pH, and an increase in the carbon dioxide level (PCO_2) cause impulses from these receptors to stimulate the respiratory center in the medulla.

During a vaginal birth, the fetal chest is compressed by the narrow birth canal. A small amount of the fetal lung fluid is forced out of the lungs into the upper air passages during birth. As the head and then the chest of the neonate emerge, recoil of the chest draws air into the lungs and helps remove some of the viscous fluid in the airways.

The temperature change that occurs during birth is also an important stimulus for the initiation of respirations. Sensors in the skin respond to the sudden change in temperature by sending impulses to the brain that stimulate the respiratory center and breathing.

Tactile stimuli that occur during birth stimulate skin sensors. Stimulation of light, sound, smell, and pain at delivery may also aid in the initiation of respiration.

Once the alveoli expand, surfactant, a liquid lipoprotein, keeps them partially open between respirations. Once the infant starts crying, pressure within the lung increases, keeping the alveoli open and causing fetal lung fluid to move into the interstitial spaces, where it is absorbed by the pulmonary circulatory and lymphatic systems. Although most fluid is absorbed within a few hours, it may take as long as 24 hours.

The transition from fetal to neonatal circulation is a major cardiovascular change and occurs simultaneously with respiratory system adaptation. During fetal life, three cardiovascular shunts—the ductus venosus, foramen ovale, and ductus arteriosus—carry blood away from the lungs and liver. Clamping of the umbilical cord allows the infant's blood to circulate to the lungs for oxygenation and to the liver for filtration.

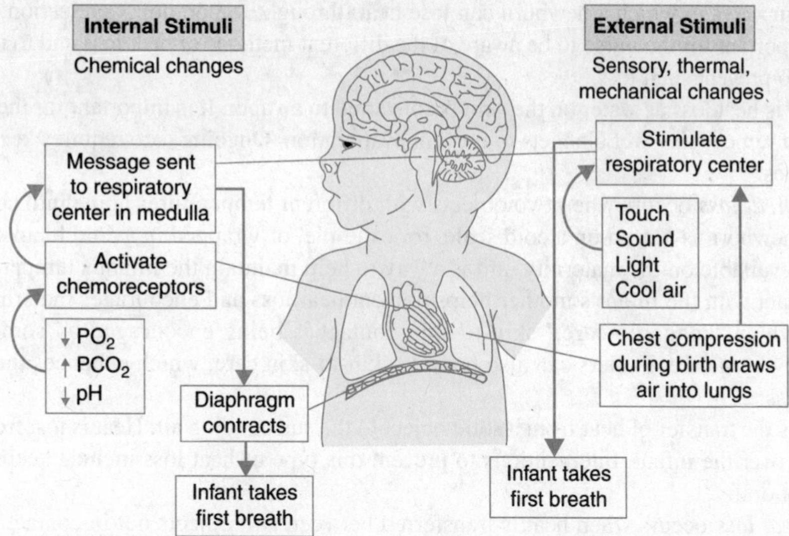

Figure 12.1 Chemical, sensory, thermal, and mechanical factors involved in respiration.

The ductus venosus, which shunts blood away from the liver prenatally, is occluded with clamping of the cord and causes blood to travel to the liver to be filtered as in adult circulation. Permanent closure is in 1 to 2 weeks.

The foramen ovale provides an opening between the right and left auricle so blood can bypass nonfunctioning lungs prenatally. Cord occlusion elevates systemic resistance and decreases pulmonary resistance, allowing free flow of blood into lungs. Permanent closure is in 3 months. After the infant begins breathing, the pulmonary blood vessels respond by dilating. This decreases the pulmonary vascular resistance that prevented blood flow into the lungs during fetal life and allows the vessels within the lungs to accommodate the sudden increase in blood flow from the pulmonary artery.

The ductus arteriosus, which is widely dilated prenatally to carry blood from the pulmonary artery to the aorta and avoids nonfunctioning lungs, constricts during delivery, preventing entrance of blood from the pulmonary artery. Blood in the pulmonary artery is directed toward the lungs for oxygenation and increases the oxygen level in the blood. Complete closure should be in 15 to 24 hours; however, permanent closure can take up to 4 weeks. A murmur may be heard in the infant as a result of blood flow through the partially opened vessel.

Neurologic System

Assessment of the central nervous system (CNS) is integrated throughout the physical exam and includes evaluation of posture, cry, muscle tone, and movement; evaluation of most cranial nerves; and evaluation of all developmental reflexes. Findings during the neurologic assessment are influenced by the gestational age and health of the newborn.

At birth infants must also assume thermoregulation. Characteristics predispose them, however, to lose heat. Along with environmental factors, a large body surface area in relation to body mass and a limited amount of subcutaneous fat predispose them to heat loss. Thin skin with blood vessels near the surface also makes newborns vulnerable to heat loss. Newborns attempt to regulate body temperature by nonshivering thermogenesis, increased metabolic rate, and increased muscle activity.

Nonshivering thermogenesis is the metabolism of brown fat. This highly vascular adipose tissue is produced between 26 and 28 weeks' gestation until approximately 5 weeks after birth. It is located in the neck, scapula, axilla, and mediastinum and around kidneys and adrenal glands. When exposed to cold stress, thermal receptors in the skin transmit messages to the CNS, activating the sympathetic nervous system and triggering metabolism of brown fat. Heat produced through voluntary muscle activity is minimal in the newborn. Full-term newborns have a flexed posture, which reduces heat loss.

There are four ways in which a newborn can lose heat: through evaporation, conduction, convection, and radiation. It is important for the nurse to be aware of the different methods of heat loss and to teach them to the parents in order to prevent such loss.

Evaporation is heat loss as water on the skin is converted to a vapor. It is important for the nurse to dry the infant at birth and remove any wet blankets to prevent evaporation. Ongoing care requires keeping the infant's skin dry at all times.

Conductive heat loss occurs when two objects with different temperatures come into contact. Heat loss can occur if the newborn is placed on a cold scale, for example, or wrapped in a cold blanket. Having warm blankets readily available on the maternity unit is a way to help maintain the infant's temperature. Providing skin-to-skin contact with the infant's mother helps prevent heat loss and encourages maternal-infant attachment. Also known as "kangaroo care," skin-to-skin contact is being encouraged by some hospitals as a regular part of newborn care. Fathers can also provide skin-to-skin care, which enhances the paternal-infant attachment process.

Convection is the transfer of heat from a solid object to the surrounding air. Heat is lost from a newborn as cooler air passes over the infant. Interventions to prevent this type of heat loss include keeping the newborn clothed and out of drafts.

Radiation heat loss occurs when heat is transferred between two objects not in contact with each other. The newborn can lose heat in a crib, near a cold window, or in a cold incubator. Interventions to prevent this type of heat loss include using a radiant warmer after birth and moving the crib or incubator away from a cold window.

Cold stress can cause many body system changes. The increased metabolic rate and metabolism of brown fat that result from cold stress increases the need for oxygen. Cold stress also causes a decrease in the production of surfactant, impeding lung expansion. Prolonged cold stress can cause respiratory distress even in an otherwise healthy full-term newborn.

Glucose is necessary in larger amounts when the metabolic rate rises to produce heat. When glycogen stores are used to produce heat, they can become depleted, which results in hypoglycemia. Metabolism of brown fat and glucose in the presence of decreased oxygen causes increased production of acids. Elevated fatty acids in the blood can prevent transport of bilirubin to the liver, increasing the risk of jaundice.

The CNS consists of the brain, spinal cord, 12 cranial nerves, and a variety of spinal nerves that come from the spinal cord. Neurologic development follows cephalocaudal (head-to-toe) and proximal-distal (center-to-outside) patterns. Myelin develops early on in sensory nerve transmitters. Therefore, the newborn has an acute sense of hearing, smell, and taste. The newborn's sensory capabilities include hearing that is well developed at birth, with the infant responding to noise by turning to sound; ability to taste sweet and sour by 72 hours of age; ability to distinguish between the mother's breast milk and milk from others; sensitivity to pain; responsiveness to tactile stimuli; ability to focus on objects close by (10 to 12 inches away) and track objects midline and beyond.

The presence and strength of reflexes are important indications of neurologic development and function. The nurse needs to assess normal newborn reflexes to evaluate neurologic function and development. Absent or weak reflexes in a newborn may indicate neurologic pathology. Normal newborn reflexes that should be present are sucking, blink, Moro, gag, tonic neck (fencing), swallow, Galant, startle, palmar grasp, and crossed extension.

Hematologic System

The average blood volume of the normal full-term infant is 85 to 100 mL/kg. The hematocrit level in the normal infant is 48% to 69% from peripheral sites during the first day, and by the third day 44% to 72%. A level > 65% is considered polycythemic and puts the infant at a greater risk for jaundice.

Hematocrit levels in the newborn range from 14.5 to 22.5 g/dL. Hemoglobin and hematocrit levels in the newborn are higher than in adults to enable fetal cells to get enough oxygen.

White blood cells, or leukocytes, range from 9000 to 30,000/mm^3. The leukocytes usually rise during the first 12 hours after birth and decrease slowly. In newborns an elevated leukocyte count does not necessarily indicate an infection. The white blood cell count may actually decrease with an infection in a newborn. Platelets range from 84,000 to 478,000/mm^3. Their number may decrease with infection.

Newborns are at risk for clotting deficiency during the first few days of life because they lack vitamin K at birth. Vitamin K is produced in the intestines, but the intestines of a newborn are sterile and unable to produce vitamin K until the infant starts to eat and pass stool. Vitamin K (1 mg intramuscularly via the vastus lateralis muscle) is given to newborns during their initial care to decrease the risk of hemorrhagic disease.

Gastrointestinal System

The full-term newborn has the ability to swallow, digest, metabolize, and absorb food taken in soon after birth. The pH of the stomach is slightly acidic.

The stomach of the newborn has a capacity ranging from 30 to 90 mL, with variable emptying time of 2 to 4 hours. The cardiac sphincter and nervous control of the stomach are immature, so frequent regurgitation is common in newborns. Term newborns lose 5% to 10% of their body weight in the first week of life. To gain weight, the newborn must consume ~120 cal/kg daily.

Bowel sounds should be heard within the first hour of life and should be assessed in all four quadrants. The frequency, consistency, and type of stool passed by newborns vary widely. The newborn's first stool, called meconium, consists of amniotic fluid, shed mucosal cells, intestinal secretions, and blood. The meconium is sterile and is thick, blackish green, and tarry. It is usually passed within 12 to 24 hours of birth.

After feedings are initiated, transitional stool develops that is greenish brown to yellowish brown, thinner in consistency, and often seedy in appearance. The last stool to be passed is the milk stool. The stools of breastfed babies are gold, loose, and often sweet smelling. The stool of the formula-fed baby is yellow to yellow-green, formed, with an unpleasant odor.

Renal System

The majority of term infants void immediately after delivery, indicating adequate renal function. The glomerular filtration rate is ~30% at birth and reaches adult values by 1 year of life. It is normal for newborns to void 6 to 10 times daily.

Hepatic System

At birth, the liver assumes functions that the placenta handled in utero. These functions include iron storage, carbohydrate metabolism, blood coagulation, and conjugation of bilirubin.

After red blood cells (RBCs) are normally broken down and replaced every 3 days after birth, the iron is released and stored by the liver. Newborn iron stores are determined by total body hemoglobin content and length of gestation. At birth, the full-term newborn has enough iron stored to last from 4 to 6 months.

When the placenta is delivered, the source of glucose is cut off, and the newborn's glucose levels decline. Initiating early feedings helps to stabilize the newborn's serum blood glucose. The liver releases glucose from glycogen stores for the first 24 hours.

The liver is responsible for the breakdown of ***bilirubin***, a yellow pigment produced by the breakdown of RBCs. The metabolic function of the liver is immature and cannot conjugate the bilirubin as it needs to. When unconjugated bilirubin is deposited in the skin and mucous membranes, jaundice results. Extremely elevated levels of bilirubin in the first week of life can cause ***kernicterus,*** a permanent and devastating form of brain damage. Treatment of newborn jaundice is discussed in Chapter 16.

Integumentary System

The epidural barrier begins to develop by 32 weeks' gestation, and although it is similar in thickness and lipid composition, skin development is not complete at birth. Therefore, the risk of injury is higher than for an adult. Careful skin care needs to be maintained with newborns. Full adult functioning is not present until the second or third year of life.

Newborns vary in appearance. Skin tones vary depending on the newborn's age, race or ethnic group, temperature, and whether or not he or she is crying. Marks from the delivery, "stork bites," and other markings may be evident and need to be investigated.

Immune System

The newborn has the ability to survive a hostile environment. The developing newborn's immune system is initiated early in gestation. The intrauterine environment usually protects the fetus from harmful microorganisms. Physical barriers (intact skin), chemical barriers (eg, gastric acids), and resident nonpathologic organisms make up the newborn's natural immune system.

The newborn depends largely on three immunoglobulins for defense mechanisms: IgG, IgA, and IgM. IgG is the major immunoglobulin and the most abundant, comprising 80% of all circulating antibodies. It is found in serum and interstitial fluid. IgG is thought to protect mucous membranes from viruses and bacteria. IgA is found in the gastrointestinal (GI) tract and respiratory tract, tears, saliva, colostrum, and breast milk. IgM is found in blood and lymph fluid and is the first immunoglobulin to respond to infection. It offers major protection to blood-borne infections.

Objective B: To Understand the Initial Assessment of the Newborn at Birth

12.2 Initial Assessment of the Newborn

Although most births result in a healthy newborn able to make the transition to extrauterine life without difficulty, perinatal nurses must be able to handle complications if they arise. The Neonatal Resuscitation program developed by the American Heart Association and the American Academy of Pediatrics has become the standard for educating health care providers involved in newborn stabilization.

Although most newborns respond successfully to oral suctioning and tactile stimulation, 5% to 10% may require additional interventions, including chest compressions or medications.

Once airway, breathing, and circulation have been established, the nurse needs to dry the infant off, wrap it in warm blankets, and put a hat on its head to prevent heat loss. Many health care providers will place the baby on the mother's chest as soon as it is delivered. This is one of the most effective ways to enhance mother–newborn attachment.

The nurse needs to do a quick assessment that includes vital signs, Apgar scores, a physical exam, and measurements. The nurse will also need to identify the infant with the mother before removing the baby. All aspects of the examination and identification should be performed in the birthing room in the parent's view.

The ***Apgar score*** was introduced in 1952 by Dr. Virginia Apgar. It provides a simple method for evaluating the infant at 1 minute and at 5 minutes of life. Five assessment criteria (heart rate, respiratory effort, muscle tone, reflex irritability, and skin color) are each scored from 0 to 2, with a maximum total score of 10 (**Table 12.1**). The American Academy of Pediatrics and the American Congress of Obstetricians and Gynecologists recommend continuing assessment every 5 minutes until the total score is > 7. The Apgar score in itself is not an accurate predictor of long-term outcome but may identify special needs the infant may have. It is the nurse who gives the baby the Apgar score, not the physician, and the nurse is superseded if there is a neonatologist at the delivery.

TABLE 12.1 Apgar Scoring

	0	1	2
Heart rate	Absent	Slow (≤ 100 beats/min)	Normal (≥ 100 beats/min)
Respirations	Absent	Irregular, slow	Regular, strong cry
Muscle tone	Limp	Some flexion	Active motion
Reflex irritability	No response	Grimace	Cough, sneeze, or cry
Skin color	Blue or pale	Body pink; extremities blue	Body and extremities pink

The infant who will be breastfed should be placed on the breast for feeding. This first period of reactivity that begins at birth and lasts for the first 30 minutes after birth allows parents to interact with their newborn and enjoy close contact with their new baby. Many newborns latch on the nipple and suck well during this first experience. Early sucking and opportunities for uninterrupted contact between mother and newborn have been shown to increase breastfeeding duration. After the newborn breastfeeds, he or she is weighed and measured. The infant is then placed under a radiant warmer.

Objective C: To Understand the Psychological Adaptation of the Newborn

12.3 Psychological Adaptation of the Newborn

In addition to adapting physiologically, the newborn adapts behaviorally. All newborns progress through a predictable pattern of behavior despite their gestational age or type of birth.

The first period, or ***period of reactivity,*** begins at birth and lasts for 30 minutes. This period is characterized by eye movements, sucking, chewing, rooting, and spontaneous Moro movements. Respirations and heart rates are elevated and gradually begin to slow with the next period.

The next period, the ***period of decreased responsiveness,*** begins at 30 minutes of age and lasts for approximately 2 hours. During this stage, the newborn enters a deep sleep. Movements are less frequent, heart and respiratory rates decline, the muscles become relaxed, and responses to external stimuli decrease. During this phase, it is difficult to arouse the newborn.

The next period, the ***second period of reactivity,*** begins as the newborn awakes and shows interest in external stimuli. This period lasts 2 to 8 hours in normal newborns. Heart rate and respiratory rates increase. Peristalsis increases, and the newborn often passes his or her first stool during this period. Interaction between parents and the newborn is encouraged.

Newborns demonstrate several predictable responses when interacting with their environment. How they respond to the world around them is termed a ***neurobehavioral response.*** Expected newborn behaviors include orientation, habituation, motor maturity, self-quieting ability, and social behaviors. The response of newborns to stimuli is termed ***orientation***. They become acutely alert when they sense a new stimulus in their environment. They face the object and stare intently.

Habituation is the newborn's ability to process and respond to visual and auditory stimuli. Newborns are also able to block out external stimuli after they have become familiar with the activity.

Motor maturity refers to posture, tone, coordination, and movements. When stimulated, newborns with good motor organization demonstrate movements that are rhythmic and spontaneous. As newborns adapt to their environment, smoother movements should be observed.

Self-quieting ability refers to newborns' ability to quiet and soothe themselves. They console themselves by hand-to-mouth movements and sucking.

Social behaviors include cuddling and snuggling into the arms of the parent when the newborn is held. Most newborns will cuddle, but some resist. Encouraging parents to assume comforting behaviors and praising them for their efforts can help foster cuddling behavior.

Objective D: To Understand Nursing Care in the Early Newborn Period

12.4 Nursing Care in the Early Newborn Period

Most states in the United States mandate that every newborn receive prophylaxis against eye infections. Erythromycin ointment is the drug of choice because of its effectiveness against gonococcal and chlamydial infections. It is also less irritating than other medications. Administration is often delayed until after the newborn has had contact with his or her mother, as erythromycin will blur the newborn's vision. Excess ointment can be wiped away. It should be applied within the first hour of life to be most effective.

Vitamin K is administered intramuscularly to all newborns to prevent hemorrhagic disease. During the first week of life, newborns are at great risk for bleeding. Vitamin K is naturally produced in the GI tract, but the GI tract is sterile and cannot produce the vitamin until the newborn starts eating, which causes colonization of bacteria in the GI tract.

The nurse should examine the umbilical cord for three vessels—two arteries and a vein. The cord should be kept dry to prevent infection.

The next step is newborn identification. Perinatal nurses must be meticulous when recording the identification band number and applying identification bands to mothers and newborns. Most hospitals use a four-band system: One is placed on the mother's wrist, two on the baby, and one on the support person who attended the delivery. Most hospitals are now employing additional security measures with central electronic monitoring, although this method is costly and controversial.

Newborn safety and security need to be discussed with parents in the labor and delivery room. Mothers need to watch as the nurse applies the identification band on their newborns. Parents need to know what security measures the hospital has in place to prevent infant abductions and should understand what they can do to increase safety. They also need to be given directions not to leave the newborn unattended and information about identification of caregivers who may transport the newborn to the nursery or other hospital departments. Once the proper identification is made, the infant can be transferred to the newborn nursery. Often the infant's father accompanies the nurse to the nursery.

The perinatal nurse in the nursery receives the newborn and places the baby under a radiant warmer. The nurse then checks identification with the labor and delivery nurse. All ID bands must match perfectly or another set of bands must be applied along with the incorrect bands. Once the newborn has been identified, the nurse performs the first detailed head-to-toe examination.

The physical examination includes the assessment skills of observation, inspection, palpation, and auscultation. Good lighting is essential. The physical assessment usually begins by observing the newborn's breathing pattern, overall skin color, general state or level of alertness, posture, and muscle tone. A full-term newborn should have extremities that are flexed at the joints.

Vital signs should be done next. Normal parameters for full-term newborns include

- Temperature: 97.7°F to 99.5°F (36.5–37°C) (axillary)
- Respiration: patterns irregular, with respiratory rates between 30 and 60 respirations per minute
- Heart rate: regular, with rates between 110 and 160 bpm
- Blood pressure is not done routinely in the newborn nursery (it is done in the neonatal intensive care unit)
- Pain scale: usually rated from 0 to 2 in newborns (0 = no pain, 1 = "fussy," and 2 = crying)

If the newborn was not weighed and measured on the labor and delivery unit, this will be the next step if the infant is stable and not in respiratory distress. Also measured are the newborn's head and chest circumferences. The head circumference is usually 2 cm greater than the chest circumference. Routine abdominal circumference is usually not obtained. Normal parameters for the full-term newborn are

- Weight: 5 lb, 8 oz to 8 lb, 13 oz (2,500–4,000 g)
- Height: 19 to 21 inches (48–53 cm)
- Head circumference: 13 to 14 inches (33–35.5 cm)
- Chest circumference: 12 to 13 inches (30.5–35.5 cm)

A gestational age assessment may be done as part of the initial newborn physical examination. This assessment evaluates physical and neuromuscular characteristics. Identifying those newborns who are preterm, term, or postterm, small for gestational age (SGA), or large for gestational age (LGA) increases the likelihood of early identification and timely interventions for complications related to gestational age. The Dubowitz Scale or Ballard Scale is used for this determination.

Newborn skin is assessed using inspection and palpation. Color, birthmarks, skin lesions, texture, and turgor are noted. At birth, some newborns may have a cheeselike coating, or vernix, on their skin. Full-term newborns should only have this in the groin and armpit area. Newborns who are preterm will have more; postterm newborns will have none.

Skin color reflects general health. The color of the skin is best observed when the newborn is quiet. Skin pigmentation depends on ethnic origin and deepens over time. In general, Caucasian newborns have pinkish red tones, African Americans have a reddish brown skin tone, and Asian and Hispanic newborns have an olive or yellow skin tone. Changes in skin color may signify illness and need to be further evaluated.

Acrocyanosis, the bluish color of a newborn's hands and feet, is related to poor circulation and is a transient condition, lasting from 24 to 48 hours. If persistent generalized or circumoral cyanosis is present, further evaluation needs to be done.

Jaundice is a yellowish discoloration of the skin resulting from deposits of unconjugated bilirubin due to the newborn's immature liver. Most newborns develop a mild case of jaundice at 3 or 4 days of age. Jaundice progresses in a cephalocaudal fashion. High levels of bilirubin need to be treated to prevent kernicterus.

Bruising is sometimes noted on newborns. Ecchymosis may occur over the head or buttocks if forceps or a vacuum extractor was used during the delivery. ***Petechiae*** (broken blood vessels; dotlike) are common over the presenting part, especially when there has been a rapid descent during the second stage of labor. Bruising may occur if there was a tight nuchal (around the neck) cord or a cord wrapped tightly around the body or body parts. Parents need an explanation when the newborn presents with a bruise. Also, the nurse must document the bruising appropriately in the newborn's medical record.

Hemangiomas are vascular skin lesions composed of dilated blood vessels. These do not pose any danger to the newborn. This is more common in females.

Cutis marmorata is a mottling, or lacelike, appearance in response to the cold, stress, or over stimulation. Parents need to know this may continue after discharge.

Nevus vasculosus, also called ***strawberry hemangioma,*** is an elevated red lesion that can occur anywhere on the body. It is usually present at birth and has a rough texture. The marks can increase in size over a couple of years and then regress. Usually no treatment is needed unless the hemangioma bleeds or becomes infected.

Nevus simplex, also called a ***"stork bite,"*** is a pink, macular lesion commonly seen in newborns. Nevi are usually seen over the eyelids or back of the head. They become darker when the infant cries. Lesions can last for a couple of years or into adulthood. These are the most common type of skin lesions seen in the newborn period.

Nevus flammeus, or ***port-wine stains,*** are permanent, flat, reddish to dark purple marks with defined borders that are present usually on the head and neck. They do not fade as the child ages and typically are benign. These marks usually can be removed with lasers.

Mongolian spots are blue-gray lesions resembling a bruise. They are most often seen over the buttocks but may be present on the back, shoulders, or legs. They are commonly seen in darker-skinned newborns and fade over time. Parents should be made aware and shown these spots on their newborn, and the nurse needs to document the marks on the infant's medical record.

Erythema toxicum, also called ***newborn rash,*** is benign and appears at about 24 to 48 hours of age in ~50% of term newborns. It is composed of small yellow papules surrounded by an erythematous area. The rash disappears and reappears over different parts of the body for several days. Most commonly seen on the face and trunk, erythema toxicum can continue to appear up to 10 days of age.

Milia, or "baby acne," are clogged sebaceous glands that appear as tiny white papules over the nose, chin, cheeks, and forehead. They disappear within 2 weeks of life.

Lanugo is fine hair that covers the fetus during intrauterine life. The term infant may still have a small amount over the body, especially on the shoulders, forehead, and side of the face.

Vernix is a thick, cheeselike coating that protects the infant's skin in utero. The full-term infant has very little left on the body except for small amounts in the creases.

Examination of the head is done for symmetry and molding. Molding may be present as the result of the delivery and usually resolves within a few weeks. Bruising may also be present. Uneven molding would be considered a **cephalohematoma**, which occurs several hours after birth from bleeding between the periosteum and skull, causing swelling that does not cross suture lines; it usually takes several weeks to resolve. ***Caput succedaneum,*** which is usually present at birth, is pitting edema of the scalp that crosses the suture line as a result of accumulation of blood or serum above the periosteum; it usually resolves in a couple of days. As part of the examination of the head, the anterior and posterior fontanelles are palpated. These are soft membranous coverings where two sutures meet. The anterior fontanelle is diamond-shaped, measures 4 to 5 cm, and closes by

18 months. The posterior fontanelle is triangular, measures 0.5 to 1 cm, and closes between 2 and 4 months. The fontanelles should never be depressed, indicating dehydration, or bulging, which indicates intracranial pressure. Further evaluation is needed if either occurs. On occasion, the anterior fontanelle moves up and down as the infant cries; the parents should be reassured that this is normal.

Next, facial features are examined. The eyes are checked for presence. The color of the iris can be slate, a deep blue, or brown. The eyelids are usually edematous immediately after birth. The pupils should be reactive to light with red reflex present. Newborns can focus on objects and follow to the midline. Mucus discharge is normal with the absence of tears. Scleral hemorrhages may be present from forceful maternal pushing during delivery.

Ears are checked next for position. The top of the pinna is horizontal with the outer canthus of the eye. The pinna is flexible and well formed, with cartilage present. Loud noises will elicit the startle reflex.

The nose is checked for patency. Newborns are obligate nose breathers.

The mouth is checked next. Mucous membranes are checked for color and should be pink. Circumoral cyanosis is indicative of heart defects. Gums should be checked for teeth before the nurse places a finger in the newborn's mouth.

Epstein pearls are sometimes present along the gum line, and are benign cysts that resemble small pearls and disappear in 1 to 2 months. The nurse places a finger in the newborn's mouth, pad side up (to prevent irritation and resultant swelling), then a finger on the roof of the mouth to check the palate for intactness. The tongue should be present with rugae. The frenulum is checked by coaxing the infant to bring the tongue forward and over the lower lip. The suck reflex is checked next, then the gag reflex by putting a finger toward the back of the newborn's throat. Cleft lip would be evident by observing. Finally, the rooting reflex is elicited. The infant should have a loud, lusty cry.

The nurse notes the newborn's hair pattern. The hair should be soft and silky. There should not be whorls or tufts of hair present. The newborn's fingernails should come to the end of the fingers or beyond.

The neck should be supple with a full range of motion and without webbing. The tonic neck reflex should be present.

The clavicles need to be assessed for tenderness, swelling, and crepitation. To assess for crepitation, the nurse uses one hand to move each of the newborn's arms through a passive range of motion while using the other hand to palpate the newborn's clavicle on that same side. Crepitus, produced when the bone slides against itself, is felt over the clavicle if a fracture exits.

The chest and lungs are assessed next. The chest should be symmetric and barrel-shaped, with equal anteroposterior and lateral diameters. Slight subcostal and intercostal retractions are common. Breast enlargement and engorgement are common in both sexes. Galactorrhea ("witch's milk") may be present.

Bilateral breath sounds should be auscultated. Fine crackles and transient hoarseness are normal.

The heart should be auscultated at the apex or point of maximal impulse (PMI) at the left or fourth intercostal space. Murmurs that are present after 12 hours of age should be evaluated to rule out underlying structural abnormalities.

The arms should be extended and checked for equal length. Much resistance from the newborn should be noted when trying to extend the arms. The hands should be inspected for five digits without webbing between the digits. The digits should have fingernails. The nail beds should be pink, or blue if there is acrocyanosis. The palm should have many creases. The creases should be inspected for a deep palmar crease known as the simian crease, common in children with Down syndrome. The grasp reflex should be elicited by placing a finger underneath the newborn's fingers. The newborn should curl his or her fingers around the nurse's finger and grasp tightly.

On examination, the abdomen should be mildly protruding. The liver is normally palpable 1 to 3 cm below the costal margin in the midclavicular line. The kidneys can be felt with deep palpation 1 to 2 cm above and to both sides of the umbilicus. Bowel sounds should be present within 1 hour of life but may be hypoactive on the first day of life. The cord should be inspected for three vessels, two arteries and a vein. Palpation around the cord often shows evidence of a hernia, which needs further evaluation.

The genitals need to be assessed next. In females, the labia and clitoris are usually edematous, and the hymenal tag is often present. The labia majora is larger than the labia minora. The urethral opening is below the clitoris. There is often vaginal discharge that is whitish or blood-tinged from the mother's hormones.

In the male newborn, the scrotum is large and covered with rugae. The testes should both be descended into the scrotal sac (palpated by the examiner with one finger on top of the scrotum and the other finger on the underside of the scrotum). The urethral opening should be at the end (tip) of the glans penis. Femoral pulses should be present and equal.

The legs should be extended and checked for equal length. Unequal lengths are usually an indication of hip abnormalities. Resistance to leg extension should be felt from a full-term infant. The nurse should examine the feet for structural and positional deformities. ***Metatarsus adductus*** (inward turning of the front part of the foot from positioning in utero) can easily be brought to midline with passive range of motion. ***Calcaneovalgus foot*** is a positional deformity in which the leg and foot form the shape of a check mark, or tick, rather than an L. Conservative treatment (usually exercises) is generally all that is needed for correction. The most serious deformity, clubfoot, has many variations and requires orthopedic correction.

The feet should be checked for five digits on each foot without webbing between the toes. The soles of the feet should be inspected for creases. The full-term infant should have creases that extend to the heel. The toes should have toenails with pink nail beds. The ***Babinski reflex*** should be elicited by taking a finger and stroking the foot from the bottom of the heel up and across the underside of the toes. The toes should fan out and return. The plantar reflex can be elicited by placing a finger underneath the newborn's toes; in response, the infant should curl his or her toes around finger.

Next, the nurse should place the newborn in the prone position and inspect the infant's back. The length of the spinal column should be palpated for masses and abnormal curvatures. The sacral area is inspected for the presence of a pilonidal dimple, tuft of hair, skin lesion, or increased pigmentation that could indicate pathology. A pilonidal dimple and tufts of hair are usually associated with kidney abnormalities. An opening at the base of the spinal column is called a ***spina bifida,*** or defective closure of the bony spine that encloses the spinal cord. Spina bifida is a type of neural tube defect.

The presence of Mongolian spots on the back needs to be documented on the medical record by the nurse, as they often look like bruises.

Gluteal folds should be inspected for symmetry. Unsymmetrical gluteal folds can indicate hip abnormalities.

The "stepping" reflex can be evaluated at this time. In a full-term, healthy newborn, the newborn will "step" if aided. To elicit this reflex, support the newborn in an upright position, with the infant "standing" on the right leg. He or she should automatically raise the left leg; once supported on the left side, the infant will then raise the right leg. This changing of legs will make it appear as if the newborn is walking.

Objective E: To Understand Continued Care of the Newborn

12.5 Continued Care of the Newborn

Nursing management of the newborn following transition will include the maintenance of cardiopulmonary function, promotion of adequate hydration and nutrition, promotion of skin integrity, promotion of safety, prevention of complications, and enhancement of parent–newborn attachment.

Nurses need to assess the newborn's vital signs every shift or more frequently, depending on the newborn's status and birth facility protocol. A bulb syringe should always be available and within easy reach on the baby's bassinet should the newborn need oral or nasal suctioning. The newborn should be observed for changes in skin color or respiration, which could signify underlying cardiorespiratory problems.

A neutral thermal environment needs to be maintained so the newborn will maintain core body temperature. He or she should be kept out of drafts and away from windows and dressed appropriately. One layer of clothing more than is necessary for an adult to maintain thermal comfort is appropriate for the newborn, and the nurse needs to instruct parents in these measures.

A newborn whose temperature falls below the normal range uses calories to maintain body heat rather than for growth. Chilling also increases oxygen use and may cause respiratory distress. Overheating will increase activity and respiratory rate in an attempt to cool the body. The newborn may also become dehydrated.

The nurse needs to promote early and frequent feedings. Early feedings promote gastric emptying and increase peristalsis, in turn promoting the excretion of bilirubin in the stool. The nurse needs to record the newborn's fluid intake and output and weigh the newborn at the same time each day. The first void should occur within the first 24 hours; the first stool should be passed within 48 hours. When they do not occur, the nurse needs to observe the newborn for bowel sounds, abdominal distention, and fluid intake. A weight loss of 10% in term newborns is considered within normal limits during the first week of life. Parents need to be told about this expected weight loss and that the infant usually regains the weight by the second week.

Proper skin care needs to be maintained for appearance of the newborn and to prevent infection. Ongoing skin care involves bathing the infant daily with a mild soap and rinsing well while maintaining a stable thermal environment. The scalp hair should be brushed with a soft bristle brush to prevent the buildup of oil and debris on the scalp, which can lead to cradle cap. Brushing also promotes brain growth. The perineal and buttock areas need to be washed with each diaper change. Avoidance of alcohol-based wipes is important to maintain skin integrity.

The umbilical cord is assessed for bleeding or signs of infection. Removal of the cord clamp in 24 to 48 hours when dry reduces the chance of tension injury and helps ease the anxiety of the parents. The cord should be kept dry and exposed to air. Recent studies disprove the practices of putting preparations and/or alcohol on the cord to keep it dry and bacteria-free. Exposing the cord to air by folding the diaper down underneath the cord can promote drying and prevent contamination. The nurse is responsible for cord care per institution protocol and is responsible for teaching the parents proper cord care.

The safety of the newborn is of upmost importance. It is vital that the nurse and other health care personnel verify the identity of the newborn by comparing the numbers and names on the identification bracelets of the mother and the newborn before giving a baby to a parent. Bands that do not match will need to be redone by the labor and delivery nurse immediately.

Nurses need to be aware of the surroundings and capabilities of the infant in order to maintain the infant's safety. Examples that demonstrate safety issues include never leaving an infant in the nursery or at a mother's bedside unattended, always supporting the infant's head, never propping bottles during feedings, always keeping a bulb syringe on the infant's bassinet, never leaving the infant alone in the middle of a bed, always placing the infant on his or her back to sleep, and being sure to follow immunization schedules. These and other safety issues need to be discussed with parents and reinforced often.

Infection can be prevented by all nursery personnel. A 3-minute scrub by all personnel who come into direct contact with newborns should be done upon entering the nursery. The hands must be washed with soap and rubbed vigorously for at least 15 seconds before and after caring for a newborn.

Parents and visitors should be instructed to practice good hand-washing technique before handling the baby. Scales, bassinets, radiant warmers, and other objects the newborn comes into contact with need to be washed before using with another infant.

In the United States, immunization for prevention of hepatitis is now included with other routine childhood immunizations. The first dose of the hepatitis vaccine is usually given to infants before they are discharged home from the birth facility. In some cases, it is given at the first pediatrician's visit. Infants infected from their mothers at birth have a very high chance of developing chronic infection, cancer, or other serious liver disease during adulthood.

Newborns of mothers with known acute or chronic hepatitis B infection should receive both the vaccine and hepatitis B immune globulin (HBIG). HBIG provides passive immunity to hepatitis to protect infants until they develop their own antibodies and should be given within 12 hours of birth. The vaccine promotes antibody formation to protect infants from further exposure to the disease.

Two types of screening tests are required by most states in the Unites States before discharge from the birth facility: hearing and screening for metabolic and genetic disorders.

Hearing screening is recommended by the American Academy of Pediatrics within the first months of life and is a continued goal of Healthy People 2020. Otoacoustic emissions (OAEs) and acoustic brainstem response (ABR) tests are used for screening. Infants who do not pass the screening should be rescreened; if they still do not pass, they are referred for further evaluation on an outpatient basis. Infants should have follow-up audiologic and medical evaluations by no later than 3 months of age, according to the American Academy of Pediatrics.

In the United States, all states require newborn screening for certain metabolic, hematologic, and genetic disorders. The conditions screened for include common disorders as well as more complex diseases and vary from state to state. The more common disorders include phenylketonuria, hypothyroidism, galactosemia, hemoglobinopathies (eg, sickle cell anemia and thalassemia), and congenital adrenal hyperplasia.

Newborn screening tests are simple and inexpensive. A heel stick is done to obtain blood from the infant, and the sample is sent to the state health department for evaluation. Only one sample of blood is needed to test for all of the indicated disorders. The test is more sensitive in infants who are more than 24 hours old, and in many cases, parents are discouraged from early discharge because of this reason.

The parents would be informed of any abnormal lab results through their pediatrician, and the infant would need further evaluation. Nurses need to be aware of the disorders tested for and be able to explain any consequences of the most common disorders that parents may ask questions about. Often, birth facilities give parents printed information about newborn screening so they will have an idea of the process. Parents need to know that they will not hear from the state health department unless there is a problem.

Circumcision care is important to prevent infection. ***Circumcision*** is a surgical procedure in which the prepuce, or skin at the tip of the penis, is separated from the glans penis and excised.

The nurse's role when a circumcision is being decided upon is that of educator. The procedure is highly controversial and only the parents can make the decision to have their newborn son circumcised. In most cases, the decision about circumcision is based on religious, cultural, and family traditions. Female circumcision is illegal in the United States and in most parts of the world.

The nurse must provide current information regarding the medical, social, and psychological aspects involved with circumcision so the parents can make an informed decision. The parents must know about the potential risks of circumcision, which include hemorrhage, infection, difficulty voiding, pain, ulcerations, adhesions, and damage to the urethra, some of which would require surgical repair.

The American Academy of Pediatrics does not recommend routine circumcision and encourages analgesia for the infant as he undergoes the procedure.

Before the procedure, the nurse must be certain that a consent form has been signed by the newborn's mother. As with any other procedure, the identification band of the infant should be checked to validate his identity before the procedure begins. The infant is placed on a circumcision board with diaper removed and restrained.

A local anesthetic ointment can be applied on the penis 30 to 60 minutes before the procedure. A 1% lidocaine block, acetaminophen, sucrose water drops, or a pacifier dipped in sucrose water can be given to the infant during the procedure to help alleviate the pain temporarily. The nurse must assess the infant's responses during the procedure. The nurse can provide other comfort measures, including lightly stroking the baby's head and talking to him during the procedure. The parents are usually discouraged from watching this procedure being performed in the health care institution; however, in many cultures, the infant is held by the father or grandfather in a ritual ceremony, often in front of the family.

Following the procedure, the nurse needs to assess the site for signs of hemorrhage or infection every 30 minutes for several hours or as per birth facility protocol. The nurse needs to assess the first void postprocedure for urinary obstruction related to edema and/or penile injury.

Vaseline gauze is applied tightly to the penis after the circumcision to prevent bleeding and protect the healing tissue. The nurse needs to clean the penis with water after diaper changes to rinse away acidic urine and apply the diaper snugly. The Vaseline gauze will fall off on its own and should not be pulled off as it starts to unravel to prevent pulling at the healing skin. Vaseline may be applied to the penis once the gauze falls off to prevent the penis from sticking to the diaper and pulling at the healing tissue. Parents need to be instructed in circumcision care and be able to perform such care prior to discharge.

Parent-newborn attachment and family-centered care are promoted by encouraging all members of the family to be involved in newborn care. The nurse can discuss ways to promote attachment, such as talking to the baby, holding the baby in an upright position, and gently swaddling the baby to increase a sense of security. The nurse needs to be aware of cultural practices and variations, such as baby naming, the involvement of only women in the infant's care, and using good luck charms. It is important for the nurse to be sensitive to the family's cultural beliefs while maintaining safe care for the infant.

Objective F: To Understand Infant Feeding

12.6 Infant Feeding

Many factors influence a woman's choice of feeding method, including support from others, culture, employment, past feeding experiences, education, age, and location.

Many women choose the method of feeding prenatally. Although breastfeeding is optimal, whichever method the mother chooses should be supported by the nursing staff. Women often equate feeding with mothering ability, so encouragement and teaching about the chosen method are appropriate.

The full-term newborn needs 110 to 120 kcal/kg of body weight each day. The infant needs to consume sufficient calories to meet energy needs, prevent use of body stores, and provide for growth.

Breast milk and formula for normal, full-term infants contain 20 kcal/oz. Although the newborn's stomach capacity is very small at birth, by the end of 1 week, the infant can take ~2 to 3 oz at each feeding. Breast milk or formula alone is sufficient to meet the neonate's dietary needs from birth until 6 months of age. Complementary solid foods are introduced in the second half of the first year, and the infant continues to receive breast milk or formula until at least 12 months of age. Supplemental water is not necessary. Cow's milk is inappropriate because the body's immune system may react to the protein in cow's milk, making it one of the most common allergies in infants.

Nutrients needed by the newborn are proteins, carbohydrates, fats, vitamins, and minerals supplied by breast milk or formula. Infants receive ~50% of their calories from fat. Fats also help the body absorb the fat-soluble vitamins A, D, E, and K. Triglycerides make up 98% to 99% of milk fat. Casein and whey are the proteins found in breast milk and formula, and are easily digested by the infant.

Carbohydrates serve as the other main source of nutrition for the infant, providing ~40% of dietary calories. In addition to providing energy, carbohydrates absorb calcium, magnesium, and zinc. In both breast milk and formula, the major carbohydrate is lactose. Lactose also promotes the normal growth of bacteria in the intestines.

Vitamins and minerals are sufficient in breast milk if the mother's diet is adequate. Vitamin D, however, is low in breast milk, and the infant may need supplementation if the mother's diet is inadequate or if she does not have much exposure to sunlight. An infant of a vegan mother may also need vitamin B_{12} supplementation.

The full-term infant who is breastfed exclusively maintains iron stores for the first 6 months of life. Breast milk also contains enzymes that aid in digestion. The addition of formula or foods may decrease the absorption of iron, so iron supplementation may be needed. For formula-fed infants, the American Academy of Pediatrics recommends iron fortification.

12.7 Breastfeeding

Breast milk is well documented as being the optimal source of nutrition for infants. There is overwhelming scientific evidence that demonstrates that breastfeeding provides newborns and infants with specific nutritional, immunologic, and psychosocial advantages over formula feeding.

In its breastfeeding policy statement, the American Academy of Pediatrics recommends breastfeeding as the preferred method for all infants for the first 6 months of life, with continued breastfeeding during the introduction of solids until the infant is 12 months or older if mutually desired. In an effort to promote breastfeeding, the World Health Organization (WHO) and the United Nations Children's Fund (UNICEF) advocate that birth facilities actively encourage breastfeeding, with policies advocating staff teaching, early feedings, avoidance of pacifiers and formula, and rooming-in.

The goals of Healthy People 2020 are for 75% of mothers to initiate breastfeeding, for 50% of mothers to be breastfeeding at 6 months of age, and for 25% to be breastfeeding at 1 year. According to the U.S. Centers for Disease Control and Prevention, in 2006 73.9% of mothers had initiated breastfeeding, 43.3% were still breastfeeding their infants at 6 months, and 22.7% were still breastfeeding at 1 year of age.

Breast milk is species-specific. Because of this, infants rarely have allergic reactions to breast milk. The macronutrients such as carbohydrates (lactose), proteins, and fats are synthesized by the mother in the alveoli of the breasts by special secretory cells. Micronutrients such as vitamins and minerals derive from the circulating maternal plasma. There are more than 200 distinct components in breast milk.

There is research supporting additional advantages for breastfeeding. Breastfed infants have a reduced risk of developing type 1 and type 2 diabetes, obesity, lymphoma, leukemia, Hodgkin disease, obesity, hypercholesterolemia, asthma, iron deficiency, atopic dermatitis, Crohn disease, ulcerative colitis, urinary and respiratory tract infections, bacterial meningitis, bacteremia, necrotizing enterocolitis, and sudden infant death syndrome (SIDS). Breastfeeding has also been associated with higher intelligence quotients later in childhood.

There are many advantages for the mother who breastfeeds as well. The oxytocin that is released to let the milk down (the ***"let-down" reflex***) causes contractions, similar to those experienced during labor. These contractions, referred to as afterpains, help keep the uterus firmly contracted and prevent hemorrhaging. The breastfeeding mother also has a decreased risk of developing breast and uterine cancers, premenopausal osteoporosis, diabetes, hypertension, hyperlipidemia, and cardiovascular diseases.

The psychosocial advantages of breastfeeding are seen in both the mother and infant. When a woman chooses to breastfeed, she often has more direct skin-to-skin contact with her infant than if she were bottle feeding.

This encourages parent–infant attachment. Infants with skin-to-skin bonding have greater physiologic stability, cry less, sleep longer, and tend to breastfeed better. Women derive satisfaction from the knowledge that they are providing their infants with the best nutritional start in life. Also, because there is less illness in breastfed babies, mortality rates and childhood medical costs for breastfed infants are lower.

Breastfeeding is economical and ecologically sound. There are significant savings for the family who chooses to breastfeed. The cost of standard formula is approximately $1200 annually per infant. Added to that is the cost of bottles, nipples, cleaning, refrigeration, and so on. The waste products from these supplies end up as more trash to pollute the environment. Breastfeeding not only helps the breastfeeding family, but also reduces health care expenditures and pollution, thereby helping society as a whole.

There are few contraindications to breastfeeding. Although most drugs penetrate breast milk to some degree (usually < 1% of the maternal dosage), very few are contraindicated for breastfeeding women. Specific medications that are contraindicated are radioactive isotopes, antimetabolites, chemotherapy drugs, and metronidazole.

Other potential contraindications to breastfeeding are

- Mother is infected with human immunodeficiency virus/acquired immunodeficiency syndrome (HIV/AIDS).
- Mother is positive for varicella.
- Mother has active tuberculosis (untreated).
- Mother has an active herpes lesion on the breast.
- Mother has leukemia (human T-lymphotropic virus 1 [HTLV–1]).
- Mother is a substance abuser (illicit drugs and/or alcohol).
- Infant has galactosemia.

There are also a few potential disadvantages to breastfeeding. Often women cite pain as a reason to supplement or discontinue breastfeeding altogether. Breastfeeding should not be painful; pain is associated with improper placement of the infant on the breast. Women experiencing pain should notify their nurse or lactation consultant for assistance in getting the baby latched on properly.

Finding time to breastfeed and returning to work or school can be very stressful for the breastfeeding mother. Worrying about pumping enough milk to give the newborn or even just having the opportunity to pump and store the milk in the work setting can also be stressful. These are common reasons as to why women prematurely discontinue breastfeeding. They should be encouraged to continue some form of breastfeeding, as receiving some breast milk is better for the infant than not receiving any.

Some women will leak milk and are embarrassed when this happens. They can be encouraged to use breast pads that prevent milk from leaking onto their clothing. Also, some women are embarrassed or afraid to breastfeed in public. Many states have laws that protect women who breastfeed in public areas. Women can be taught how to breastfeed discreetly in public by using blankets or shawls to cover the breast.

One of the main reasons for early weaning to formula is mothers' perception of insufficient milk supply. Women with positive attitudes and confidence are less likely to wean early. Nurses need to give positive feedback and encouragement to women to continue breastfeeding. Referrals to lactation consultants are helpful in helping new mothers breastfeed.

Some women have perceived diet restrictions and think they have to give up certain foods when they breastfeed, as they will make the baby gassy or colicky. For the most part, this is not true. There are no particular foods that will cause GI upset in an infant. Women just need to be aware of what they ate at the time their baby became fussy or had some GI upset. It is a trial-and-error process.

Many women feel they have very limited hormonal birth control options. Some think they cannot take oral contraceptives if they are breastfeeding. Contraceptives that contain both estrogen and progesterone can decrease milk supply; progestin-only mini-pills, however, are compatible with breastfeeding. It is recommended that the woman wait 6 to 8 weeks after birth before starting on a hormonal medication in order to ensure a good milk supply.

Some women report vaginal dryness related to low levels of estrogen while breastfeeding. They should be reassured that this is temporary and encouraged to use K-Y jelly or other lubricant during intercourse.

New fathers report feeling "left out" of the feeding responsibilities and want to take a more active role. Parents need to be informed that it is advisable for the father to wait to feed the infant with expressed breast milk in a bottle until the breastfeeding pattern has been established. In the meantime, the father can do other things to share in infant care responsibilities, such as bathing and changing the baby.

Objective G: To Understand the Mechanism of Lactation

12.8 Lactation

During pregnancy, increased levels of estrogen stimulate breast duct proliferation and development, and elevated progesterone levels promote the development of lobules and alveoli. When the placenta is delivered, progesterone levels drop and trigger milk production.

The hormone prolactin is released from the anterior pituitary in response to suckling or the use of a breast pump. Prolactin stimulates the milk-secreting cells in the alveoli to produce milk. In addition to prolactin release, stretching of the nipple and compression of the areola signal the hypothalamus to trigger the posterior pituitary gland to release oxytocin. Oxytocin acts on the myoepithelial cells surrounding the alveoli in the breast tissue to contract, ejecting milk into the ducts. This process is called the milk-ejection or let-down reflex.

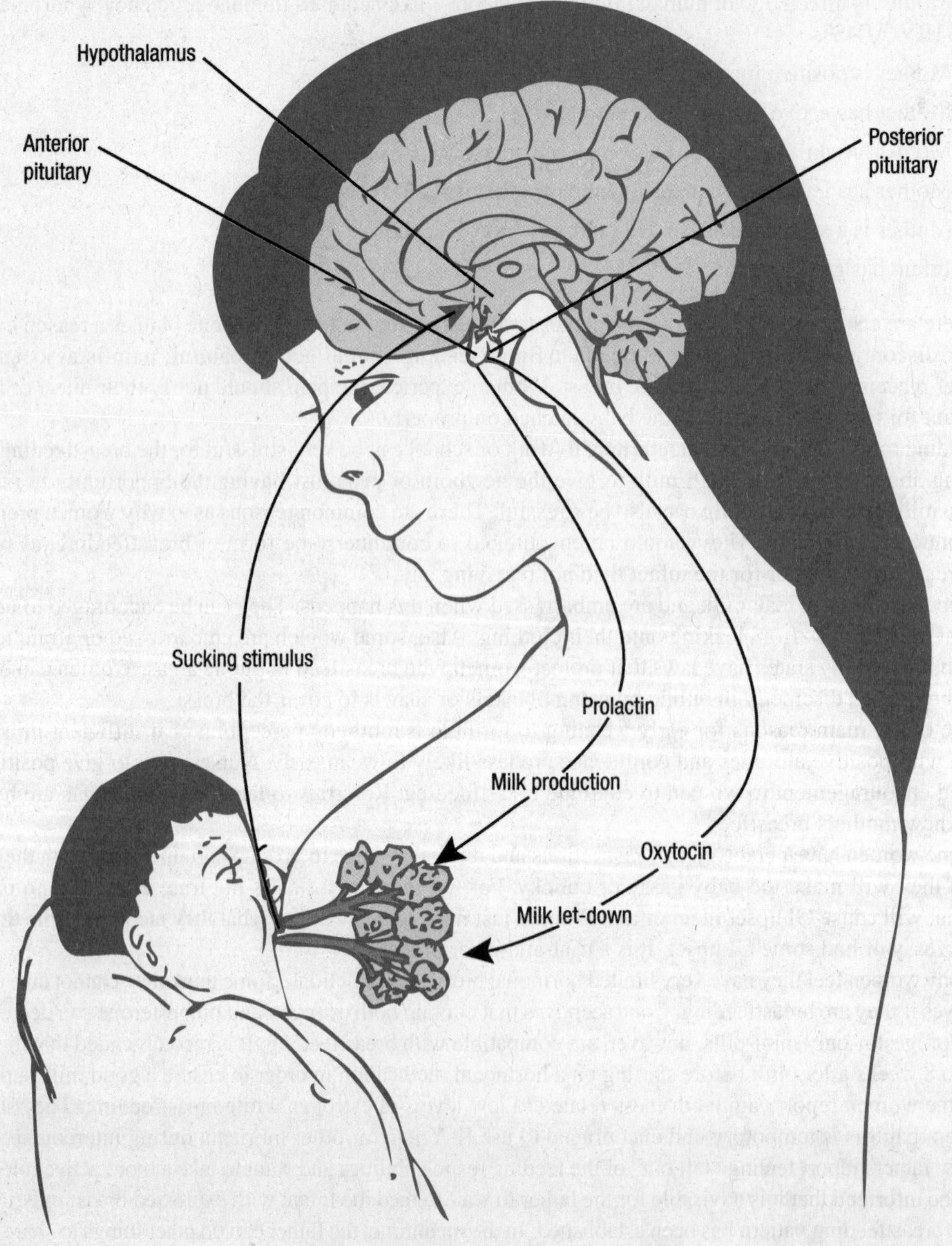

Figure 12.2 Mechanism for milk production.

The milk that flows from the breast at the start of a feeding is called foremilk. This milk is watery, high in protein, and low in fat. The milk that flows during let-down is called hindmilk. It is rich in fat (can exceed 10%) and high in calories. The average total fat concentration in breast milk is ~4 %, and the total caloric intake is ~20 calories/oz. It takes about 2 weeks to establish a good milk supply. Women need to be encouraged to stimulate their breasts, whether or not they are separated from their babies, to establish the milk supply.

Objective H: To Understand the Stages of Human Milk

12.9 Stages of Human Milk

During the establishment of lactation, there are three stages of human milk: colostrum, transitional milk, and mature milk.

Colostrum is the initial milk that is immediately available to the baby at delivery. It provides the newborn with sufficient nutrition until the mother's milk supply comes in within a few days. A thick, creamy yellowish fluid, colostrum has concentrated amounts of protein, fat-soluble vitamins, and minerals, as well as lower amounts of fat and lactose compared with mature milk. It also contains antioxidants and high levels of lactoferrin and secretory IgA. Colostrum helps establish normal bacterial flora in the digestive tract that helps protect the infant from illness and disease. Because it has a laxative effect, it helps the baby pass meconium. It is sometimes referred to as ***"liquid gold."***

Transitional milk is produced between days 2 and 5 (frequently referred to as "coming in") and becomes more abundant. It is still yellowish in color but is more copious than colostrum and contains more fat, lactose, water-soluble vitamins, and calories.

Mature milk, which is white or slightly blue-tinged, is present by 2 weeks postpartum and continues until breastfeeding ceases. It is composed of ~13% solids (carbohydrates, protein, and fats) and 87% water. Infants receiving sufficient amounts of breast milk do not need supplemental water.

Oxytocin-producing neurons throughout the brain are thought to be associated with social behavior and attachment. In addition to being released in the maternal brain tissue, oxytocin is released into the newborn brain by means of milk transfer and is thought to modulate attachment behavior between the mother and newborn. Separating mothers and newborns should be discouraged unless there is a medical indication.

Objective I: To Understand the Process of Breastfeeding

12.10 Process of Breastfeeding

Women should be encouraged to attend prenatal breastfeeding classes. The typically short length of stay at birth facilities today puts pressure on new mothers to demonstrate effective breastfeeding before some mother–baby dyads are ready. Twenty-four-hour rooming-in supports breastfeeding. Contact with the newborn enables a woman to recognize and respond to his or her needs and begin to develop confidence in her mothering role. Rooming-in provides opportunities for identifying hunger cues and to respond with a feeding.

There is no scientific research that demonstrates physical preparation of the breasts for breastfeeding. Some women believe that prenatal nipple rolling, applications of creams, or rubbing a rough towel across the nipples to "toughen them up" will help decrease nipple pain caused by breastfeeding. If the infant is latched on correctly, however, nipples should not hurt. If they do, the mother should be encouraged to remove the infant from the breast and try to get him or her to latch on again.

Hunger cues the mother should look for to initiate a feeding include sucking movements of the mouth and tongue, hand-to-mouth movements, rooting, small sounds, body movement, smacking of lips, mouth opening in response to tactile stimulation, and rapid eye movements under the eyelids.

The new mother should begin breastfeeding within 1 hour of birth. She should be assisted into a comfortable position. The most comfortable are the cradle hold, cross-cradle hold, clutch hold (or football hold), and side-lying position (frequently used by women who underwent cesarean sections).

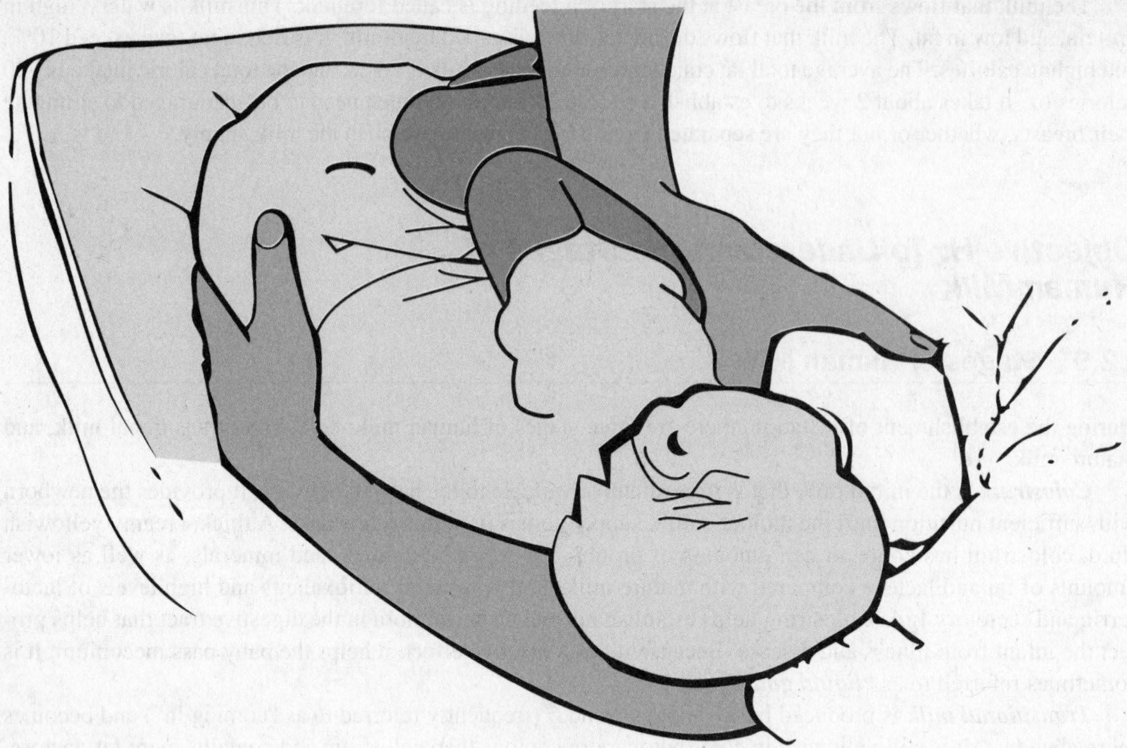

Figure 12.3 Cradle hold.

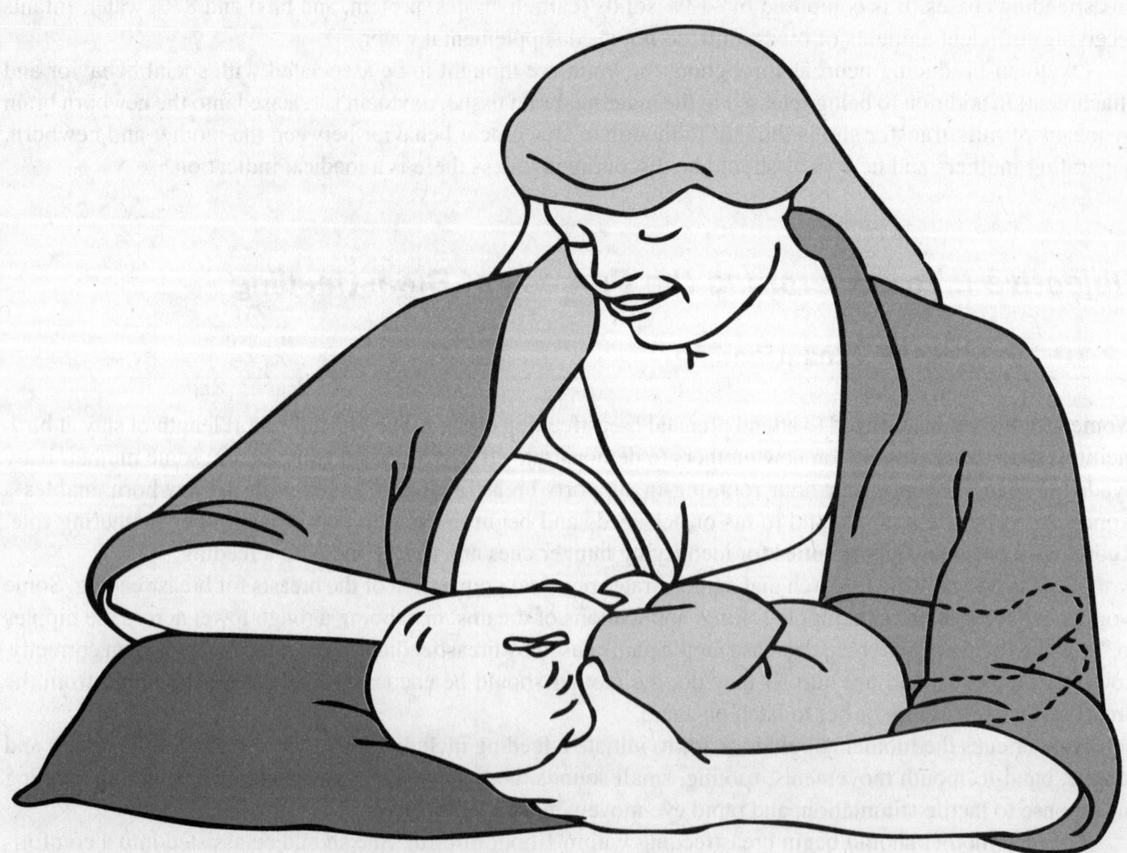

Figure 12.4 Modified cradle hold (cross-cradle hold).

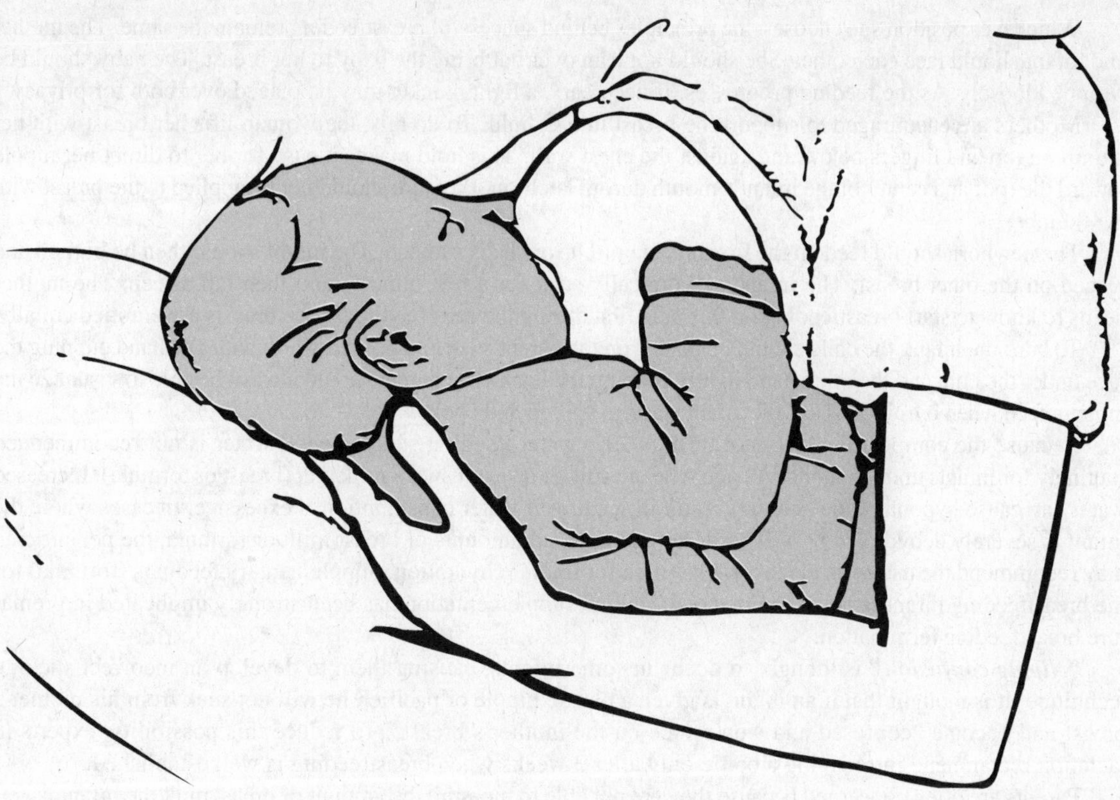

Figure 12.5 Clutch hold (football hold).

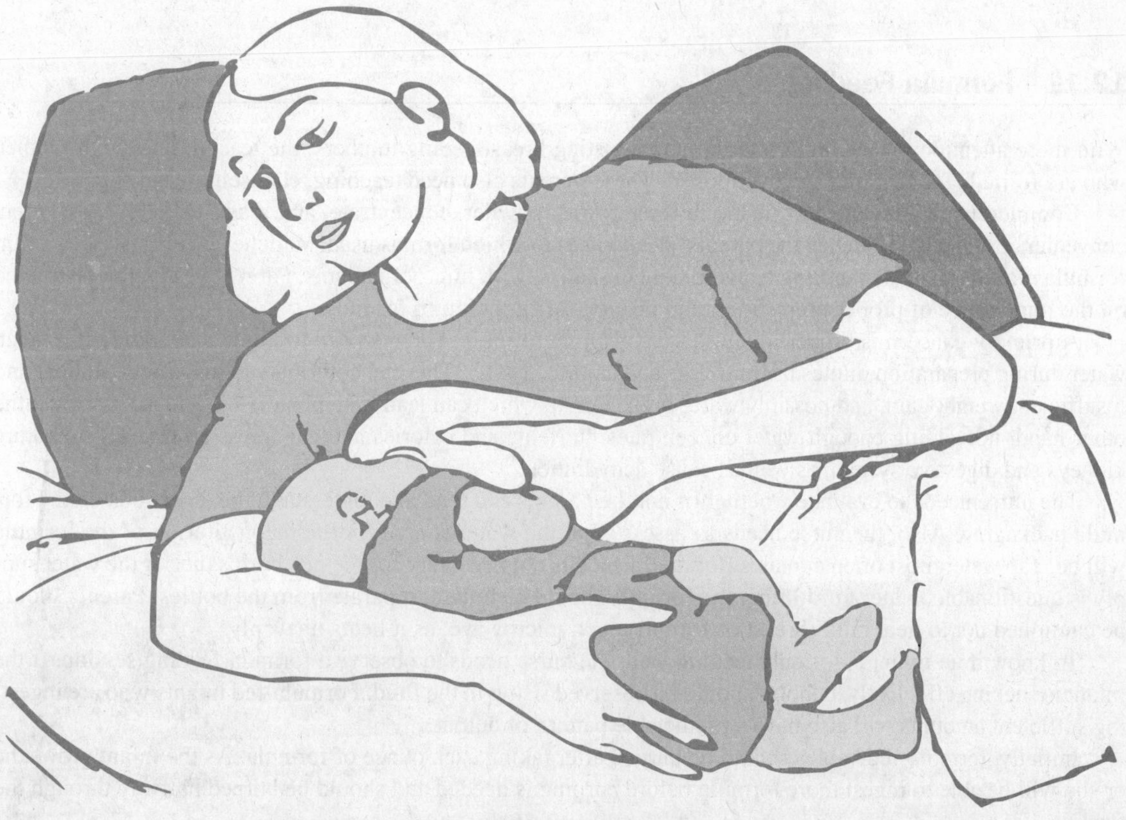

Figure 12.6 Side lying.

Whichever position she chooses, the principles behind successful breastfeeding remain the same. The mother and infant should face each other. She should not lean over but bring the baby to her breast. The baby should be wrapped loosely. As the feeding progresses, if necessary, a light blanket may be placed over both for privacy.

Mothers are encouraged to support the breast in a C hold. To do this, the woman lifts her breast with her thumb on top and fingers below and against the chest wall. This hold makes it easy for her to direct her nipple toward the roof and center of the infant's mouth during latch-on. Pressure should not be applied to the breast with the thumb.

The newborn should feed on the first breast until he or she is satiated. The infant should then be burped and placed on the other breast. The infant will typically suck for a few minutes and then fall asleep. The mother needs to know to start breastfeeding on this side first during the next feeding so the breasts are emptied equally.

To burp the infant, the child should be placed on the parent's lap and held forward, with one hand cupping the face under the chin and the other hand lightly rubbing the back. The parent should always be able to visualize the infant's face when burping in case the infant starts to spit up and choke.

Because the composition of breast milk is 90% water, feeding supplemental water is not recommended routinely for infants under 6 months of age who are still on an exclusively milk diet (breast or formula). Increased water can cause hyponatremia and may result in seizures if water consumption is excessive. In cases where the infant is severely dehydrated or will not tolerate increased amounts of breast milk or formula, the pediatrician may recommend the use of an electrolyte solution for initial rehydration. Supplementary feedings (formula) for the breastfeeding infant is not recommended; routine supplementation has been strongly implicated in premature breastfeeding termination.

"Nipple confusion" is thought to occur in some infants, causing them to develop an incorrect sucking technique. It is thought that if an infant is given a plastic nipple or pacifier, he will not suck from his mother's breast and become "confused and won't suck on the mother's breast." To reduce this possibility, experts in lactation recommend introducing a bottle only after 3 weeks when breastfeeding is well established.

Parents are often concerned because they are not able to measure the amount of breast milk the infant is getting when breastfeeding. When satiated, the infant will either pull away from the breast or fall asleep. The infant will be relaxed and will often sleep until the next feeding. As the infant matures, the feedings will lengthen. Infants will also have a predictable pattern of output when feeding properly.

12.11 Formula Feeding

With more attention placed on promoting and assisting breastfeeding mothers, the teaching needs of women who are formula feeding may get overlooked. These parents also need teaching, counseling, and support.

Commercial formulas are available in three forms: powder, concentrate, and ready-to-feed. Most often, convenience and cost influence the parents' decision as to which form is used. Whichever form is used, infant formula requires careful handling to avoid contamination with microorganisms. Parents need to be instructed on the importance of proper preparation and prompt refrigeration of formula.

A primary concern is proper mixing to reconstitute formula. Parents need to know that adding too much water during preparation dilutes the nutrients and caloric density. This can contribute to undernourishment and insufficient weight gain, and possibly water intoxication, which can lead to hyponatremia and seizures. On the other hand, not adding enough water concentrates nutrients and calories and can stress an infant's immature kidneys and digestive system, as well as cause dehydration.

The nurse needs to evaluate whether or not the parents can read and understand the directions on the formula packaging. Also, the nurse needs to assess what the water source for the reconstitution of the formula will be. Tap water most often contains fluoride, which is not necessary for the newborn's diet. If the water supply is questionable, water for diluting the formula should be boiled, separate from the bottles. Parents should be cautioned not to heat milk (breast or formula) in a microwave, as it heats unevenly.

To know if an infant is formula feeding well, the nurse needs to observe a formula-feeding session. If the infant is sucking effectively, bubbles should be observed rising in the fluid. Formula-fed infants who are ingesting sufficient amounts will also have a predictable pattern of output.

Initially, formula-fed babies should be burped after taking each ounce of formula. As the infant grows, he or she will be able to ingest more formula before burping is needed and should be burped halfway through the feeding.

Safety issues during bath time should be addressed. If parents need to turn away, for example, they should be instructed to leave one hand on the infant. Infants should never be left alone in even 1 inch of water because of the danger of drowning. If parents must leave the room, they need to take the infant out of the water and bring the child with them. It should be suggested that parents ignore the phone or the doorbell when bathing the infant.

Animals are another safety issue. Pets can become jealous of the new baby, and parents need to take precautions. To familiarize a pet with the child before discharge, it may be helpful if the parents bring home an article of clothing the baby wore in the hospital and allow the animal to sniff it. This allows the animal to become familiar with the baby's scent. Once home, the parents should never leave the baby unattended with a cat or dog that could jump up and into a crib.

Many parents are concerned about immunizations. They need to be made aware that immunizations safeguard infants and communities from the spread of communicable diseases. The nurse should discuss the age at which each immunization is given and when boosters are needed. Because recommendations for immunizations change from time to time, parents should be referred to their pediatrician or clinic for the latest information.

Well-baby checkups are an important opportunity for the health care provider to assess the infant's growth and development, answer questions about feeding and infant care, and give immunizations. Infants usually have their first checkup within the first 2 weeks of life and typically at 1, 2, 4, 6, 9, and 12 months of age.

Parents need to be taught the common signs and symptoms of illness in the infant, including temperature > 100°F (37.8°C); vomiting all of a feeding once or twice in 1 day; watery stools or an increased number of stools than is usual for the infant; rashes; coughing, frequent sneezing, or runny nose; and pulling or rubbing an ear or drainage from an ear. The nurse should explain that any time parents think the infant looks sick or believe there is something wrong, they should contact their health care provider. Most importantly, parents need to know that in an emergency situation, they should take the infant immediately to the emergency room.

Review Questions

True/False

1. _______ The anterior fontanelle is triangular-shaped and closes within 2 to 4 months.
2. _______ The Moro reflex is also known as the "startle" reflex.
3. _______ The full-term newborn should urinate 6 to 10 times in a 24-hour period.
4. _______ Newborns generate heat through nonshivering thermogenesis.
5. _______ Vitamin K is given to newborns on the day of discharge.
6. _______ In males, the urethra is located at the tip of the penis.
7. _______ The Apgar score evaluates the condition of the newborn at 1 and 5 minutes of life.
8. _______ Erythema toxicum is common in newborns.
9. _______ Providing the opportunity to breastfeed soon after birth supports the attachment process.
10. _______ Transition from fetal to neonatal circulation is a major cardiovascular change and occurs simultaneously with respiratory system adaptation.
11. _______ Everyone on the maternity unit is responsible for safety and security of newborns on the unit.
12. _______ The newborn umbilical cord stump should be bathed daily.
13. _______ A cephalohematoma crosses the suture line.
14. _______ Newborns are nose breathers.

Bottles should never be propped during feeding. Propping increases the likelihood of choking if regurgitation occurs and eliminates the closeness between the infant and parent when the child is held close. The infant should not be coaxed to drink the whole bottle once he or she pushes it away, as this can result in regurgitation and overweight.

Any formula that is not ingested within 1 hour should be discarded. Formula should not be kept for the next feeding because of the growth of bacteria in the bottle.

Objective J: To Understand the Discharge Responsibilities of the Nurse

12.12 Discharge Responsibilities of the Nurse

Nurses must be sure that new mothers are capable of performing basic self- and infant care activities prior to discharge. Documentation needs to be reviewed by the discharging nurse for evidence of these capabilities. Also of importance is maternal-infant interaction. The nurse needs to be sure the mother is exhibiting appropriate maternal-infant attachment behaviors and participating in the infant's care even if she will have help when she is discharged home with the infant.

In the birth facility, parents receive much more information than they can absorb in the short stay. New mothers' anxieties often interfere with their ability to learn. It is more common today that family members, particularly grandparents, who were once the major support for new parents, live far away. Many younger parents rely on information gathered from magazines, TV, or the Internet. They need to be cautioned about receiving information from these sources, as it often is not accurate or reliable.

Part of the discharge instructions should include phone numbers of both the mother's and infant's health care providers, as well as community support numbers. Often the birth facility has a "warm line" setup for new parents to call if they have questions regarding their or their infant's care. It is often just the phone number to the postpartum unit, but the parents have the security of knowing that someone is available 24 hours a day to receive their call. Parents also need to know that in an emergency, it is important to go to an emergency room rather than make phone calls to "warm lines" or their health care provider.

Many birth facilities offer telephone follow-up calls after discharge, especially to breastfeeding mothers. The nurse can ask a series of questions to determine the physical and psychosocial condition of the mother and her infant and identify any needs or problems they may be having. The nurse should use open-ended questions or statements to elicit responses from the mother in her own order of priority. If problems are discovered, there may be more follow-up calls or a home visit, or a referral to the woman's primary health care provider or pediatrician may be warranted.

Most mothers and infants are discharged from the birth facility within 48 to 96 hours, but some women will ask to be discharged earlier. Infants discharged earlier than 48 hours should have a follow-up visit within 48 hours after they go home. Breastfeeding infants should be seen by the health care provider 3 to 5 days after birth and again at 2 weeks to assess for weight gain and any problems that may occur after discharge. Mothers need to be made aware of these time limits and encouraged to make appointments to take the infant to the pediatrician's office or clinic before they are discharged home. Often appointments are made for patients who attend the birth facility's antenatal clinics.

Most birth facilities have a printed discharge form that lists important instructions and contact phone numbers. During discharge, the nurse should encourage the parents to ask any questions they may have regarding care for the baby and themselves in the immediate postdischarge period.

The day before discharge, the parents should be told to bring an outfit for the baby that is appropriate for the season. The infant should wear one layer more of clothing as an adult.

They should also be reminded to bring the infant car seat to the maternity unit on the morning of discharge. The discharging nurse commonly inspects the car seat for the appropriate size and observes the parents as they secure the infant in it. Children under 1 year old and 20 lb must ride in a rear-facing car seat in the center of the back seat of the car. The incline of the seat should be at 45 degrees. Parents using public transportation are still expected by law in most states in the United States to place the infant in a car seat. They need to be made aware of this requirement.

The harness of the car seat should firmly restrain the infant but should release quickly. For the rear-facing newborn, shoulder straps should be in the lowest position and at or slightly below the shoulder level. The restraint clip should be placed at midchest or the axillary level to keep the straps in place on the infant's shoulders.

Blankets should never be placed under the infant or behind the infant's back or head. If a blanket is needed for warmth, it should be placed over the infant after he or she has been secured in the car seat.

As part of discharge preparation, the nurse needs to talk with parents about ***shaken baby syndrome (SBS).*** SBS results from shaking an infant vigorously enough to cause the soft tissue of the brain to bounce against the skull. Symptoms include subdural or subarachnoid hemorrhage, retinal hemorrhage, skull fractures, and damage to the spinal cord. The nurse should discuss this danger with parents and help them identify ways to cope with a fussy or crying baby. Many birth facilities provide pamphlets on this topic.

Some of the concerns commonly voiced by parents are infant crying, colic, sleep patterns, breastfeeding, voiding and stool patterns, sucking needs, bathing, accident prevention, immunizations, and signs and symptoms of illness.

Infants cry for many reasons, and parents need to be aware that they should check on a crying infant. The infant can be hungry, cold, tired, bored, or just need to be held. Often parents voice their concern about "spoiling" the infant. Infants cannot signal that they have unmet needs in any other way but crying, and they are not spoiled when parents meet those needs. The infants' needs must be met in a consistent manner for the development of trust to occur. Changing a wet diaper or soothing the infant may be all that is needed to quiet it.

Colic is characterized by irritable crying for no obvious reason for 3 hours or more per day. Although there are many theories about why infants develop colic, the cause remains unknown.

Approximately 10% to 25% of infants have symptoms of colic. The condition peaks at about 6 weeks and usually disappears by the sixth month. Parents need to be reassured that the infant will recover and that the episodes of crying do not mean they are "bad" parents. They should be encouraged to try to soothe the baby by gently rocking or singing to the baby, playing soothing music, giving the baby a bath, or taking the baby for a ride in the stroller or car. The nurse needs to advise the health care provider if crying or colic persists.

Parents need to be instructed that although newborns sleep approximately 20 hours daily, there are wide variations in sleep patterns. Some infants sleep during the day and are up all night. Mothers are encouraged to nap when the baby naps during the day.

Parents need to be instructed to position their infants on their backs to sleep in order to prevent SIDS. No pillows or stuffed animals should be put in the crib with the infant, as they pose a suffocation risk.

By 12 weeks of age, many infants sleep at least 5 hours at night, and most sleep that long by 4 months. By 12 months, infants take two naps during the day and sleep about 10 hours at night.

The infant should have at least six wet diapers by the fourth day of life. Breastfed infants may have a bowel movement after each feeding. Formula-fed infants generally pass at least one stool daily.

Breastfed infants should be fed 8 to 12 times daily (every 2 or 3 hours), and formula-fed infants should be fed six to eight times daily (every 3 or 4 hours). Breastfeeding mothers who are returning to work need to be instructed on the use of a breast pump and storage of breast milk prior to discharge.

The discharging nurse should explain to parents that all infants have the need to suck, although this need varies among individuals. Pacifiers are recommended for sleep by the American Academy of Pediatrics to help prevent SIDS. The nurse should reassure parents that sucking that ends before the secondary teeth erupt is unlikely to cause malocclusion of the teeth.

Bathing the infant every day is not necessary if the infant is washed well at diaper changes and when milk is regurgitated. When bathing, it is important to keep the infant warm. A tub bath is preferable to sponge bathing, as infants maintain their temperature better if immersed in the tub. Studies show that immersion in a tub does not add risk of infection or decrease cord healing. The infant should be immersed so the water covers his or her shoulders. Bath water temperature should be ~100.4°F (38°C). The bath should be performed quickly and the infant dried off thoroughly. The hair should be washed and brushed afterward to stimulate the scalp (aids in brain development) and to remove oils, perspiration, and debris that can collect on the scalp in order to prevent "cradle cap."

Parents need to be made aware of safety issues before discharge. For example, they should be taught about the dangers of leaving the infant alone for any length of time. An infant left unattended on an unprotected surface can wiggle from the middle to the edge and fall. Crib sides should always be up when the infant is in the bed. The crib should be positioned away from a window and from the cords of blinds or drapes. Additionally, nothing with strings or cords should be on the bed because the infant could become entangled in them and strangulated.

15. _______ The umbilical cord contains one artery and one vein.
16. _______ Acrocyanosis in a newborn 4 hours old is within normal limits.
17. _______ Kangaroo care is a method for use only with fathers of newborns.
18. _______ The full-term infant's posture should demonstrate tightly flexed joints.
19. _______ The newborn's eyelids are usually edematous immediately after birth.
20. _______ Newborns should be placed on their backs to sleep.
21. _______ A murmur may be heard in a partially open ductus arteriosus in the newborn.
22. _______ Convection is the transfer of heat from a solid object to surrounding air.
23. _______ The presence and strength of reflexes in the newborn are important indicators of neurologic development and function.
24. _______ Term newborns normally lose 5% to 10% of their body weight in the first week of life.
25. _______ The majority of newborns do not void immediately after delivery.

Matching Columns

1. Heat loss from being wet _______________
2. Infant turns face when a cheek is stroked ____________
3. Keeps newborn's lungs partially open between respirations _______________
4. Metabolism of brown fat ___________
5. Evaluation of newborn at 1 and 5 minutes of life ________
6. The newborn's ability to respond to visual and auditory stimuli ____________
7. Administered to all newborns to prevent hemorrhagic disease _____________
8. Bluish discoloration of the newborn's hands and feet _______
9. Pink macular lesion commonly seen in newborns over the eyelids and back of the head _____________
10. Thick, cheeselike coating that protects the infant's skin in utero _____________

A. Nonshivering thermogenesis

B. Rooting

C. Acrocyanosis

D. Vitamin K

E. Stork bite

F. Surfactant

G. Evaporation

H. Apgar score

I. Vernix

J. Habituation

Multiple Choice

1. When listening to the newborn's heart, all of the following are true except

   A. The heart rate should be auscultated at the point of maximal impulse.

   B. Murmurs heard after 12 hours of age need to be investigated further.

   C. The heart rate should be auscultated for 60 seconds.

   D. The heart rate can be auscultated for 15 seconds and multiplied by 4.

2. Newborns attempt to regulate body temperature by

   A. Nonshivering thermogenesis

   B. Lowering heart rate

   C. Decreasing need for oxygen

   D. Decreasing their metabolism

3. The best area to place a newborn's crib would be

   A. Against the far wall of a room

   B. In the corner of a room

   C. In the center of a room

   D. Against a sunny window

4. Glycogen stores, which are used by the newborn to produce heat, can become depleted and cause

   A. The infant to cry

   B. Jaundice

   C. Blood in the urine

   D. Hypoglycemia

5. At birth, the full-term infant has enough iron stores to last approximately

   A. One year

   B. One week

   C. Four to 6 months

   D. Three months

6. To enhance attachment behavior, the best intervention on the part of the nurse would be

   A. Have the mother breastfeed immediately in the delivery room

   B. Send the infant to the nursery immediately after birth so the mother can rest

   C. Encourage grandparents to visit the mother and infant in the hospital

   D. Have siblings meet the newborn once the baby is discharged home

7. Extremely elevated levels of bilirubin in the first week of life can cause a permanent and devastating form of brain damage called

   A. Hypospadias

   B. Epispadias

   C. Jaundice

   D. Kernicterus

8. The first period of reactivity in the newborn

   A. Lasts 24 hours

   B. Lasts 1 week

   C. Lasts 30 minutes

   D. Lasts 1 year

9. Self-quieting ability refers to the newborn's ability to quiet and soothe himself or herself by

   A. Hand-to-mouth movements and sucking

   B. Crying

   C. Latching onto the breast

   D. Passing meconium

10. Identification bands should be placed on the mother and her infant

    A. In the labor and delivery room before the newborn is transferred to the nursery

    B. When the father arrives in the delivery room after the birth

    C. Upon admission to the newborn nursery

    D. Prior to discharge

11. The nurse in the newborn nursery knows that the polycythemic infant is at risk to develop which condition?

    A. Hair loss

    B. Rh incompatibility

    C. Sepsis

    D. Jaundice

12. When assessing the clavicles in a newborn, crepitus would be a sign of

    A. A fracture

    B. Blood loss

    C. Tonic neck

    D. Rooting reflex

13. When assessing breath sounds in the newborn, fine crackles and transient hoarseness are

    A. A sign that the newborn should be transferred to the neonatal intensive care unit

    B. Normal

    C. A sign of a worsening condition

    D. A sign that the infant should not be fed

14. Full-term infants should be placed in which position to sleep?

    A. Prone

    B. Supine

    C. On their side

    D. In an upright position

15. Tufts of hair located in the sacral area are associated with what type of abnormalities?

A. Cardiac

B. Kidney

C. Respiratory

D. Abdominal

16. Parents should be instructed upon discharge that they need to go to the hospital emergency room in which scenario?

A. The newborn has respiratory distress.

B. The baby is fussy.

C. The baby cries for 2-hour-long periods.

D. The baby has erythema toxicum.

17. Unsymmetrical gluteal folds can indicate what type of abnormalities?

A. Hip

B. Buttock

C. Leg

D. Feet

18. To be sure the infant is breastfeeding successfully, the nurse must

A. Check the number of feeding episodes per day

B. Observe the newborn's latch, suck, and swallow

C. Weigh the newborn's dirty diapers

D. Ask the mother how well she thinks the infant is feeding

19. Newborns receive approximately 50% of their calories from

A. Carbohydrates

B. Fat

C. Protein

D. Lactose

20. The parents of an uncircumcised male infant require information about

A. Surgery

B. Counseling

C. Good hygiene practices

D. Teenage sexual practices

21. Newborns should go home from the birthing unit in

A. A federally approved car seat adapted to fit newborns

B. In their mother's arms in the back seat of a car

C. In their older brother's toddler car seat

D. In a taxicab, on the seat between the parents

22. The nurse can demonstrate sensitivity to the cultural beliefs and values of the family by
    A. Incorporating cultural preferences, health beliefs and behaviors, and traditional practices into the management plan
    B. Enforcing the one-person-at the-bedside rule for laboring patients
    C. Playing music during the patient's stay
    D. Finding a nurse to take care of the patient from the same culture
23. The newborn's cry should be
    A. Shrill and high-pitched
    B. Strong, lusty, and of medium pitch
    C. Catlike
    D. Low-pitched
24. A bulging fontanelle in a newborn usually signifies
    A. Dehydration
    B. Jaundice
    C. Increased intracranial pressure
    D. That the baby has to pass meconium
25. A single umbilical artery is frequently associated with
    A. Small for gestational age infant
    B. Large for gestational age infant
    C. Congenital anomalies
    D. Jaundice

Answers

True/False

1. False. The anterior fontanelle is diamond-shaped and closes at approximately 18 months.
2. True
3. True
4. True
5. False. Vitamin K is given to the newborn in the delivery room immediately after birth.
6. True
7. True
8. True
9. True
10. True
11. True
12. False. The umbilical cord stump needs to be kept as dry as possible.
13. False. A cephalohematoma does not cross the suture line.
14. True
15. False. The umbilical cord contains two arteries and one vein.
16. True

17. False. Kangaroo care can be used with either parent.
18. True
19. True
20. True
21. True
22. True
23. True
24. False. The majority of newborns do void immediately after birth.

Matching Columns

1. G
2. B
3. F
4. A
5. H
6. J
7. D
8. C
9. E
10. I

Multiple Choice

1. D
2. A
3. C
4. D
5. C
6. A
7. D
8. C
9. A
10. A
11. D
12. A
13. B
14. B
15. B
16. A
17. A
18. B
19. B
20. C
21. A
22. A
23. B
24. C
25. C

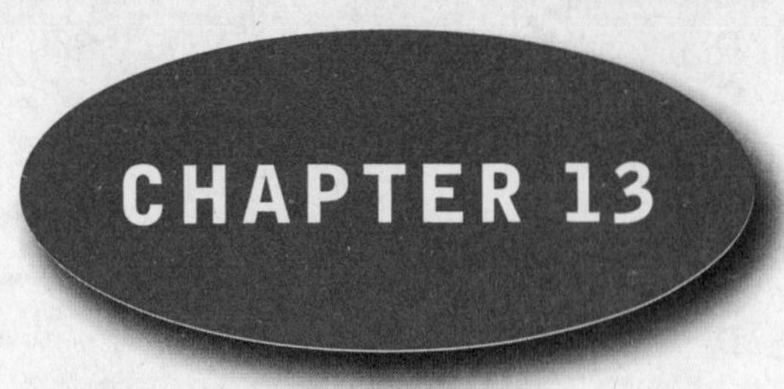

Nursing Management of the Pregnancy at Risk

Objective A: To Identify the High-Risk Pregnancy

13.1 High-Risk Pregnancy

The goal of risk assessment during pregnancy is to identify women and fetuses at risk for developing antepartum, intrapartum, or neonatal complications to promote risk-appropriate care and enhance perinatal outcomes.

13.2 Preexisting Conditions

Pregnancy is psychologically and physiologically stressful, even for healthy women, and for those with preexisting (pregestational) conditions, it may be life threatening. For these women, pregestational counseling is especially important to identify early interventions designed to diminish the adverse effects of pregnancy on both the mother and the fetus. In some cases, interventions before conception may be critical.

The responsibilities of the nurse when taking care of the woman with a high-risk pregnancy include conducting accurate assessment taking to identify changes in conditions, educating, and providing emotional support as the patient progresses through pregnancy.

Objective B: To Understand the Woman with a Preexisting Condition

13.3 Hematologic Disorders and Pregnancy

Anemia indicates inadequate levels of hemoglobin in the blood. It is defined as hemoglobin < 12 g/dL in nonpregnant women and < 11 g/dL in pregnant women. The common anemias of pregnancy are due to either nutritional deficiency in iron or folic acid or to hemoglobin destruction in inherited disorders, specifically sickle cell anemia and thalassemia.

Iron deficiency anemia is the most common medical complication of pregnancy, primarily as a consequence of expansion of plasma volume without normal expansion of maternal hemoglobin mass. A pregnant woman needs ~1000 mg more iron intake during pregnancy. The greatest need for increased iron intake occurs in the second half of pregnancy.

The woman with iron deficiency anemia may be asymptomatic, but she is more susceptible to infection, may tire easily, and has an increased risk for preeclampsia and postpartal hemorrhage and may not be able to tolerate even a minimal amount of blood loss at delivery. Fetal-neonatal risks include low birth weight, prematurity, stillbirth, and neonatal death in infants with severe deficiency.

If anemia is diagnosed during pregnancy, the dosage of iron is increased to 60 to 120 mg daily. With a multiple gestation pregnancy, a higher dosage is needed.

Folate deficiency is the most common cause of megaloblastic anemia during pregnancy and affects between 1% and 4% of pregnant women in the United States. Folate is needed for DNA and RNA synthesis and cell duplication. In its absence, immature red blood cells (RBCs) fail to divide, become enlarged, and are fewer in number. An inadequate intake of folate is associated with neural tube defects in the fetus or newborn.

The diagnosis of folic acid deficiency anemia is difficult, so it is usually not detected until late in pregnancy or the early puerperium. Women who have true folic acid deficiency present with nausea, vomiting, and anorexia. Folic acid deficiency in pregnancy is treated with 0.4 mg of folate daily. The nurse needs to recommend dietary sources of folic acid and encourage the patient to increase her intake of these food sources. The best sources of folic acid are fresh green leafy vegetables, orange juice, red meats, fish, poultry, and legumes.

Because half of all pregnancies in the United States are unplanned, nurses need to teach women of child-bearing age to include sufficient quantities of folic acid in their diets. Many women have passed the stage of neural tube development before they realize they are pregnant.

Sickle Cell Anemia

Sickle cell anemia is a recessive autosomal disorder in which the normal adult hemoglobin, hemoglobin A (HbA), is abnormally formed. The anemia is characterized by acute, recurring episodes of tissue, abdominal, and joint pain. RBCs sickle, or become crescent shaped, and are called HbS. In conditions of low oxygenation, these cells become semisolid and interlock, clogging capillaries, particularly in organs characterized by slow flow and high oxygen extraction, such as the spleen, bone marrow, and placenta.

Women with sickle cell anemia have a good prognosis with pregnancy if they have adequate nutrition and prenatal care. However, they have considerably more risks during pregnancy, including nephritis, bacteriuria, hematuria, and anemia, as well as sudden attacks of pain that may be general or localized in bones or joints, lungs, abdominal organs, or the spinal cord. Maternal mortality due to sickle cell anemia is rare. Fifty percent to 67% of pregnant women with sickle cell anemia develop infections, usually urinary tract or pulmonary. Congestive heart failure or acute renal failure may also occur. Prematurity and intrauterine growth retardation (IUGR) are associated with sickle cell anemia. The incidence of fetal death during and immediately following an attack is estimated to be 18%.

Nursing goals for a pregnant woman with sickle cell disease is to provide effective health teaching to prevent a crisis, improve the anemia, and to prevent infection. Treatment with a folic acid supplement (1mg/d) is needed. Infections should be treated promptly. For those in crisis, intravenous (IV) hydration, administration of oxygen, antibiotics, analgesics, and fetal monitoring are all important aspects of care. Antiembolism stockings are used postpartum.

If crisis occurs later in pregnancy, the woman is kept in the left lateral position, and pitocin may be used to promote labor. An episiotomy or outlet forceps may be used to shorten the second stage of labor.

Sickle cell anemia affects people primarily of African descent and occasionally in people of Southeast Asian or Mediterranean origin.

Thalassemia

The thalassemias are a group of autosomal recessive disorders characterized by a synthesis of the alpha or beta chains in the hemoglobin molecule. Symptoms are caused by the shortened life span of the RBCs, which results in active erythropoiesis in the liver, spleen, and bones. This produces hepatosplenomegaly and sometimes bony malformations. Prenatal genetic diagnosing is now available for these disorders.

The woman with thalassemia has mild anemia and small blood cells. This must be distinguished from iron deficiency anemia, because a patient with thalassemia must not be treated with iron unless she is also deficient in it. Folic acid supplements are indicated, but iron supplements are not given.

Because newborns have fetal hemoglobin (HbF), which does not have beta chains, symptoms are present for several months. Once infants start to produce adult-type hemoglobin (HbA), they develop severe anemia and require transfusions, which results in iron overload. Chelating therapy must be instituted to prevent liver and heart damage from excess iron.

Hepatitis

Hepatitis B is caused by a virus that is transmitted via blood, saliva, vaginal secretions, semen, or breast milk and readily crosses the placenta. Chronic hepatitis B develops in 10% of infected adults, who can continue to transmit the disease to others.

The incidence of prematurity, low birth weight, and neonatal death increases when the mother has hepatitis B infection during pregnancy. Infants born to mothers who have hepatitis B or who are chronic carriers of hepatitis B surface antigen (HBsAg) are at risk for the development of acute infection at birth. Chronic hepatitis infection will develop in ~90% of newborns.

No specific treatment exists for acute hepatitis B. Recommended supportive treatment includes bed rest and a high-protein, low-fat diet.

Human Immunodeficiency Virus/Acquired Immunodeficiency Syndrome

Acquired immunodeficiency syndrome (AIDS) is a breakdown in the immune function caused by the retrovirus human immunodeficiency virus (HIV). The infected person develops opportunistic infections. Transmission of HIV is predominantly via three modes:

1. Sexual exposure to genital secretions of an infected person
2. Parenteral exposure to infected blood or tissue
3. Perinatal exposure of an infant to infected maternal secretions during birth (vertical transmission)

An infant born to an HIV-positive mother who did not have antiretroviral treatment during pregnancy has a higher risk of becoming infected. Prevention remains the only way to control HIV infection. To reduce vertical transmission to the newborn, zidovudine (ZDV) is recommended for pregnant women who are HIV positive. Additional drugs are used for greatest effectiveness for the woman, but ZDV is included because of the drug's effectiveness in reducing HIV transmission to the fetus.

The woman should be given reassurance that her right to privacy will not be violated. She will be anxious, especially if newly diagnosed with HIV. She will also be anxious wondering if her baby will become infected. The nurse's response should be one of encouragement and assisting her in selecting those in her family who will provide committed love and emotional support.

The nurse can help a woman who is HIV positive maintain the highest level of wellness by teaching the patient that adequate, high-quality nutrition decreases the risk of opportunistic infections and promotes vitality. A daily regimen should include sufficient rest and activity. Avoiding large crowds, travel to areas with poor sanitation, and exposure to infected individuals is important. Meticulous skin care is also important.

The nurse needs to reinforce with the patient at each prenatal visit that most infants do not get the virus if the medication regimen is followed carefully.

13.4 Cardiac Disease

Cardiac disease complicates 1% of all pregnancies. Although the overall mortality rate of heart disease has decreased, it remains a major cause of maternal mortality. Pregnancy may aggravate a known cardiac condition or may unmask a previously unknown cardiac condition.

The cardiovascular system consists of the heart and circulatory system. Assessment of cardiovascular risk factors related to pregnancy and subsequent preconception (optimally) or antenatal counseling are traditionally based on three factors:

1. Type of cardiovascular disorder
2. Degree of the woman's functional ability
3. Incidence of pregnancy complications

Women with congenital heart disease are more likely to survive reproductive age, with the possibility of adding cardiac risk to their pregnancies. A third category, mitral valve prolapse, is a common but benign condition that usually does not cause problems during pregnancy. Myocardial infarction and conduction defects also may occur in women of childbearing age, especially with the increase of obesity.

Signs and symptoms of heart disease include dyspnea, syncope (fainting) with exertion, hemoptysis, paroxysmal nocturnal dyspnea, and chest pain with exertion. Additional signs that confirm the diagnosis are cyanosis; clubbing; diastolic, presystolic, or continuous heart murmur; cardiac enlargement; a loud, harsh systolic murmur associated with a thrill; and serious dysrhythmias.

The diagnosis of heart disease may be made from clinical signs and symptoms and by physical examination. It is usually confirmed by heart imaging studies. Once the diagnosis is made, the severity of the disease is determined by the client's ability to endure physical activity. A clinical classification based on the effect of exercise on the heart has been developed by the New York Heart Association. In general, maternal and fetal risks with classes I and II are low but greatly increased with classes III and IV.

- Class I: Uncompromised; no limits on physical activity
- Class II: Slightly compromised, requiring slight alteration of physical activity; comfortable at rest, but ordinary activity causes fatigue, dyspnea, palpitations, or anginal pain
- Class III: Markedly compromised with limitation of physical activity; comfortable at rest, but less than ordinary activity causes excessive fatigue, dyspnea, palpitation, or anginal pain
- Class IV: Inability to perform any physical activity without discomfort

Symptoms of Cardiac Insufficiency Even at Rest

The primary goal of management is to prevent cardiac decompensation and the development of congestive heart failure.

The nurse must carefully assess vital signs at each prenatal visit, identifying even subtle changes since the last appointment, as well as levels of fatigue. He or she must observe for signs and symptoms of congestive heart failure. The woman's weight must be assessed for pattern of weight gain to detect excessive weight gain and fluid overload. The nurse also needs to assess the woman's knowledge of the prescribed regime and her ability to comply with it.

The nurse needs to note other factors that may increase the cardiac workload, such as anemia, infections, anxiety, and lack of support, and report these to the patient's physician. Topics for teaching include avoiding excessive weight gain and anemia, as they both increase the cardiac workload of the heart. A well-balanced diet of ~2200 calories is recommended, which includes high-quality protein. The woman should be instructed to regulate energy expenditure and take frequent rest periods. All women with cardiac disease require 8 to 10 hours of sleep each night.

The patient should be instructed to avoid exposure to environmental extremes. This includes dressing warmly in the winter and avoiding travel to places with extremes in temperature, as this places additional demands on the heart.

Stress management should be discussed with women with heart disease. Emotional stress increases blood pressure, heart rate, and respiratory rate. Various methods for stress management, such as meditation, biofeedback, and progressive relaxation of the muscles, should be discussed. The patient should be taught that smoking and the use of illicit drugs such as cocaine greatly increase the stress on the heart and are associated with hypertension, which further adds to the cardiac workload and fetal compromise.

Hypertensive Disorders

Hypertensive disorders are the most common medical complications during pregnancy, labor, birth, and the postpartum period. Four categories of hypertensive disorders that occur during pregnancy are

1. ***Gestational hypertension***—blood pressure elevation after 20 weeks' gestation that is not accompanied by proteinuria
2. ***Preeclampsia***—a systolic blood pressure ≥140 mm Hg or a diastolic blood pressure ≥90 mm Hg occurring after 20 weeks of pregnancy that is accompanied by significant proteinuria (> 0.3 in a 24-hour period; edema, common in preeclampsia, is now considered nonspecific because it occurs in many pregnancies not complicated by hypertension)

3. ***Eclampsia***—progression of preeclampsia to generalized seizures that cannot be attributed to other causes
4. ***Chronic hypertension***—blood pressure that was known to exist before pregnancy

Unrecognized chronic hypertension may not be diagnosed until well after the end of pregnancy when the blood pressure remains high.

In the United States, pregnancy-associated hypertension is a leading cause of maternal death. Maternal race influences the rate of hypertension complicating pregnancy, with the highest rates seen in Native American and African-American women, and the lowest rates in Asian and Pacific Islander. Age distribution graphs demonstrate women younger than 20 years and older than 40 years are at highest risk for developing hypertension during pregnancy.

Hypertension during pregnancy predisposes the pregnant woman to potentially lethal complications, such as abruptio placentae, disseminated intravascular coagulation (DIC), hepatic failure, cerebral hemorrhage, cerebral vascular accident, and acute renal failure. Leading causes of maternal death from hypertension complicating pregnancy include complications from abruptio placentae, hepatic rupture, and eclampsia. Maternal hypertension contributes to intrauterine fetal death and perinatal mortality. The main causes of neonatal death are placental insufficiency and abruptio placentae. IUGR is common in infants of women with preeclampsia.

13.5 Respiratory Disease

Pulmonary diseases have become more prevalent in general, and during pregnancy.

Pregnant women are more susceptible to injury to the respiratory tract for several reasons, including alterations in the immune system that involve cell-mediated immunity and mechanical and anatomical changes involving the chest and abdominal cavities. The cumulative effect is decreased tolerance to hypoxia and acute changes in pulmonary mechanics.

Increased circulating levels of progesterone during pregnancy result in maternal hyperventilation, causing a state of chronic compensated respiratory alkalosis. Normal maternal hyperventilation during pregnancy lowers the maternal carbon dioxide level and minimally increases blood pH. The increase in blood pH in turn increases the oxygen affinity of maternal hemoglobin and facilitates elimination of fetal carbon dioxide, but it appears to impair release of maternal oxygen to the fetus. The high levels of estrogen and progesterone during pregnancy facilitate a shift of the oxygen dissociation, stimulating a shift of oxygen back to the fetus. This shift ensures that the fetus has increased oxygen release and adequate blood gas exchange.

Asthma

Asthma, an obstructive lung condition, is the most common respiratory disease found in pregnancy, complicating as much as 10% of all pregnancies. Typical symptoms include wheezing, dyspnea, and episodic coughing. During pregnancy, in approximately one third of women the asthma improves, in one third it remains unchanged, and in one third the condition worsens. The highest incidence of exacerbation occurs between 24 and 36 weeks' gestation.

Asthma has been linked with higher rates of hyperemesis gravidarum, preeclampsia, uterine hemorrhage, and perinatal mortality. Prematurity and low birth weight are more common among infants of women who have asthma. The goal of therapy is to prevent maternal exacerbations that can cause severe hypoxia-related complications in the fetus. If an exacerbation occurs, it should be treated in the same way as for a nonpregnant woman because the asthma drugs used are less of a threat to the fetus than a serious asthma attack.

Asthma is managed by long-term comprehensive drug therapy to prevent airway inflammation, combined with drug treatment to manage attacks or exacerbations. The nurse needs to educate the patient about triggers, such as cold air, dust, smoke, exercise, and food additives, along with methods of prevention and treatment options.

A severe asthma attack often requires hospitalization.

Tuberculosis

Tuberculosis (TB), caused by *Mycobacterium tuberculosis,* produces an inflammatory process that results in destruction of lung tissue, increased sputum, and coughing. It is transmitted by droplets that are inhaled by a noninfected individual and taken into the lungs. TB is associated primarily with poverty and malnutrition and in the United States may be found among immigrants from countries where TB is prevalent. It is also increasingly associated with HIV infection.

Women at risk should be screened for TB when obtaining prenatal care if they are not already known to be positive. This screening involves an intradermal injection of mycobacterial protein. If the reaction is positive or the woman is already known to have a positive reaction, a chest radiograph should be taken, preferably after the first trimester, with a lead shield covering the abdomen. Diagnosis is confirmed by isolating and identifying the bacterium in the sputum.

Signs and symptoms include general malaise, fatigue, loss of appetite, weight loss, fever, and night sweats. As the disease progresses, a chronic cough develops, and a mucopurulent sputum is produced.

Although perinatal infection is uncommon, it may result from a fetus swallowing or aspirating infected amniotic fluid. Signs of congenital TB include failure to thrive, lethargy, respiratory distress, fever, and enlargement of the spleen, liver, and lymph nodes. If the mother remains untreated, the newborn is at high risk for acquiring TB by inhalation of infectious respiratory droplets from the mother.

Treatment is with isoniazid and either rifampin or ethambutol, or both. The pregnant woman should also take supplemental pyridoxine (vitamin B_6). Extra rest and limited contact with others are required until the disease becomes inactive.

If maternal TB is inactive at the time of delivery, the mother may breastfeed and take care of her infant. If TB is active, the newborn should not have direct contact with the mother until she is noninfectious.

Nursing care includes teaching the patient and at least one other responsible individual information on the mode of transmission of TB, the importance of medications, the duration of treatment, and the possible side effects of the medications. The nurse should teach the patient essential facts about TB, such as

- Urine may turn orange as a result of the medications.
- Contact lenses may turn orange.
- It is important not to skip medications or double up on medications.
- Medications should be taken at the same time every day.
- Alcohol can increase liver toxicity and should not be used.
- Nausea, heartburn, diarrhea, and flatulence are common side effects.
- Oral contraceptives are less effective with rifampin.

13.6 Neurologic Disorders

Seizure disorders are the most common form of epilepsy, which is a recurrent disorder of cerebral function. Seizures may occur in pregnancy even though the woman has been seizure-free for many years. The effect of pregnancy on the course of epilepsy is variable and unpredictable. In general, the longer the woman has been seizure-free before pregnancy, the less likely she is to develop seizures during pregnancy. Those with partial (focal) seizures are more likely to have an increased frequency. Seizures that occur only during pregnancy have been reported as well.

Women with epilepsy have a higher than normal incidence of stillbirth and preterm labors. Maternal bleeding may occur because of a deficiency of clotting factors associated with anticonvulsant drugs such as Dilantin and phenobarbital. Anticonvulsant drugs also compete with folate for absorption, which may result in folate deficiency. Use of any anticonvulsant drugs during pregnancy is controversial, and patients considering a pregnancy should be advised to consult with a neurologist before becoming pregnant.

Anticonvulsant drugs have been associated with craniofacial deformities, limb reduction defects, growth restriction, mental retardation, and cardiac anomalies in newborns. The patient and family need to be made aware that these medications cannot be stopped abruptly when a pregnancy is confirmed. Generalized seizures cause hypoxia and acidosis in the fetus.

The goals of treatment are to prevent generalized seizures and reduce the adverse effects of anticonvulsant medications on the fetus. The nurse needs to be supportive of the family and provide teaching, especially about the use of over-the-counter medications that should be avoided when taking anticonvulsant medications.

Bell's palsy is a sudden unilateral neuropathy of the seventh cranial nerve (facial) that causes facial paralysis with weakness of the forehead and face. No specific cause is usually identified. It is three times more common during pregnancy, and 90% of women will recover in the first few weeks after delivery. Patients report feeling a stiff face, having difficulty closing an eye and eating, and sometimes losing the ability to taste.

Treatment is controversial. Some physicians prescribe steroids during the first few days. Care includes covering the affected eye with a patch, applying eye drops, and offering psychological support. The nurse needs to instruct the patient to cut food into small pieces and to chew slowly and carefully.

13.7 Autoimmune Disorders

Systemic lupus erythematosus (SLE) is a chronic, inflammatory autoimmune disease that can affect any organ system in the body. The cause is unknown, and females are affected 10 times more often than males. Because pregnancy can worsen SLE, women must be carefully observed for signs that the disease has progressed.

Signs and symptoms result from inflammation of multiple organ systems, especially the joints, kidneys, skin, and nervous system. The most common symptoms are a butterfly rash over the face, joint pain, and photosensitivity. Women whose disease is under good control at the time of pregnancy are likely to have a favorable outcome.

SLE is associated with increased incidence of abortion and fetal death during the first trimester. After the first trimester, the prognosis for a live birth is higher if no active disease exists. Newborn risks include preterm births, growth restriction, and congenital heart block. Nurses need to give supportive care to patients with SLE.

Rheumatoid arthritis is a chronic inflammatory disease that usually affects the synovial joints. The cause is unknown and affects females two to four times more frequently than males.

Marked improvement in symptoms of rheumatoid arthritis often occurs during pregnancy. The exact reason is unknown but thought to be due to the increase in hormones during pregnancy. A relapse often occurs, though, 6 weeks to 6 months after birth. In most instances, obstetric problems do not occur unless the hips or cervical spine is significantly deteriorated.

Multiple sclerosis (MS) is a neurologic disease characterized by destruction of the myelin sheath of nerve fibers. The condition occurs primarily in younger adults, more commonly in females, and is marked by periods of remission. It progresses to marked physical disability in 10 to 20 years. MS is associated with remission during pregnancy, but with a slightly increased relapse rate postpartum. A patient with MS needs extra rest, and help with child care activities should be arranged.

13.8 Endocrine System

Hashimoto thyroiditis, characterized by antithyroid antibodies, causes most cases of ***hypothyroidism.*** Symptoms include lack of energy, excessive weight gain, cold intolerance, dry skin, and constipation. Women with hypothyroidism have a higher incidence of preeclampsia, abruptio placentae, and low birth weight or stillborn infants. Treatment is with levothyroxine. Nurses need to reinforce the medication regime and give accurate information regarding the disease process.

Hyperthyroidism produces an overactive, enlarged thyroid gland that is difficult to diagnose because the normal changes of pregnancy increase the metabolic rate and mimic hyperthyroidism. Women with hyperthyroidism have an increased incidence of preeclampsia and postpartum hemorrhage if not well controlled during pregnancy. Treatment is with propylthiouracil. Additional drugs, such as iodides and beta blockers, may be needed, particularly in thyroid crisis.

Diabetes mellitus, an endocrine disorder of carbohydrate metabolism, results from inadequate production or utilization of insulin. Patients with diabetes during pregnancy can be divided into two groups. The first group consists of women who have preexisting or pregestational diabetes (type 1 or 2). The second group is those women who develop gestational diabetes mellitus (GDM), defined as carbohydrate intolerance of any degree with onset or first recognition during pregnancy. GDM is subdivided further to designate those women who are diet controlled or insulin controlled.

The pregnancy of a woman who has diabetes carries a higher risk of complications, including hydramnios, preeclampsia/eclampsia, hyperglycemia, labor dystocia, kidney infection, and retinopathy. The incidence of congenital anomalies in diabetic pregnancies is 5% to 10% and is the major cause of death of infants of diabetic mothers. The anomalies often involve the heart, central nervous system (CNS), and skeletal system. Septal defects, coarctation of the aorta, and transposition of the great vessels are the most common heart lesions seen. CNS anomalies include hydrocephalus, meningomyelocele, and anencephaly.

The major goals of care for a pregnant woman with diabetes are to maintain a physiologic equilibrium of insulin availability and glucose utilization during pregnancy, and to ensure an optimally healthy mother and newborn. Specifically, goals of treatment are to decrease the likelihood of fetal macrosomia, shoulder dystocia, birth trauma, and cesarean birth.

To achieve these goals, good prenatal care using a team approach is the top priority. Education of the woman and her significant other and their active involvement in managing her care are essential for a good outcome. For the woman with GDM, the diagnosis may be a shock and leave her frightened and anxious. This anxiety may cause an inability to adhere to specific regimens. The woman newly diagnosed will need clear explanations and teaching by the nurse to enlist her participation in ensuring a good outcome. Diet therapy and regular exercise are the essential interventions for the gestational diabetic woman. Insulin therapy is indicated when dietary management is unable to achieve a 1-hour postprandial blood glucose level value < 130 to 140 mg/dL, a 2-hour postprandial level < 120 mg/dL, or a fasting glucose < 95 mg/dL.

Whether or not the woman with GDM needs insulin or not depends on how well her glucose levels can be maintained by diet alone. Oral hypoglycemic medications are rarely used during pregnancy because they cross the placenta. Glyburide, a second-generation sulfonylurea, does not cross the placenta and has been found to be comparable to insulin without evidence of adverse effects in the mother or the fetus.

Information about the well-being, maturation, and size of the fetus is important for planning the course of the pregnancy and the timing of birth. Because pregnancies complicated by diabetes are at increased risk of neural tube defects, maternal serum alpha fetoprotein (AFP) screening is offered at 16 to 20 weeks' gestation. Daily maternal evaluation of fetal activity is encouraged beginning at 28 weeks. Fetal kick counting should be taught, and the patient should be asked to keep a log, which she brings to each prenatal visit. Nonstress tests (NSTs) are also begun at this time and done weekly. If an NST is nonreactive, a fetal biophysical profile may be performed. If the woman requires hospitalization, NSTs may be done daily.

13.9 Cancer During Pregnancy

Cancer is rare during pregnancy, occurring in ~1 per 1,000 live births. More than half the cases are tumors of the uterine cervix, breast, or thyroid, which can metastasize to the placenta, but not to the fetus. Breast cancer is the most common cancer in pregnant women.

Treatment for cancer during pregnancy means deciding what the best approach for the mother is as opposed to the possible risks to the fetus. The type of treatment depends on many factors, including how far along the pregnancy is; the type, location, size, and stage of the cancer; and the wishes of the woman and her family. Because some of the treatments can be harmful to the fetus, treatment is often delayed until the second or third trimester. When cancer is diagnosed late in pregnancy, treatment may be delayed until the pregnancy is over, or labor may be induced early in order to start treatment. Treatment used during pregnancy may include surgery, chemotherapy, and sometimes radiation therapy, but only after careful consideration and planning are given to ensure the safety of the mother and the fetus.

The prognosis for a pregnant woman with cancer is often the same as for another woman of the same age with the same type and stage of cancer. If treatment is delayed during pregnancy, her prognosis will be worse overall than for that of a nonpregnant woman diagnosed with cancer.

Cancer rarely affects the fetus directly. Although some cancers can spread to the placenta, most cancers cannot spread to the fetus itself. Although cancer cells cannot pass to the fetus in breast milk, women who are being treated for cancer are usually advised not to breastfeed. Chemotherapy can be especially harmful, as it builds up in breast milk and can harm the infant.

Because radiation therapy can harm the fetus, particularly during the first trimester, this treatment is generally not recommended. The use of radiation therapy in the second or third trimester depends on the dose of radiation and the area of the body being treated. Radioactive components that are taken internally, such as radioactive iodine used for treating thyroid cancer, also cross into breast milk and can harm the infant.

13.10 Mental Illness and Pregnancy

Despite the notion that pregnancy is a time of happiness and emotional well-being, evidence demonstrates that pregnancy does not protect women from mental illness.

Maternal mental illness poses a huge human, social, and economic burden to women, their infants, their families, and society and constitutes a major public health challenge. All women can have or develop mental disorders during pregnancy or in the first year after pregnancy, but poverty, migration, extreme stress, exposure to violence, emergency and conflict situations, natural disasters, and low social support generally increase risks for specific disorders.

Depression and anxiety in women are seen at their highest rates in women of childbearing years. Studies of depression and anxiety show their incidence to be ~5% in nonpregnant women, ~8% to 10% during pregnancy, and highest (13%) in the year following delivery. In developed countries, suicide is one of the most common causes of maternal death in the year following delivery. Psychosis is relatively rare and occurs in one or two women for every 1,000 giving birth. During pregnancy the affected woman is less likely to eat and sleep well and may fail to adequately gain weight. She is less likely to attend prenatal care and may even fail to seek help for the birth. She is more likely to use harmful substances such as alcohol, cigarettes, and drugs and may even try to injure or kill herself.

In addition, stress hormones are elevated during maternal mental illness and can predispose her to high blood pressure, preeclampsia, early and/or difficult delivery, and increased incidence of postpartum depression. As for the fetus, depression during pregnancy has been associated with preterm birth, smaller head circumferences, low birth weights, and lower Apgar scores.

Patients with mild to moderate illness should be referred for psychotherapy. Patients who are more severely ill might require additional treatment with medication.

Medication during pregnancy is a controversial issue, given the fact that psychotropic drugs cross the placenta. No conclusive evidence exists for or against the use of psychotropic drugs. For each patient, the risk of treatment with medication needs to be compared with the risk of not treating the illness. Medication already being taken by the patient should not be stopped abruptly, as that could cause an exacerbation or relapse of the condition. The most common antidepressants used during pregnancy are the serotonin reuptake inhibitors and the norepinephrine reuptake inhibitor venlafaxine.

Untreated maternal mental illness can impair mother–infant attachments and have cognitive, emotional, and behavioral consequences for children of affected mothers.

The nurse needs to be emotionally supportive of the patient with a mental illness during pregnancy. Teaching about self-care, appropriate drug dosages and side effects, and the importance of regular prenatal care needs to be reinforced by the nurse.

Support by the woman's significant other and family is important in the treatment of a mental illness during pregnancy. Family members should be incorporated into the treatment plan.

13.11 Obesity and Pregnancy

The prevalence of being overweight and obesity is a major health concern in the United States. While the overall occurrence of obesity and being overweight in the U.S. population has dramatically increased during the past 2 decades, some women of childbearing age (ages 20–34) have had the fastest increase of being overweight and obesity compared with any other group.

Research has demonstrated that obesity increases the risk of adverse outcomes for both mother and infant. Complications include hypertension, preeclampsia, GDM, neural tube defects, labor and delivery complications, delivery of a large-for-gestational-age infant, fetal and neonatal death, and infertility. Women of childbearing age and their health care providers should work together to address this important health issue before, during, and after pregnancy.

Treatment would include encouraging a healthy diet, as outlined by the U.S. Department of Agriculture; encouraging a weight gain of 15 to 25 lb (6.8 to 11.4 kg) as recommended by the Institute of Medicine for overweight patients; encouraging the patient to take prenatal vitamins; counseling the woman to consume adequate amounts of folic acid, iron, and calcium; screening for hypertension and diabetes mellitus; encouraging regular exercise (at least 30 minutes of moderate physical activity daily); counseling the patient to quit smoking; and counseling the woman to avoid consuming alcohol during pregnancy.

The nurse needs to teach the patient about a healthy lifestyle and provide emotional support. Further counseling by a nutritionist may be warranted, as well as counseling for smoking cessation.

13.12 Teen Pregnancy

Adolescent pregnancy is a multifaceted issue. Although the birth rate for adolescents in the United States has declined in the past decade, it remains the highest of any industrialized nation.

For a teenager, pregnancy comes at a time when she is still developing herself. She may not be prepared emotionally, physically, or economically for parenthood. As a result, she and her child are at high risk. Teen mothers are less likely to finish high school, are more likely to end up on welfare, and are more likely to deliver a premature or low birth weight baby. Preeclampsia is the most prevalent medical condition of pregnant adolescents. In addition, children of teen mothers are at an increased risk for mental retardation, poverty, welfare dependency, and poor school performance. They are more likely to grow up without a father and are more likely to suffer higher rates of abuse and neglect than would occur if their mothers had delayed childbearing.

In working with adolescents, the nurse has to remember that they often think differently than adults. Adolescents are concrete thinkers and often do not plan ahead more than a few days at a time. It is important to assess the individual teen's level of maturity, her self-concept, her attitude about the pregnancy, her coping methods, and her support system. The nurse needs to develop a trusting relationship with the pregnant adolescent. When adolesçents are treated positively, they value the experience and respond by asking more questions and seeking more assistance.

The nurse also needs to keep in mind that there are federal laws that give minors in certain situations the rights of adults. Pregnancy is one such instance. The pregnant adolescent, even if very young, is considered an "emancipated minor" and has the right and responsibility to consent for treatment for herself and that of her child. She is entitled to respect and confidentiality in her dealings with health care providers.

Often the adolescent has little understanding of pregnancy, childbirth, or pregnancy. The nurse's primary responsibility is education of the adolescent patient.

Objective C: To Understand the Woman Who Develops a Complication of Pregnancy

13.13 Bleeding

During the first and second trimesters of pregnancy, the most common cause of bleeding is ***abortion***. This is the expulsion of the fetus prior to viability. Viability is considered 20 weeks' gestation or a weight < 500 g. Abortions can be spontaneous or induced as a result of mechanical or artificial interruption of the pregnancy.

Other complications that can cause bleeding in the first half of the pregnancy are ectopic pregnancy and gestational trophoblastic disease. During the third trimester of pregnancy, the two major causes of bleeding are placenta previa and abruptio placentae.

Many pregnancies end in the first trimester as a result of a spontaneous abortion. Up to 60% of first trimester spontaneous abortions are due to chromosomal abnormalities. Other causes include teratogenic drugs, faulty implantation, a weakened cervix, placental abnormalities, chronic maternal diseases, endocrine imbalances, and maternal infections. Spontaneous abortions are subdivided into the following categories:

- Threatened abortion
- Inevitable abortion
- Incomplete abortion
- Complete abortion
- Missed abortion

In cases of ***threatened abortion,*** there is unexplained bleeding, cramping, or backache indicating that the fetus may be in jeopardy. The cervical os remains closed, and bleeding may persist for days. The bleeding may resolve or end with partial or complete expulsion of the fetus.

With ***inevitable abortion,*** bleeding and cramping may increase. The internal cervical ȯs dilates, and membranes may rupture.

With ***incomplete abortion,*** the internal os is dilated, and products of the pregnancy (often the placenta) are retained.

With ***complete abortion,*** all of the products of conception are expelled. The uterus is contracted, and the cervical os may be closed.

In ***missed abortion,*** the fetus dies in utero but is not expelled. The cervix is closed, and the woman may complain of some brown discharge. Diagnosis is made based on history, pelvic exam, a drop in human chorionic gonadotropin (hCG) levels, and an ultrasound. If the fetus is retained for more than 4 weeks, fetal autolysis results in thromboplastin, and DIC may develop.

Recurrent pregnancy loss, formally called habitual abortions, occurs consecutively in three or more pregnancies.

In ***septic abortion,*** there is the presence of infection. This may occur with prolonged, unrecognized rupture of the membranes, pregnancy with an intrauterine device (IUD) in place, or in cases of self-induced abortion. Treatment includes bed rest, abstinence from coitus, and, at times, sedation. If bleeding persists and abortion is inevitable, the woman may be hospitalized and given IV therapy and blood transfusions. Dilatation and curettage (D&C) may be done, or suction evacuation may be required to remove the remainder of the products of conception. In the case of a missed abortion past 12 weeks' gestation, labor may be induced.

If the woman is Rh negative and not sensitized, and there has been documentation of a fetal heart rate, Rh immune globulin (RhoGAM) is given within 72 hours.

Nursing care includes assessment of the amount of bleeding, monitoring of vital signs, and assessment of degree of discomfort. The nurse can also offer psychological support to the woman and family by encouraging them to verbalize their feelings. Referrals can be made to support groups for all of the family members to help them with the grieving process.

An ***ectopic pregnancy*** is one where there is an implantation of a fertilized ovum in a site other than in the endometrial lining of the uterus. The most common location for implantation of an ectopic pregnancy is the ampulla of the tube. Risk factors for ectopic pregnancy include tubal damage caused by pelvic inflammatory disease, previous tubal pregnancy or tubal surgery, congenital anomalies of the tube, use of ovulation-inducing drugs, smoking, and advanced maternal age. Initially, it appears as though the patient has a normal pregnancy, but there is internal hemorrhaging. The woman may experience one-sided lower abdominal pain or diffuse lower abdominal pain and vasomotor disturbances, such as fainting or dizziness. It is important to differentiate an ectopic pregnancy from other disorders with similar presenting symptoms.

Treatment is with methotrexate given intramuscularly (IM) for the woman who desires a future pregnancy, whose ectopic pregnancy is not ruptured, whose condition is stable, and when there is no fetal cardiac activity, maternal thrombocytopenia, or kidney or liver disease. The woman is monitored on an outpatient basis for pain and decreasing beta hCG (b-hCG) levels. If surgery is needed and the woman desires a future pregnancy, a laparoscopic salpingostomy will be performed to evacuate the pregnancy. If the tube is ruptured or a future pregnancy is not an issue, removal of the tube (laparoscopic salpingectomy) is performed.

Gestational trophoblastic disease (GTD) is the pathologic proliferation of trophoblastic cells and includes partial or complete hydatidiform mole, invasive mole, and choriocarcinoma. Hydatidiform mole, or molar pregnancy, is a condition in which a proliferation of trophoblastic cells results in the formation of a placenta characterized by grapelike clusters. The significance of this disease is the loss of the pregnancy, but also the remote possibility of carcinoma. Often the fetus lasts 8 or 9 weeks and in other cases never grows (is an empty egg).

The diagnosis of hydatidiform mole is often suspected in the presence of vaginal bleeding (often brown and prune juice–like), the passage of clusters of fluid-filled grapelike tissue, uterine enlargement greater than expected for gestational age (classic sign), absence of fetal heart sounds, markedly elevated serum hCG, and very low levels of maternal serum AFP.

Treatment begins with the suction evacuation of the mole and curettage of the uterus to remove all fragments of the placenta. If there is excessive bleeding, hysterectomy may be the treatment of choice to reduce the incidence of malignant sequelae.

Because carcinoma develops in ~20% of women after having a molar pregnancy, follow-up for a woman who has had a molar pregnancy is very important. Patients are advised not to become pregnant for 1 year until the follow-up program is completed, so teaching about effective contraception is an important aspect of nursing care.

In ***placenta previa,*** the placenta is improperly implanted in the lower uterine segment, sometimes over the cervical os. The classic sign of placenta previa is painless vaginal bleeding (usually bright red) occurring after 20 weeks of pregnancy. Abdominal exam generally shows a nontender, soft uterus with normal tone. Leopold maneuvers often reveal the fetus to be in a breech or oblique position or transverse lie because of the abnormal location of the placenta.

Because of the risk of placental perforation, vaginal exams are not done, and the nurse instructs the patient to alert all medical personnel that vaginal exams are prohibited.

The cause of placenta previa is unknown. Factors associated with placenta previa are multiparity, increasing age, placenta accreta, defective development of blood vessels in the deciduas, prior cesarean birth, smoking, a recent abortion, cocaine use, a prior history of placenta previa, closely spaced pregnancies, African or Asian ethnicity, and a large placenta.

Maternal risks associated with placenta previa include shock, the potential for a hysterectomy, and death. Fetal risks include premature delivery, preterm premature rupture of the membranes (PROM), IUGR, malpresentation, congenital anomalies, and vasa previa. ***Vasa previa*** is a condition where the umbilical cord is implanted into the membranes and not the placenta. The appearance of blood with the rupture of membranes should alert the nurse to the possibility of a vasa previa.

There are three recognized variations of placenta previa.

1. A ***complete, or total, placenta previa*** covers the entire cervical os. Because it is associated with the greatest amount of blood loss, a complete previa presents the most serious risk.
2. A ***partial previa*** describes a placenta that partially occludes the cervical os.
3. A ***marginal previa*** is characterized by the encroachment of the placenta to the margins of the cervical os.

Placenta accreta is an abnormally firm attachment to the uterine wall. Unusual placental adherence may accompany a placenta previa. Placenta previa should be suspected in all patients who present with bleeding after 24 completed weeks of gestation.

Management of the patient with bleeding placenta previa requires acute assessment skills so there is no delay in treatment. Stabilization involves the administration of IV fluids and a laboratory workup that includes a complete blood count (CBC), prothrombin time (PT), partial thromboplastin time (PTT), fibrin split products, and fibrinogen. A blood type and cross-match should be obtained in anticipation of the need for a transfusion. A maternal Kleihauer-Betke blood test may be ordered to determine if there has been a transfer of fetal blood cells into the maternal circulation. If the patient is Rh negative and unsensitized, RhoGAM should be administered. The patient is placed on bed rest, and the fetus is continuously assessed by electronic fetal monitoring. If time permits, betamethasone (a long-acting corticosteroid) may be administered (to the woman) to promote fetal lung maturity. Labor that cannot be halted, fetal compromise, and life-threatening maternal hemorrhaging are all indications for immediate delivery by cesarean section.

Abruptio placentae is the separation of the normally implanted placenta from the uterine wall. An abruption results in hemorrhage between the uterine wall and the placenta.

The classic presenting sign is bleeding during the third trimester with severe abdominal pain. Other signs include abdominal tenderness, back pain, a boardlike abdomen with no bleeding, abnormal contractions and increased uterine tone, fetal compromise as evidenced by late fetal heart rate decelerations, bradycardia and lack of variability on the electronic fetal monitoring, and fetal demise.

Maternal mortality from abruptio placentae is as much as 5%. The maternal risks include anemia, shock, acute renal failure, and maternal death. Thirty-five percent of infants whose mother requires a transfusion will be anemic as well and require a transfusion. Fetal mortality occurs in 35% of cases and can be as high as 80% in cases of severe abruption. Death results from hypoxia that is related to the decreased placental surface area and maternal hemorrhage.

The potential for rapid deterioration due to hemorrhage, DIC, or hypoxia necessitates emergency delivery in some cases of abruptio placentae. However, most abruptions are small and do not require immediate delivery. Management would include hospitalization, laboratory studies, continuous monitoring, and ongoing patient support.

13.14 Hyperemesis Gravidarum

Hyperemesis gravidarum is characterized by persistent, uncontrolled nausea and vomiting before the 20th week of gestation. This complication can lead to dehydration, acid–base imbalances, electrolyte imbalances, and weight loss. It can also jeopardize fetal well-being.

This condition affects 1% of pregnant women who report feeling "very uncomfortable." Symptoms include disturbed nutrition, severe vomiting, electrolyte imbalance, ketosis, acetonuria, and weight loss > 5% of body mass. Other common symptoms are ptyalism, fatigue, weakness, dizziness, sleep disturbances, depression, anxiety, irritability, mood changes, and decreased ability to concentrate. If the condition progresses without treatment, it may cause neurologic disturbance, renal damage, retinal hemorrhage, or even death.

Conservative treatment in the home is the first line of treatment for a woman with hyperemesis gravidarum. The focus is on lifestyle and dietary changes. If conservative management fails to alleviate the patient's symptoms, hospitalization is warranted.

On admission to the hospital, blood tests are ordered to assess the severity of dehydration, electrolyte imbalance, ketosis, and malnutrition. IV fluids and drug therapy are begun to rehydrate and reduce symptoms. Food is usually withheld for 24 to 36 hours to give the gastrointestinal tract a rest. Antiemetics may be ordered and administered orally, rectally, or intravenously to control the nausea and vomiting. If symptoms do not improve within a few days, total parenteral nutrition (TPN) may be provided or a percutaneous endoscopic gastrostomy (PEG) tube may be placed to prevent malnutrition.

Nursing care focuses on providing comfort and emotional support to the anxious and exhausted patient. Providing information about the plan of care and attempting to provide the patient with a "sense of control" over her condition may alleviate much anxiety.

13.15 Preterm Labor

Preterm labor is cervical changes and regular uterine contractions that occur between 20 and 37 weeks' gestation.

Preterm birth, which is a birth that occurs before the completion of the 37th week of gestation, is considered the most acute problem in maternal-fetal health. Despite the advances in obstetric care, the rate of prematurity has not decreased over the past 40 years, and in most industrialized countries, it has slightly increased. The preterm delivery rate in the United States is 11%; in Europe, the rates vary between 5% and 7%.

The defining physiologic mechanism that triggers premature labor is unknown. Various risk factors are associated with preterm labor and birth and include a history of previous preterm birth, cervical or uterine abnormalities, multiple gestation, hypertension, diabetes, obesity, clotting factor deficiencies, urinary tract infections, fetal anomalies, PROM, late or no prenatal care, illicit drug use, smoking, alcohol use, domestic violence, low socioeconomic status, stress, periodontal disease, and long working hours with long periods of standing.

The sequelae of preterm birth have a profound effect on the survival and health of those born prematurely. With appropriate medical care, neonatal survival dramatically improves as gestational age increases.

Short-term neonatal morbidities associated with preterm birth are numerous and include respiratory distress syndrome, intraventricular hemorrhage, periventricular leukomalacia, necrotizing enterocolitis, bronchopulmonary dysplasia, sepsis, and patent ductus arteriosus. Long-term morbidities include cerebral palsy, mental retardation, and retinopathy of prematurity. The risk of these morbidities is directly related to the infant's gestational age and birth weight.

The diagnosis of preterm labor can be very challenging, as many of the symptoms are subtle and common during pregnancy. A diagnosis of preterm labor is made when the following criteria are met: gestation of 20 to 37 weeks, documented persistent uterine contractions, documented cervical effacement ≥80%, cervical dilation > 1 cm, and a documented change in dilation.

The two major goals of management of preterm labor are to inhibit or reduce the strength and frequency of contractions and to optimize the fetal status before preterm delivery. To achieve these goals, tocolysis and administration of antenatal corticosteroids are the recommended treatments. Tocolysis is the use of medications to inhibit uterine contractions. Drugs used for this purpose include beta-adrenergic agonists and magnesium sulfate. The most commonly used tocolytics are ritodrine and terbutaline sulfate. By delaying the birth, corticosteroids can be given to accelerate fetal lung maturity. Delaying the birth also allows time to transfer the mother to a tertiary care center equipped with a neonatal intensive care unit (NICU).

The nurse caring for the patient in preterm labor needs to monitor the administration of tocolytics carefully and safely and to provide emotional support to the woman and family during this period of stress and uncertainty.

13.16 Premature Rupture of the Membranes

PROM is rupture of the membranes before the onset of labor at any gestational age. ***Preterm rupture of the membranes*** is rupture of the membranes before 37 completed weeks of gestation. It is a common cause of preterm birth. ***Preterm premature rupture of the membranes (PPROM)*** is a combination of both terms: rupture that occurs before 37 weeks of gestation and in the absence of labor.

PROM is thought to be the result of multifactorial problems. Risk factors include inflammatory processes, decreased amniotic fluid membrane collagen, lower socioeconomic status, cigarette smoking, sexually transmitted infections, prior preterm delivery, prior preterm labor during the current pregnancy, uterine distention, cervical cerclage, amniocentesis, and vaginal bleeding in pregnancy. In many cases, the cause is unknown.

When diagnosing PROM, the patient will often report a gush or leakage of fluid from the vagina; however, sometimes there is only an increase in vaginal fluid. Patients should be taught that any increase in fluidlike discharge from the vagina should be evaluated. Nitrazine and ferning tests done on the leaking fluid will confirm the diagnosis.

The risk of perinatal complications varies according to the gestational age of the fetus when rupture of the membranes occurs.

Management is controversial. An ultrasound should be performed to accurately assess gestational age, assessment of fetal growth should be done, assessment of residual amniotic fluid needs to ascertained, and the woman needs to be assessed for evidence of infection, fetal distress, and abruptio placentae. Frequent ultrasounds will be done to monitor the amniotic fluid level. Corticosteroids will be administered to the woman to enhance fetal lung maturity.

Patients with advanced labor, intrauterine infections, significant vaginal bleeding, or nonreassuring fetal testing should be delivered promptly, regardless of gestational age.

Conservative management for those who are stable includes inpatient observation, continuous fetal and maternal monitoring, and modified bed rest.

The nurse's duties in taking care of a patient with PROM include explaining to her that she will be on bed rest and that her vital signs will be checked every 4 hours to detect early signs of a developing infection. An important part of nursing care is providing emotional support to the woman who is worried about the outcome for her baby. The nurse should encourage the woman and her family members to ask questions and verbalize their concerns and fears.

13.17 Preeclampsia

Preeclampsia is a multisystem, vasopressive disease process that targets the cardiovascular, hematologic, hepatic, renal, and central nervous systems. It is a pregnancy-specific syndrome clinically defined as an increase in blood pressure (140/90) after 20 weeks' gestation accompanied by proteinuria. The condition can be devastating to both mother and child. With severe preeclampsia, blood pressure is > 160/110 mm Hg on two occasions at least 6 hours apart. Proteinuria is > 500 mg in 24-hour urine collection, and oliguria (≤500 mL in 24 h) is present. Other symptoms that present in severe preeclampsia are pulmonary edema, thrombocytopenia with or without liver damage, cerebral or visual disturbances, epigastric or visual disturbances, epigastric or right upper quadrant pain, and fetal growth restriction.

Eclampsia is the onset of seizure activity or coma in the woman diagnosed with preeclampsia, with no history of preexisting pathology that can result in seizure activity.

The cause of preeclampsia remains a mystery. Decades of research have not proven any theories of the etiology of the condition. Factors associated with an increased risk of developing it include primigravida status; history of preeclampsia with a previous pregnancy; excessive placental tissue; a close family history of preeclampsia (mother or sister); lower socioeconomic group; history of diabetes, hypertension, or renal disease; poor nutrition; Mexican American ethnicity; age extremes (younger than 17 years and older than 35 years); and obesity.

Vasospasm and hypoperfusion are the underlying mechanisms involved in this disorder. The condition is characterized by generalized vasospasm, a decrease in circulating blood volume, and activation of the coagulation system. Generalized vasospasm results in elevation of blood pressure and reduced blood flow to the brain, liver, kidneys, placenta, and lung. Clinically, these changes present as hypertension and decreased perfusion to the placenta, kidneys, and brain.

Decreased liver perfusion leads to impaired liver function and subcapsular hemorrhage. This presents as epigastric pain and elevated liver enzymes in the maternal serum.

Decreased brain perfusion leads to small cerebral hemorrhages and symptoms of arterial vasospasm and presents as headaches, visual disturbances, blurred vision, and hyperactive deep tendon reflexes (DTRs).

Decreased kidney perfusion reduces the glomerular filtration rate (GFR), resulting in decreased urine output and increased serum levels of sodium, BUN (blood urea nitrogen), uric acid, and creatinine, which further increase extracellular fluid and edema. Increased capillary permeability in the kidneys allows albumin to escape, which reduces plasma colloid osmotic pressure and moves more fluid into the extracellular spaces, and leads to pulmonary edema and generalized edema.

Poor placental perfusion resulting from prolonged vasoconstriction helps to contribute to IUGR, premature separation of the placenta (abruptio placentae), persistent fetal hypoxia, and acidosis.

Hemoconcentration of the blood causes increased blood viscosity and elevated hematocrit.

Preeclampsia is categorized as mild or severe, or as complicated by HELLP syndrome (see discussion below).

Although preeclampsia is not preventable, theoretically, eclampsia should be preventable by identifying preeclampsia and swiftly delivering the newborn before seizures start. The only known cure for preeclampsia is delivery of the fetus.

Antepartum management includes conservative management for the patient with mild preeclampsia who exhibits no sign of renal or hepatic dysfunctions or coagulopathy. A woman with mild elevations in blood pressure may be placed on bed rest at home. Rest as much as possible in the lateral recumbent position to improve uteroplacental blood flow, reduce blood pressure, and promote diuresis should be encouraged.

In addition, frequent antepartal visits will need to be made for diagnostic testing, which includes CBCs, clotting studies, liver enzyme studies, and platelet counts. NSTs may be instituted in the latter part of pregnancy. Kick counting will be taught to the patient, and any decrease in fetal movement needs to be evaluated by the provider the same day. The woman will be asked to monitor her blood pressure every 4 to 6 hours daily while awake.

A balanced, nutritious diet with no sodium restriction is encouraged. Also, the woman needs to be encouraged to drink 6 to 8 glasses (8 oz) of water daily. If home management fails to reduce blood pressure, admission to the hospital is warranted, and the treatment is individualized based on the severity of the condition. Expectant management is continued until the pregnancy reaches term, the fetal lung maturity is documented, or complications develop that warrant immediate birth.

Severe preeclampsia can develop suddenly and is treated aggressively. The goal of care is to stabilize the mother–fetus dyad and prepare for birth. Therapy is focused on reducing blood pressure and preventing seizures, long-term morbidity, and maternal, fetal, or newborn death. IV fluid is given at a rate to replace urine output and additional insensible losses. Fetal heart rate is monitored continuously. Magnesium sulfate is given intravenously to prevent or decrease seizure activity. Hypertension is controlled with antihypertensive medications. Birth via induction or cesarean section may be planned if the condition worsens.

Eclamptic seizures are a life-threatening emergency and require immediate treatment to prevent maternal morbidity and mortality. In the woman who develops eclamptic seizures, the convulsive activity begins with facial twitching followed by generalized muscle rigidity. The woman may have one or more seizures, usually lasting 60 to 75 seconds. Severe headache and hyperreflexia are typically clinical precursors of eclamptic seizures.

Preventing hypertension-induced complications during pregnancy requires the nurse to use assessment, counseling, and advocacy skills. Assessment begins with the accurate assessment of the patient's blood pressure and of subjective complaints from the patient that may indicate a worsening of the condition.

At every prenatal visit, the nurse needs to assess the fetal heart rate, obtain maternal blood pressure, check a clean-catch urine specimen for protein using a dipstick, obtain the patient's weight, and assess for the amount and location of edema. The nurse needs to instruct the patient on the signs and symptoms of preeclampsia worsening and direct her to contact her health care provider for emergency evaluation if needed.

For the patient who is hospitalized, the nurse needs to make frequent assessments of maternal-fetal well-being by evaluating for disease progression and the patient's response to therapy. These include assessments for edema, the overall health status of the woman, DTRs, and results of laboratory studies.

Assessment of edema should be done, looking for distribution, degree, and pitting. Dependent edema is located in the lower half of the body. It is usually observed in the feet and ankles or in the sacral area if the patient is on bed rest. Assessment of the woman for pulmonary edema is also done. Signs and symptoms include crackles and wheezing heard on auscultation, dyspnea, decreased oxygen saturation, cough, neck vein distention, anxiety, and restlessness.

If the woman is receiving magnesium sulfate therapy, assessment of DTRs is done to check for adequacy of treatment. Hyperreflexia is usually present in patients with preeclampsia. Brisk reflexes reflect CNS involvement. Diminished reflexes indicate magnesium toxicity. A scale for reporting reflexes from 0 to 4 is used, with 2+ and 3+ indicating normal reflexes. Calcium gluconate is the antidote for magnesium sulfate toxicity and should be on hand to give in an emergency situation (10 mg).

Assessment for clonus needs to done. ***Clonus*** is the presence of rhythmic involuntary contractions, most often at the foot or ankle. Sustained clonus confirms CNS involvement.

Serum magnesium levels ranging from 4 to 8 mg/dL are considered therapeutic. Levels > 8 mg/dL are considered toxic. Symptoms of toxicity include absent or weak DTRs, respirations < 12 breaths/min, diminished levels of consciousness, drowsiness, and urinary output < 30 mL/h.

Lab tests that can be performed to monitor the disease process and to determine if it is progressing into HELLP syndrome (see below) include liver enzymes (lactate dehydrogenase [LDH], alanine transaminase [ALT], and aspartate transaminase [AST]), creatinine, BUN, uric acid, glucose, CBC with platelet count, coagulation studies, and 24-hour urine collection for protein and creatinine clearance.

13.18 HELLP Syndrome

HELLP is an acronym for hemolysis, elevated liver enzymes, and low platelets. HELLP syndrome occurs in ~20% of pregnant women diagnosed with severe preeclampsia. It is usually diagnosed between 22 and 36 weeks' gestation. This devastating maternal complication can result in multiorgan failure and death.

The exact cause of HELLP syndrome is unclear. It is thought to happen when RBCs become fragmented as they pass through small damaged blood vessels. Elevated liver enzymes are the result of reduced blood flow to the liver secondary to obstruction from fibrin deposits. Hyperbilirubinemia and jaundice may result from liver impairment. Low platelets result from vascular damage, which is the result of vasospasm, and platelet aggregation at the sites of damage, resulting in thrombocytopenia in multiple sites.

Signs and symptoms of HELLP syndrome include nausea, vomiting, malaise, epigastric pain, upper right quadrant pain, demonstrable edema, hyperbilirubinemia, low hematocrit not explained by any blood loss, elevated LDH, elevated AST, elevated ALT, elevated BUN, elevated bilirubin level, elevated uric acid and creatinine levels, and low platelet count ($< 100{,}000$ cell/mm^3). HELLP syndrome is diagnosed based on lab results.

The treatment for HELLP syndrome is based on the severity of the disease, the gestational age of the fetus, and the condition of the mother and the fetus. The client should be admitted to a tertiary care center with NICU. Magnesium sulfate is used prophylactically to prevent seizures. Hydralazine is given to control blood pressure. Blood component therapy (eg, fresh frozen plasma, packed RBCs, or platelets) is transfused to address the microangiopathic hemolytic anemia. Fluid replacement is managed to avoid worsening of the woman's condition and must be regulated by an infusion pump. Cervical ripening with labor induction is done if the gestation is at least 34 weeks. Delivery may be delayed up to 96 hours so steroids can be given to stimulate fetal lung maturity.

Nursing management of the patient with HELLP syndrome is the same for the woman with severe preeclampsia. Frequent maternal and fetal assessments need to be done and their frequency is related to the severity of the condition. After delivery, most women begin recovering within 72 hours.

13.19 Blood Incompatibility

Rhesus (Rh) factor incompatibility during pregnancy is possible only when the expectant mother is Rh negative and the fetus is Rh positive. For such a circumstance to occur, the father of the baby must be Rh positive. Rh incompatibility is a problem that affects only the fetus and poses no problems for the mother. It occurs in ~15% of Caucasian mothers in the United States, with a lower incidence in African American and Asian populations. It is an autosomal recessive trait.

People who are Rh positive have the antigen on their RBCs, whereas those who are Rh negative do not have the antigen. When blood from an Rh-positive person enters the bloodstream of someone who is Rh negative, the body reacts by producing antibodies to destroy the invading antigen.

Theoretically, maternal and fetal blood do not mix during pregnancy; however, small placental accidents may occur that allow a drop or two of fetal blood to enter the maternal circulation and initiate the production of antibodies to destroy the Rh-positive blood.

Sensitization can also occur during a spontaneous or elective abortion or during antenatal procedures, such as an amniocentesis or chorionic villus sampling. Most exposure happens during the third stage of labor or in complications such as abruptio placentae and placenta previa.

If antibodies are present in the pregnant woman's blood, they cross the placenta and destroy fetal erythrocytes. The fetus becomes deficient in RBCs, which are needed to transport oxygen to fetal tissue. As fetal blood cells are destroyed, fetal bilirubin levels increase, which can lead to neurologic disease. This hemolytic process results in the rapid production of immature RBCs, which cannot carry oxygen. The entire syndrome is called ***erythroblastosis fetalis.*** The fetus may become so anemic that generalized fetal edema results, which may cause fetal congestive heart failure.

At the initial prenatal visit, patients have blood tests to determine their blood type and Rh factor. Anyone who is Rh negative should also have an indirect Coombs test to determine whether she is sensitized (has developed antibodies) as a result of previous exposure to Rh-positive blood. If the indirect Coombs test is negative, it is repeated at 28 weeks' gestation to check if the patient has become sensitized.

Rh(D) immune globulin (RhoGAM) is administered to the unsensitized Rh-negative woman at 28 weeks' gestation to prevent sensitization, which may occur from small leaks in the placenta. RhoGAM effectively prevents the formation of active antibodies against Rh-positive erythrocytes if a small amount of fetal Rh-negative blood enters the circulation of the Rh-negative mother during the remainder of the pregnancy.

Administration of RhoGAM is repeated after birth if the woman delivers an Rh-positive infant. If the indirect Coombs test is positive, indicating maternal sensitization and the presence of antibodies, it is repeated at frequent intervals during the remainder of the pregnancy to determine whether the antibody titer is rising. An increasing titer indicates that the fetus will be in jeopardy.

Ultrasound examination of the fetus will be done. Generalized fetal edema, ascites, enlarged heart, or hydramnios indicates fetal compromise. A cordocentesis may be performed to evaluate the fetal hematocrit, and an intrauterine transfusion may follow if the preterm infant is anemic.

ABO incompatibility occurs when the mother is blood type O and the fetus's blood type is A, B, or AB. Types A, B, and AB have a protein component (antigen) that is not present in type O blood. People with blood type O develop anti-A or anti-B antibodies naturally occurring as a result of exposure to antigens in the foods that they eat or to infection by gram-positive bacteria.

No specific prenatal care is required; however, the patient should be made aware that ABO incompatibility may occur. ABO incompatibility can result in hyperbilirubinemia in the infant. It usually poses no serious health threat to the child.

13.20 Infections During Pregnancy

A number of different infections can adversely affect the health of the fetus, the mother, or both when acquired during pregnancy.

Pregnancy does not worsen the effects of most viral infections in the woman, but they can be lethal for the fetus. Maternal infection with cytomegalovirus (CMV), rubella, varicella-zoster virus, herpes simplex, hepatitis B, and HIV have the greatest potential for harm to the fetus or newborn.

CMV is a member of the herpes group. It is widespread and eventually affects most humans. It has been isolated from urine, saliva, cervical mucus, semen, breast milk, and stool. The greatest rate of infection is seen during the childbearing years. Day care centers are a common place for transmission of CMV among children, especially toddlers, so mothers who may have a child in day care need to be aware that their child can acquire an infection and transmit it to someone who has not had a primary infection.

If a woman develops a primary CMV infection during pregnancy, her fetus has a 40% to 50% chance of being infected. Of affected fetuses, 5% to 18% are symptomatic at birth, having problems such as an enlarged spleen and liver, CNS abnormalities, jaundice, chorioretinitis, hearing loss, and IUGR. Another 10% to 15% will develop manifestations within the first 2 years of life. No effective therapy exists. Primary prevention, such as hand washing, warning of the risks of having several sexual partners, and transfusing filtered CMV-free blood, is most effective.

Rubella is caused by a virus transmitted from person to person by droplets or through direct contact with articles containing contaminated nasopharyngeal secretions. Rubella is a mild disease. Major symptoms include fever, general malaise, and a characteristic maculopapular rash that begins on the face and migrates over the body.

Rubella virus from the mother can cross the placenta and affect the fetus at any time. The greatest risk to the fetus is during the first trimester, when fetal organs are developing. If maternal infection occurs at this time, approximately one third of these cases will end in spontaneous abortions, and the remaining fetuses may be seriously compromised. Deafness, mental retardation, cataracts, cardiac defects, IUGR, and microcephaly are the most common fetal complications.

Prevention is the only effective protection for the fetus. Women who are immune do not become infected, so determining the immune status of women of childbearing age is important. Immune status assays such as ELISA (enzyme-linked immunosorbent assay) have replaced older serologic tests to determine rubella immunity.

Women who are not immune should be vaccinated before they become pregnant; furthermore, they should be advised not to become pregnant for 4 weeks after the immunization because it is a live virus and can do damage to a fetus. Pregnant women who are not immune will be given the vaccine on the postpartum unit before discharge.

Varicella-zoster virus (chickenpox) is caused by the varicella-zoster virus, a herpes virus that is transmitted by direct contact or through the respiratory tract. After the primary infection, the virus can become latent in the nerve ganglia. If the virus is reactivated, shingles may erupt.

Maternal complications of acute varicella infection include preterm labor, encephalitis, and varicella pneumonia. Fetal and neonatal effects depend on the time of maternal infection. If the infection occurs during the first trimester, the fetus has a small risk of congenital varicella syndrome. Clinical findings include limb hypoplasia, cutaneous scars, chorioretinitis, cataracts, microcephaly, and IUGR. In later pregnancy, transplacental passage usually protects the fetus. However, in the period from 5 days before to 2 days after birth, if the infant is infected, he or she will not have the benefit of the maternal antibodies and is at risk for life-threatening varicella infection.

Immune testing may be recommended for a pregnant woman at risk. Varicella-zoster immune globulin (VZIG) should be administered to women who have been exposed. Those infected with varicella-zoster during pregnancy should be instructed to report pulmonary symptoms immediately. Hospitalization and hemodynamic monitoring should be available for women with varicella pneumonia because it may become severe in a short time. Acyclovir is the primary drug used to treat varicella pneumonia.

For infants born to mothers infected with varicella during the perinatal period, immunization with VZIG as soon as possible but within 96 hours of birth provides passive immunity against varicella. Women and infants with varicella are very contagious and should be placed in strict isolation. Only staff members known to be immune should come in contact with these patients.

If a female of childbearing age is to be vaccinated, she should be instructed not to become pregnant for at least 1 month after the two vaccinations, which are given 4 to 8 weeks apart. Nonimmune health care workers should be immunized also.

Genital herpes is one of the most common sexually transmitted diseases in the herpes simplex virus (HSV) group. It may be caused by HSV type 1 or 2. HSV infection occurs as a result of direct contact with the skin or mucous membranes with an active lesion.

Vertical transmission of the virus from mother to child occurs either by the virus ascending to the fetus after rupture of membranes or during birth, when the fetus comes into contact with infectious genital secretions or the fetal skin is punctured, such as with a scalp electrode.

Diagnosis is based on clinical signs and symptoms. Definitive diagnosis requires a culture for the virus from an active lesion. Complication in pregnancy from a recurrent infection is rare. Primary infection is more serious. The rates of spontaneous abortion, IUGR, and preterm labor increase. Neonatal herpes infection is rare but can be lethal. The infant may have an infection that is limited to skin lesions or can be systemic. Symptoms usually appear during the first week, but the disease progresses rapidly. The likelihood of death or serious sequelae for infants who have systemic herpes infection is ~50%.

No known cure for herpes exists, although antiviral medication (acyclovir) is prescribed to reduce symptoms and shorten the duration of the lesions. Acyclovir may be given during late pregnancy to a woman with recurrent outbreaks to reduce the possibility that she will have an active lesion at birth.

For women with a history of genital herpes, vaginal delivery is allowed as long as there are no genital lesions at the time of labor. Cesarean birth is recommended for women with active lesions at the time of labor.

Isolation of the mother from her infant is not necessary after birth if the mother uses careful hand washing, and the infant is not in direct contact with any lesions. The baby may breastfeed if there are no lesions on the breasts. The infant must be monitored carefully for signs of infection, including temperature regulation instability, lethargy, poor suck, jaundice, seizures, and lesions. Acyclovir therapy is prescribed for neonatal infection with herpes.

Parvovirus 19 (erythema infectiosum), also known as ***Fifth disease,*** is an acute communicable disease characterized by a highly distinctive rash. The rash starts on the face with a "slapped cheek" appearance, followed by a maculopapular rash. Other symptoms are fever, malaise, and joint pain.

When infection occurs during pregnancy, fetal death can occur, usually from failure of fetal RBC production, followed by severe fetal anemia, hydrops (generalized edema), and heart failure.

Intrauterine transfusion is an option to treat severe fetal anemia if it does not spontaneously resolve. The affected infant will be followed closely to identify delayed complications. No specific treatment exists. Starch baths may help the pruritis. Analgesics may be needed for relief of joint pain.

Toxoplasmosis is a nonviral infection transmitted though organisms in raw and undercooked meat, through infected cat feces, and across the placental barrier to the fetus if the expectant mother acquires the infection during pregnancy.

Toxoplasmosis is often subclinical. The mother may experience a few days of malaise, fatigue, muscle pains, and swollen glands but be unaware of the disease. Diagnosis is confirmed by positive serologic tests. Although the mother experiences mild symptoms, toxoplasmosis may cause abortion or result in the birth of a live born infant infected with the disease. Approximately 40% of infants born to mothers with an acute primary infection during pregnancy acquire congenital toxoplasmosis. About 50% of infants are asymptomatic at birth, but others have serious effects, such as low birth weight, enlarged liver and spleen, jaundice, anemia, and coagulation disorders. Severe complications may develop several years after birth, including blindness, deafness, seizures, hydrocephalus, and microcephaly. Maternal treatment of toxoplasmosis during pregnancy is essential to reduce the risk of congenital infection. Sulfonamides are used to treat toxoplasmosis.

Group B streptococcus (GBS) is a cause of life-threatening perinatal infection in the United States. The gram-positive bacterium colonizes the rectum, vagina, cervix, and urethra of pregnant and nonpregnant women. Approximately 10% to 30% of pregnant women are colonized with GBS in the vaginal or rectal area, but isolating the organism is difficult.

Early-onset GBS disease occurs during the first week after birth, often within 48 hours. Women who have a positive GBS status at the time of birth have a 60% chance of transmitting the organism to the infant at birth. One percent to 2% of these infants will develop early-onset GBS disease. Sepsis, pneumonia, and meningitis are the primary infections in early-onset disease. Late-onset disease happens after the first week of life, and meningitis is the most common clinical manifestation.

Identification of GBS status is by prenatal screening cultures (vaginal and rectal) obtained between 35 and 37 weeks' gestation.

Penicillin is the drug of choice to treat the infection during labor. Ampicillin is an acceptable alternative. Typically, the first dose of ampicillin (2 g) is given intravenously upon admission to the labor and delivery room. The patient then receives 1 g of ampicillin every 4 hours until she delivers, according to the Centers for Disease Control and Prevention and the American Academy of Pediatric guidelines. The newborn's vital signs are monitored closely every 4 hours, along with close observation for signs and symptoms of infection.

13.21 Sexually Transmitted Infections

Syphilis, caused by *Treponema pallidum,* in a pregnant woman increases the risk of premature labor and birth. Newborns may be born with congenital syphilis, which includes jaundice, rhinitis, anemia, IUGR, and CNS involvement. All pregnant women should be screened for this sexually transmitted infection (STI) and treated with benzathine penicillin G, 2.4 million units intramuscularly (IM), to prevent placental transmission. It is important that partners of the pregnant woman be treated as well to prevent reinfection.

Pregnant women with ***gonorrhea,*** caused by *Neisseria gonorrhoeae,* are asymptomatic. All patients are screened at the first prenatal visit, with repeat screening in the third trimester. Those who test positive are treated with ceftriaxone (Rocephin), 125 mg IM, in a single dose. All infants in the United States receive mandatory eye prophylaxis (erythromycin ointment) within the first hour of life. The nurse should postpone the administration of the eye medication for a short period after delivery, however, so the infant can bond with the parents. If untreated, gonorrhea causes ophthalmia neonatorum in the newborn.

The pregnant woman with a ***chlamydia*** (*Chlamydia trachomatis*) infection is usually asymptomatic. This infection is associated with infertility and ectopic pregnancy, spontaneous abortions, preterm labor, PROM, low birth weight, stillbirth, and neonatal mortality. Infection is transmitted to the infant through vaginal birth. A neonate may develop conjunctivitis or pneumonia. All pregnant women are screened at the first prenatal visit and treated with erythromycin.

Human papilloma virus (HPV), also known as condylomata acuminata, infection causes warts in the anogenital area. These warts may grow large enough to block a vaginal birth. Fetal exposure to HPV during birth is associated with laryngeal papillomas. Warts are treated with trichloroacetic acid, liquid nitrogen, or laser therapy under colposcopy.

A ***Trichomonas*** (*Trichomonas vaginalis*) infection causes burning, itching, dysuria, strawberry patches on the cervix, and a foul-smelling green discharge. Infection is associated with PROM and premature birth. Treatment is with a single 2 g dose of metronidazole (Flagyl).

The nurse should provide information to the client with an STI in a nonjudgmental fashion. Many women may be embarrassed, angry, anxious, or fearful that something may happen to the fetus. The nurse can provide teaching and emotional support. It is important for the nurse to emphasize that the woman needs to tell any sexual partners she may have had so that they may be screened and treated, and to prevent reinfection.

13.22 Hydramnios

Hydramnios, also called polyhydramnios, is a condition in which there is too much amniotic fluid (≥2,000 mL) surrounding the fetus between 32 and 36 weeks' gestation. It occurs in ~3% to 4% of all pregnancies and is associated with fetal anomalies of development. It is associated with poor fetal outcomes because of the increased incidence of preterm birth, fetal malpresentation, and cord prolapse.

There are several causes of hydramnios. Common factors associated with hydramnios are maternal diabetes, fetal esophageal atresia, fetal intestinal atresia, neural tube defects, multiple gestation, chromosomal deviations, fetal hydrops, CNS defects, cardiovascular anomalies, and hydrocephaly.

Diagnosis is made after a thorough history and physical exam, as well as an ultrasound exam in which amniotic fluid pockets are measured. In hydramnios there is a discrepancy between fundal height measurements and weeks of gestation. The patient may complain of shortness of breath and of her abdomen being severely stretched or "tight," and she may have edema in the lower extremities.

Treatment includes close monitoring and frequent visits to the health care provider. In severe cases, an amniocentesis may be ordered, or rupture of the membranes may be done to relieve pressure and lower the amount of fluid.

Nursing care includes teaching the patient that this condition can cause her uterus to become overdistended and may lead to premature labor and PROM. The patient needs to be instructed to look for the signs and symptoms of both conditions and to call the health care provider if they do occur.

13.23 Oligohydramnios

Oligohydramnios is a decreased amount of amniotic fluid (≤500 mL) between 32 and 36 weeks' gestation. This condition predisposes the fetus to increased risk of perinatal mortality and morbidity. Reduction in amniotic fluid reduces the ability of the fetus to move freely and without risk of cord compression, which increases the risk of fetal death and intrapartal hypoxia.

Factors associated with oligohydramnios include uteroplacental insufficiency, PROM prior to the onset of labor, hypertension of pregnancy, maternal diabetes, intrauterine growth restriction, postterm pregnancy, fetal renal agenesis, polycystic kidneys, and urinary tract obstructions.

Diagnosis is often made by ultrasound, as the woman may not present with any symptoms.

The woman with oligohydramnios is often managed on an outpatient basis with serial ultrasounds and fetal surveillance through NSTs and biophysical profiles. As long as there is no fetal compromise, no intervention is needed. If fetal well-being is compromised, delivery is planned, along with amnioinfusion (the transvaginal infusion of crystalloid fluid to compensate for the loss of amniotic fluid).

Nursing care for the woman with oligohydramnios includes continuous monitoring of fetal well-being during NSTs or during labor and birth. After birth, the nurse needs to assess the newborn for signs of postmaturity, congenital anomalies, and respiratory difficulty.

13.24 Multiple Gestation

Multiple gestation is defined as more than one fetus developing in the uterus. It is a concern because women who are expecting more than one infant are at a higher risk for preterm labor, hydramnios, hyperemesis gravidarum, anemia, preeclampsia, and antepartum hemorrhage. Fetal/newborn risks include prematurity, respiratory distress syndrome, birth asphyxia, congenital anomalies, twin-to-twin transfusion syndrome, IUGR, and becoming conjoined twins.

Clinically, the woman's uterus will be larger than that associated with her estimated date of birth. Anemia, fatigue, and severe nausea and vomiting also may be present. The diagnosis of multiple gestation is made by ultrasound early in the pregnancy.

The treatment for a woman with multiple gestation begins from diagnosis with serial ultrasounds to determine fetal growth patterns and development of the fetuses. Biophysical profiles as well as NSTs will be instituted to determine fetal well-being. Operative birth is often needed due to malpresentation.

Care for the patient with a multiple gestation pregnancy includes education and support for the woman and family. The nurse needs to teach the patient about nutritional needs, encourage increased rest periods, and observe closely for pregnancy complications.

The woman should be alerted to the signs and symptoms of preterm labor, including contractions, low back pain, increased vaginal discharge, loss of the mucus plug, pelvic pain, and pressure. She should be instructed to call her health care provider if any of these conditions occur.

13.25 Intimate Partner Violence

Intimate partner violence is actual or threatened physical or sexual violence or psychological/emotional abuse. It includes threats of physical or sexual violence when the threat is used to control a person's actions.

Women are at risk for being abused at every stage of their lives, and no one group of women escapes intimate partner violence. Pregnancy does not protect women from being abused, and it often exacerbates tension between the victim and abuser. The strongest predictor for being abused during pregnancy is prior abuse.

Millions of women are abused annually, and this has far-reaching consequences for all of society. One in four women in the United States has been physically or sexually abused by an intimate partner. In some parts of the world, it is considered normal behavior.

The long-term effects of violence on victims and children can be profound. Children who witness one parent abuse the other are more likely to become delinquent or to become batterers themselves.

In 50% to 75% of cases where a parent is abused, the children will be also. Exposure to violence has a negative impact on children's physical, mental, emotional, and cognitive well-being. Most children grow up with feelings of anger, anxiety, fear, inadequacy, hostility, rage, and guilt. They often lack impulse control, blame others, and generally struggle with authority. Violence is a learned behavior and cyclic in nature. Unless the cycle is broken, more than half of abused people become abusers themselves.

In an abusive relationship, the cycle of violence includes three distinct phases:

1. Tension-building phase
2. Acute battering phase
3. "Honeymoon" phase

The nurse may be the first health care professional to discover the signs and symptoms of intimate partner violence and can have a profound impact on a woman's decision to seek help. It is important for nurses to be able to identify abuse and help the victim. Often a woman who has been the victim of violence will complain about physical ailments that will give her the opportunity to visit a health care setting. Because nurses are viewed as trustworthy and sensitive about very personal subjects, women often feel confident in discussing these issues with them.

The nurse needs to isolate the patient if abuse is suspected. Assisting the woman in acknowledging what has happened to her helps her begin to deal with the situation. The nurse needs to emphasize to the patient that she has the right not to be abused. Direct and indirect questioning can be appropriate in assessing the patient's needs.

Communicating support through a nonjudgmental attitude is the next step in establishing trust and rapport. Accurate documentation is critical because this evidence may be used to support the woman in a court case. Documentation must include details as to the frequency of abuse; the severity of the abuse; the location, extent, and outcome of injuries; and a description of treatments. When documenting, use direct quotes made by the victim. Laws in many states require that health care providers alert the police to any injuries that involve knives, firearms, or other deadly weapons or that present life-threatening emergencies.

The goal of intervention is to enable the victim to gain control of her life. The nurse should be aware of support opportunities in the community and encourage the patient to take advantage of them. Support may include counseling, legal advice, social services, support groups, hotlines, crisis intervention services, housing, and vocational training.

The choice to leave an abuser must rest with the victim. The nurse cannot force the woman to leave an unsafe situation. Instead, the nurse can help the woman formulate a "safety plan" by which the victim can leave in an emergency situation. Having a bag packed with an extra set of keys, putting money away, keeping an extra set of clothing in a separate location, and having a friend or neighbor who can be "on call" for the woman are steps in such a plan.

13.26 Female Genital Mutilation

Female genital mutilation, also known as ***female circumcision,*** is a cultural practice carried out in Africa, the Middle East, and Asia. Female circumcision is not practiced in most parts of the world.

The World Health Organization (WHO) defines female genital mutilation as all procedures involving the partial or total removal or other injury to the female genital organs, whether for cultural or other nontherapeutic purposes. Reasons for performing the ritual reflect the ideology and cultural values of each community that practices it and are not part of any religious texts.

Female genital mutilation is usually performed when the girl is a minor, often between the ages of 4 and 10 years. In its mildest form, the clitoris is partially or totally removed. In the most extreme case, called infibulation, the clitoris, labia majora, labia minora, and urethral and vaginal openings are cut away and then stitched tightly, leaving a small hole for menstruation and urination.

Untrained practitioners often perform the procedure, done without anesthesia. In addition to experiencing extreme pain, the procedure puts the girl at risk for many health problems, including pelvic infection; hemorrhage; HIV infection; damage to the urethra, vagina, and anus; incontinence; dermoid cysts; vulvar abscesses; keloid formation; dysmenorrhea; dyspareunia; panic attacks; posttraumatic stress disorder; and increased morbidity and mortality.

Helping the woman who has had one of these procedures done requires good communication skills and often an interpreter, as the patient may not speak English. The nurse should remember to look at the patient, not the interpreter, and encourage her to express herself freely. The nurse needs to remember to maintain strict confidentiality and provide culturally competent care to all women.

13.27 Trauma and Pregnancy

Two types of trauma may affect the pregnant woman—blunt force injuries and penetrating injuries.

Automobile accidents cause the majority of ***blunt force injuries***. Maternal deaths are usually caused by head injury or intra-abdominal hemorrhage. Fetal death may be secondary to maternal death or may follow sudden premature separation of the placenta or rupture of the uterus. During the first trimester, the fetus is protected from external forces by the bony pelvis, amniotic fluid, and soft tissue surrounding the pelvis. Later in pregnancy, the fetal compartment extends beyond the bony pelvis, and the fetus is more susceptible to damage from blunt force.

Use of a seat belt significantly improves maternal and fetal outcomes in automobile accidents. The nurse needs to instruct the pregnant patient on how to wear a seat belt restraint. Current recommendations advise using a three-point restraint seat belt, with the lap belt under the woman's protruding abdomen.

Gunshots and knife wounds are the most common ***penetrating injuries*** and may be associated with assaults or suicide attempts. The abdomen acts as a protective shield for the pregnant woman; however, the fetus does poorly with this type of injury.

Initial management of trauma in pregnancy is similar to that in the nonpregnant state. Primary goals are evaluation and stabilization of maternal injuries. Because placental abruption occurs soon after trauma, electronic monitoring is begun as soon as possible. Ultrasonography provides additional information about the fetal condition. The need for cesarean delivery of a live fetus depends on several factors, including the age of the fetus, fetal condition, and extent of uterine damage. Antibiotics, RhoGAM, and tetanus immunizations are given as indicated.

The nurse needs to provide emotional support to the patient experiencing trauma, as she will be anxious and fearful of losing her baby. Explaining what is happening and allowing the patient to ask questions are essential to the care of the pregnant woman at this time.

13.28 Substance Abuse

Drug use in pregnancy, with its associated problems, has become a major public health issue. Polydrug use, such as alcohol and tobacco with marijuana or cocaine, has become more common. Illegal drugs are used by over 9 million women in the United States. Half of the women of childbearing age have taken illegal drugs at least once in their lifetime. The incidence of substance abuse during pregnancy is estimated at 5% to 15% and occurs in women of all ages, races, ethnicities, and social groups. A disproportionately high incidence of teen pregnancy associated with substance abuse is especially prevalent among those who live in poverty.

The first 8 weeks of pregnancy are the most critical time in terms of embryonic development. During the third trimester, drug use has the greatest potential for impairing fetal growth. Drugs taken orally might reduce the drug's ability to cross the placenta. Drugs taken intravenously or intranasally more readily cross the placenta. IV drug use increases maternal and fetal exposure to HIV.

Many medical conditions, including anemia, bacteremia/septicemia, cardiac disease, cellulitis, depression, diabetes, edema, hepatitis B and C, TB, hypertension, phlebitis, STIs, urinary tract infections, and vitamin deficiency, compromise many drug-involved pregnancies. Obstetric complications include abruptio placentae, placenta previa, intrauterine death, spontaneous abortion, premature labor and delivery, PROM, polyhydramnios, and IUGR.

Effects on the fetus include generalized growth restriction and its associated complications, along with an increase in sudden infant death syndrome (SIDS). Signs of withdrawal that can occur from birth to 6 days of life include a high-pitched or shrill cry, gastrointestinal disturbances (vomiting, diarrhea, and excessive sucking), tremulousness, excoriation of the knees and elbows from increased restlessness and sleeplessness, perianal excoriation (chemical dermatitis due to acidic stool), respiratory restlessness (tachypnea, nasal congestion, frequent yawning, and sneezing), and seizure activity.

Specific drugs and their effects to the fetus are as follows:

Marijuana (also known as pot, weed, grass, reefer, herb, Mary Jane, or MJ) is the most commonly used illicit drug. Marijuana causes tachycardia and decreased blood pressure, resulting in orthostatic hypotension. Research has shown that babies born to women who used marijuana during pregnancy display altered responses to visual stimuli, increased tremulousness, and a high-pitched cry, which might indicate problems with neurologic development.

Cocaine use is second only to marijuana in pregnant women who used an illicit drug during pregnancy. The incidence of cocaine exposure is 1 to 10 per 1,000 live births. Cocaine readily crosses the placenta by diffusion. It blocks the reuptake of catecholamines at nerve terminals, which increases the level of catecholamines in the blood, resulting in vasoconstriction, tachycardia, hypertension, and uterine contractions.

Hypertension, myocardial ischemia, sudden death, dysrhythmias, subarachnoid hemorrhage, and seizures have been described among women who abuse cocaine. Acute cocaine use during the third trimester can result in PROM, preterm labor, abruptio placentae, an increased incidence of meconium staining, and precipitous delivery.

Fetal anomalies involving the upper limbs and neurologic (myelomeningocele, microcephaly, and growth restriction), cardiovascular (congenital heart defects), genitourinary ("prune belly" syndrome, hydronephrosis, and ambiguous genitalia), and gastrointestinal (ilea atresia and necrotizing enterocolitis) systems have been attributed to cocaine use in early pregnancy.

Heroin easily crosses the placenta via simple diffusion. Signs and symptoms of early pregnancy might be confused with heroin use (fatigue, nausea, vomiting, and pelvic cramping)

Heroin causes analgesia, sedation, a feeling of well-being, and euphoria in the woman. Users typically do not attend to early prenatal care because of fear of detection or because of the absence of regular menstrual periods as an effect of the drug. There is also an increased incidence of STIs in women who abuse heroin.

Heroin is not thought to be a teratogen capable of producing congenital malformation. Hazards of heroin to the fetus include severe neonatal abstinence syndrome, with a possibility of withdrawal symptoms lasting up to 6 months; increased incidence of meconium staining at birth; an increased incidence of neonatal sepsis; symmetric IUGR; and neurobehavioral problems (tremulousness and irritability, poor responses to stimuli, poor motor control, difficulty in consoling, and poor suck and swallow coordination, which leads to poor feeding tolerance).

Methadone is frequently used to treat pregnant heroin-dependent women to prevent repeated episodes of heroin withdrawal in the fetus. In the woman it acts to block the craving of withdrawal. It helps decrease maternal complications and prematurity and low birth weight.

Methadone treatment requires enrollment in a drug-treatment program, thereby increasing the likelihood of prenatal care. Women on methadone may breastfeed if not infected with HIV, hepatitis, or TB. The long-term effects on the neonate have not been determined.

Alcohol is the most commonly used drug overall and is the drug of choice for teenagers. Fetal alcohol syndrome (FAS) is estimated to occur at the rate of 1 to 2 in 1000 live births in the United States, and fetal alcohol effects are seen in 4 in 1000 live births.

Prenatal exposure to alcohol is one of the leading preventable causes of birth defects, mental retardation, and neurodevelopment disorders. Alcohol in a pregnant woman's bloodstream circulates to the fetus by crossing the placenta and interferes with the ability of the fetus to receive sufficient oxygen and nourishment for normal cell development in the brain and other body organs.

Current data do not support the concept of a "safe level" of alcohol consumption by pregnant women below which no damage to the fetus will occur. The American Academy of Pediatrics recommends that all pregnant women and women who are planning to become pregnant not drink alcohol.

FAS refers to a constellation of physical, behavioral, and cognitive abnormalities. The exact mechanism by which alcohol damages the fetus and critical times of exposure are not known. However, exposure during the first trimester results in the structural defects characteristic of FAS, whereas growth and CNS disturbances could occur from alcohol use at any time.

Possible FAS manifestations include attention deficits, cardiac defects, cleft lip or palate, delayed motor and speech development, flat midface, fusion of cerebral vertebrae, hyperactivity, kidney defects, learning disabilities, microcephaly, mild to moderate mental retardation, poor coordination, poor suck, prenatal and postnatal growth restriction, retarded bone growth, small eye openings, sleep disturbances, small stature, strabismus, ptosis, myopia, and thin upper lip.

Cigarette smoking is the chief, single avoidable cause of death. Tobacco use occurs in ~25% of all pregnancies in the United States.

Nicotine is linked to dependency in the woman and increased spontaneous abortions. The vasoconstrictive property of nicotine causes increased maternal heart rate and blood pressure. Also, poor nutritional states are associated with cigarette smoking due to the known anorexigenic effect of nicotine. Smoking also increases the mother's risk of hemorrhage, sepsis, bronchitis, lung cancer, and depletion of vitamin C, which is needed to produce collagen and enhances absorption of iron.

For the fetus, there is blood flow restriction to the placenta, which results in decreased oxygen. Research has established that maternal smoking during pregnancy adversely affects prenatal and postnatal growth and cognitive development and is linked to SIDS, stillbirth, low birth weight, low Apgar scores, increased frequency of apnea, and neurobehavioral effects.

The nurse needs to provide a nonjudgmental, concerned, and empathetic environment for the patient abusing drugs. He or she should encourage the patient to express her feelings and concerns about herself, her drug use, and her unborn child. The nurse can dispel myths that drugs, alcohol, and smoking are harmless and can educate the patient on the potential dangers to both mother and baby. The health care facility should provide easily understood printed information for patients to take home for referral. Additionally, patients should be referred to specialized programs that address their medical, obstetric, psychological, neonatal, and pediatric needs. Involvement of a patient's family and friends can help a patient during the pregnancy and recovery process. Most importantly, the nurse should emphasize that quitting or decreasing drug use at any time during pregnancy improves obstetric outcomes.

13.29 Surgery During Pregnancy

The incidence of ***nonobstetric surgery*** performed during pregnancy ranges from 1% to 2% in the United States. Laparoscopy for appendicitis is the most common first-trimester procedure. Other situations that may result in surgery during pregnancy are acute cholecystitis, intestinal obstruction, trauma with visceral injury, ruptured aneurysms, peptic ulcer, rectal cancer, breast tumors or other malignancies, and cardiac or neurologic conditions. Gynecologic reasons for surgery include incompetent cervix, ovarian cyst, torsion of a fallopian tube, ovarian abscess, and uterine myoma. Intrauterine fetal surgery as an intervention for certain prenatal congenital defects may be done.

Surgery puts the pregnant woman at a higher risk for spontaneous abortion in the first trimester and at a higher risk for preterm labor in the second trimester. The increased risks for the fetus include effects of maternal disease or treatment modalities, possible teratogenicity of anesthetic agents, intraoperative decrease in uteroplacental flow, and increased risk of preterm delivery.

The nurse should take special precautions with the pregnant patient during surgery. Placing the woman in a left lateral position, if at all possible, or placing the woman with a wedge under the right hip, displacing the uterus to the left, would be appropriate to prevent venacaval compression (can lead to uteroplacental insufficiency). If feasible, fetal heart rate monitoring in the operating room should be done and in the immediate postoperative period to detect any need for administration of tocolytic agents. Normal postoperative care should be followed with periodic obstetric evaluation.

13.30 Perinatal Loss

When perinatal loss occurs, women are especially vulnerable. Not only do they experience psychological trauma, but they must also cope with physiologic changes. Perinatal loss can be divided into two major types: death of the fetus or newborn and birth of a "less than perfect" child.

Death occurring before the onset of labor is referred to as fetal death or stillbirth. Neonatal death occurs in the period from birth to 28 days of life.

Before the diagnosis of fetal death, parents often know that "something isn't right." There may be no fetal movement, or tests may show adverse results. This allows parents time for anticipatory grief, or time to begin the grieving process before the event. Anticipatory grief also occurs when the infant is critically ill.

If the death occurs before birth, it is often only the woman who has bonded to the child. If the death occurs several days after birth, people other than the mother have an opportunity to become attached to the newborn. The father of the neonate, the grandparents, siblings, and other family members may feel a tremendous sense of loss.

Bereavement is not limited to death or pregnancy loss. It can be experienced when the pregnancy results in a newborn who is seriously ill. In such a situation, the parents grieve the loss of the fantasized perfect infant. They may have difficulty attaching to the newborn until there is evidence that the baby will survive. The nurse must understand this process and support the parents in their emotional work of bonding to a sick newborn. A similar process may occur if the newborn has anomalies.

It is not uncommon for parents to have definite ideas and fantasies about the preferred sex of their child. In some ethnic groups, it is essential to produce male children. When a child of the "wrong sex" is born, parents may need time to adjust to the idea. Some parents become permanently estranged from the child, creating significant psychological problems.

When the nurse becomes aware that the sex of the baby is a critical issue, he or she needs to encourage the parents to become involved in the care of the child. This include offering positive feedback on their caretaking. By demonstrating acceptance, the nurse can promote attitudinal change toward acceptance of the child. Not all situations can be corrected, but most can be improved.

Placing a newborn up for adoption involves issues of loss and bereavement. This process, called relinquishment, contains aspects of the general bereavement process and of chronic sorrow. The nurses should be nonjudgmental and convey an understanding that this decision takes great courage and is based on the best interests of the child. Appropriate nursing care during this period allows a woman to sort through her feelings and accept the decision she is making.

Ectopic pregnancy is an example of multiple losses occurring in a single event. Even though it is an early loss, the pregnancy may have been planned and highly desired, and the subsequent grief can be significant. Also, a tubal pregnancy sometimes results in the loss of the tube and a possible loss of fertility. This combination of losses can be extremely difficult for a woman.

With the death of a newborn, the parents' needs and strengths must be assessed. This is followed by establishing priorities and nursing interventions. Physical comfort and support measures are necessary throughout the grieving process. The nurse can encourage the parents to see and hold the dead newborn and to take photographs if they so desire. Family members should be provided a chance to see and hold the newborn, if the parents permit. However, the parents should not be forced to do any of these things. The patient should be allowed to make the choice as to whether or not she would like to be placed on the postpartum unit or be discharged from the labor and delivery unit, providing there is room for her there. The nurse should speak of the newborn by its intended name and should encourage the support of family and friends for the grieving parents.

Mementos can help in the process of grief and healing. Footprints, ID bands, a photo, and a lock of the baby's hair should be assembled and placed in a memory box. The parents can be offered this box upon discharge. Many parents refuse initially, but they will often call a birth facility months later to ask about these remembrances. Generally, birth facilities keep these memory boxes for 1 year in case parents request them at a later date.

Spiritual counseling should be provided for the parents and family. A clergy person should be contacted to meet with the family. A social worker should be contacted to alert parents to various support groups and community resources available to them.

The parents should be encouraged to acknowledge with other children their feelings of sadness and fear. They should assure the siblings that they in no way caused the death of the baby.

The nurse can provide for follow-up care for the mother to ensure ongoing assessment and support after birth facility discharge. For example, the nurse can schedule the postpartum physician appointment on a day when general gynecologic patients are being seen so the mother is not exposed to many pregnant women in the office. The nurse can also alert parents to be prepared for what may seem like thoughtless comments by some people on learning of the death of the newborn. Follow-up phone calls after discharge may be beneficial to the patient.

Review Questions

True/False

1. _______ The goal of risk assessment during pregnancy is to identify women and fetuses at risk in order to provide appropriate care and enhance perinatal outcomes.

2. _______ Anemia indicates inadequate hemoglobin in the blood.

3. _______ Iron deficiency anemia is the most common medical complication of pregnancy.

4. _______ A pregnant woman needs to take an extra 500 mg of iron daily.

5. _______ An inadequate intake of folic acid is associated with neural tube defects in the newborn.

6. _______ The best sources of folic acid are orange juice, green leafy vegetables, red meats, poultry, and legumes.

7. _______ Sickle cell anemia is an autosomal dominant disorder.

8. _______ Pregnant women with sickle cell anemia have a poor prognosis even if they have adequate nutrition and prenatal care.

9. _______ The incidence of prematurity, low birth weight, and neonatal death increases when the mother has hepatitis B.

10. _______ Mothers who are HIV positive will automatically infect their newborns.

11. _______ Prevention is the only way to control HIV infection.

12. _______ Although the overall mortality rate of heart disease has decreased, it remains a major cause of maternal mortality.

13. _______ All women with cardiac disease require 8 to 10 hours of sleep nightly.

14. _______ Stress management should be discussed with women with heart disease.

15. _______ Intrauterine growth restriction is common in infants of women with preeclampsia.

16. _______ Asthma complicates 10% of pregnancies.

17. _______ All mothers with tuberculosis (TB) cannot breastfeed their newborns.

18. _______ Seizures may occur in pregnancy even if the woman has been seizure-free for many years.

19. _______ Women with epilepsy have a higher than normal incidence of stillbirth and preterm labors.

20. _______ Women with multiple sclerosis usually have an exacerbation of the condition during pregnancy.

21. _______ Marked improvement in symptoms of rheumatoid arthritis often occurs during pregnancy.

22. _______ Depression and anxiety in women are seen at their highest rates during the childbearing years.

23. _______ Untreated maternal mental illness can impair mother–infant attachment.

24. _______ Research demonstrates that obesity increases the risk of adverse outcomes for both mother and infant.

25. _______ The rate of teenage pregnancy in the United States is currently the highest of any industrialized nation.

26. _______ In cases of spontaneous abortion, there is unexplained bleeding, cramping, and backache.

27. _______ The classic sign of placenta previa is painful vaginal bleeding occurring after 20 weeks' gestation.

28. _______ The defining physiologic mechanism that triggers premature labor is unknown.

29. _______ Vasospasm and hyperperfusion are the underlying mechanisms of preeclampsia.

30. _______ Severe preeclampsia can develop suddenly.

31. _______ Clonus confirms central nervous system involvement in the patient with preeclampsia.

32. _______ The HELLP syndrome is diagnosed based on lab findings.

33. _______ Rubella can cause mental retardation in fetuses.

34. _______ Acyclovir is the primary drug used to treat varicella pneumonia.

35. _______ Isolation of the mother with active herpes lesions from her infant is necessary.

36. _______ Toxoplasmosis is a nonviral infection transmitted through undercooked meat and infected cat feces.

37. _______ Group B streptococcus (GBS) in the newborn is not dangerous.

38. _______ Chlamydia infections are associated with infertility.

39. _______ Polyhydramnios is associated with diabetes in pregnancy.

40. _______ Intimate partner violence only affects only low-income women.

41. _______ Female circumcision is not practiced in most parts of the world.

42. _______ Use of seat belts by pregnant women significantly improves maternal and fetal outcomes in automobile accidents.

43. _______ The fetus usually does well in cases of penetrating injuries.

44. _______ Drug abuse is not a major problem for pregnant women in the United States.

45. _______ Cocaine use causes tachycardia, hypertension, and uterine contractions in the pregnant woman.

46. _______ Heroin is not thought to be a teratogen capable of producing congenital malformation.

47. _______ A woman on methadone cannot breastfeed.

48. _______ Prenatal exposure to alcohol is one of the leading preventable causes of birth defects.

49. _______ Infants born to mothers who smoke are at a greater risk for sudden infant death syndrome (SIDS).

50. _______ Mothers who relinquish their infants to adoption experience grief.

Completion

1. Women need approximately _______________ more iron intake during pregnancy.

2. _______________ and _____________ in newborns are associated with sickle cell anemia.

3. Thalassemia is an autosomal _______________ disorder.

4. _______________is recommended for preventing transmission of HIV to the newborn.

5. When teaching the pregnant woman with cardiac disease, the nurse needs to encourage the patient to avoid_______________ and _______________.

6. __________________________ is high blood pressure seen after 20 weeks' gestation, without accompanying proteinuria.

7. ______________________ is a sudden unilateral neuropathy of the seventh cranial nerve seen three times more frequently in pregnant women.

8. Because pregnancy may exacerbate this autoimmune disease, ______________, women must be monitored carefully for signs that the disease has progressed.

9. ________________ and ______________ are the interventions for gestational diabetes.

10. The pregnant teenager, although she may be very young, is considered a(n) ______________ ______________ and has the right and responsibility to consent for treatment for herself and that of her child.

Matching Columns

1. Diabetes ____________
2. Placenta previa ____________
3. Ectopic pregnancy ____________
4. Betamethasone ____________
5. Preterm birth ____________
6. Hyperemesis gravidarum ____________
7. Cure for preeclampsia ____________
8. Placenta accreta ____________
9. Preeclampsia ____________
10. Human papilloma virus (HPV) ____________

A. Drug used to stimulate fetal lung maturity

B. Persistent, uncontrolled vomiting before the 20th week of gestation

C. Usually occurs in ampulla of the fallopian tube

D. The most acute problem in maternal-newborn health

E. Multisystem vasopressive disease process that is pregnancy specific

F. Delivery of the fetus

G. Placenta improperly implanted in lower uterine segment

H. Placenta abnormally firmly attached to uterine wall

I. Disorder of carbohydrate metabolism

J. Warts in anogenital area

Multiple Choice

1. A teenager arrives at the labor and delivery unit in labor. The nurse notices the patient has periorbital edema, a round face, and swollen hands. These findings are typical in a patient with what condition?

   A. Gestational diabetes

   B. Obesity

C. Preeclampsia

D. Placenta previa

2. The best treatment for a woman in labor with a positive group B streptococcus (GBS) status would be to

A. Give betamethasone

B. Give prophylactic ampicillin

C. Start on intravenous pitocin

D. Give the rubella vaccine

3. A woman who arrives at the hospital in labor has suspicious bruises on the upper portion of her body. The nurse's first response would be

A. To isolate the patient from family member(s) to interview her alone

B. Call the police

C. Ask family member(s) how she got the bruises

D. Call for a consult with a psychiatrist

4. What complications is a woman with a multiple gestation pregnancy at risk for?

A. Hyperemesis gravidarum, anemïa, preeclampsia, and postpartum hemorrhage

B. Poor weight gain, positive GBS status, anemia

C. Precipitous delivery, large for gestational age infants, Bell palsy

D. Intimate partner violence, drug abuse, insomnia

5. The "honeymoon" phase is associated with

A. First pregnancies

B. Intimate partner violence

C. Women with preeclampsia

D. Female circumcision

6. The nurse knows that when taking care of the pregnant patient with rheumatoid arthritis,

A. Pregnancy exacerbates the condition.

B. The patient usually feels better during pregnancy.

C. The patient will need a referral to a counselor.

D. The patient will have a difficult delivery.

7. When a mother uses this drug during pregnancy, the infant can have severe withdrawal symptoms for up to 6 months.

A. Marijuana

B. Cocaine

C. Heroin

D. Methadone

8. Cigarette smoking during pregnancy is associated with a higher rate of this in the newborn.

   A. Large for gestational age infant

   B. Diarrhea

   C. Sudden infant death syndrome

   D. Colic

9. When a mother experiences a full-term perinatal loss, what is an appropriate nursing care measure?

   A. Tell her you are sorry and that you know what she is feeling.

   B. Encourage her to hold the newborn.

   C. Force her to hold the newborn.

   D. Give her privacy by leaving her alone in her room.

10. Which of the following is the drug of choice to prevent seizures in a patient with preeclampsia?

    A. Calcium gluconate

    B. Magnesium sulfate

    C. RhoGAM

    D. (Flagyl) metronidazole

Answers

True/False

1. True
2. True
3. True
4. False. Pregnant women need 1000 mg of extra iron daily.
5. True
6. True
7. False. Sickle cell disease is an autosomal recessive disorder.
8. False. Sickle cell patients have good prognoses during pregnancy with good nutrition and antepartal care.
9. True
10. False. If the woman takes zidovudine (ZDV) during pregnancy, the chance of transmitting HIV to her newborn is decreased.
11. True
12. True
13. True
14. True
15. True
16. True
17. False. If a woman does not have active TB, she can breastfeed.
18. True
19. True

20. False. Multiple sclerosis is associated with remission during pregnancy.
21. True
22. True
23. True
24. True
25. True
26. True
27. True
28. True
29. True
30. True
31. True
32. True
33. True
34. True
35. False. A woman with herpes does not have to be isolated from her baby if she takes proper precautions, specifically, avoidance of lesions and strict hand washing.
36. True
37. False. Untreated GBS in the newborn can be lethal.
38. True
39. True
40. False. Intimate partner violence affects people in all socioeconomic groups.
41. True
42. True
43. False. The fetus does poorly in cases of penetrating injuries to a pregnant woman.
44. True
45. True
46. False. Heroin is not thought to be a teratogen to fetuses.
47. False. Women on methadone can breastfeed if they are not infected with HIV, hepatitis, or active TB.
48. True
49. True
50. True

Completion

1. 1000 mg
2. prematurity, IUGR (intrauterine growth restriction instead of retardation)
3. recessive
4. ZDV (zidovudine)
5. gaining too much weight, anemia
6. gestational hypertension
7. Bell's palsy
8. systemic lupus erythematosus
9. diet, exercise
10. emancipated minor

Matching Columns

1. I
2. G
3. C
4. A
5. D
6. B
7. F
8. H

9. **E**

10. **J**

Multiple Choice

1. **C**

2. **B**

3. **A**

4. **A**

5. **B**

6. **B**

7. **C**

8. **C**

9. **B**

10. **B**

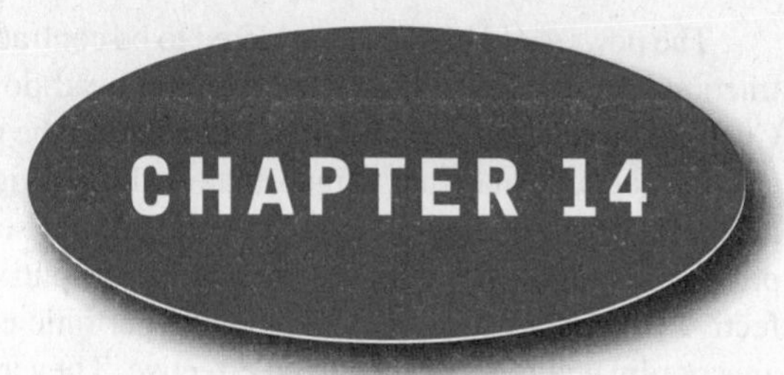

High-Risk Labor and Childbirth

Objective A: To Understand Risk Assessment and Identification of High-Risk Labor and Childbirth

14.1 Risk Assessment and Identification

For most women, labor and birth are normal processes and free of complications. However, complications sometimes arise that make labor and birth difficult and even hazardous for the mother, baby, or both. Regular prenatal care is important so high-risk patients can be identified and the appropriate counseling, guidance, and treatment can be rendered. Proper identification of risk also allows for support systems to be in place when the woman does come in to deliver. Sometimes, though, the patient who has had a normal course of pregnancy will have difficulty during labor and delivery and become high risk during this time.

Once a high-risk patient is admitted to the labor and delivery unit, or once a patient becomes high risk during the course of labor, the nurse must alert the appropriate staff so all the support systems will be at the delivery or in place to accept the infant. This includes notifying the nurse manager so proper staffing is obtained in relation to the acuity on the unit, readying the operating room in case a cesarean birth becomes necessary, notifying the neonatologist to be available to examine the infant as soon as delivery is completed, and having the neonatal intensive care unit (NICU) on alert in case the infant needs to be admitted.

Careful, accurate documentation is necessary when a high-risk obstetric patient is admitted to the labor and delivery unit. The nurse's notes should accurately describe the patient's journey from admission to the birth of the infant and should give details about any problems encountered and how they were addressed by the nurse and support staff. It is important for the nurse to keep the staff informed of the progress of the high-risk labor patient so everyone and everything needed will be in place and available to the patient and her infant.

Objective B: To Understand Dysfunctional Labor

14.2 Dysfunctional Labor

Normal labor is characterized by progressive changes in cervical effacement and dilation. A ***dysfunctional labor*** is one that does not produce these changes. Most often dysfunctional labor is caused by problems with the powers of labor (contractions and/or maternal pushing), the passenger (the fetus), the passage (the birth canal), the psyche, or any combination of these. Dysfunctional labor is often long but can also be short and intense.

The powers of labor are considered to be contractions and maternal pushing efforts. Strong, coordinated contractions are needed to help push the fetal head down, putting pressure on the cervix and helping it to dilate. Contractions also help to push the fetus through the pelvis and expel the fetus at birth. Causes of ineffective contractions include maternal fatigue, maternal inactivity, fluid and electrolyte imbalance, hypoglycemia, excessive analgesia or anesthesia, maternal catecholamines secreted in response to pain, disproportion between maternal pelvis and presenting fetal part, and uterine distention (multiple gestation or hydramnios). Two patterns of ineffective contractions are hypotonic and hypertonic contractions. With ***hypotonic contractions,*** the contractions are coordinated but too weak to be effective. They are often seen during the active phase of labor when contractions should be getting quicker and stronger.

Treatment of hypotonic contractions depends on the cause. For dehydration or hypoglycemia, an intravenous (IV) line would be inserted. Position changes or increased activity, such as walking, may promote more effective contractions. In some cases, an amniotomy (artificial rupture of the membranes) may be done to hasten the labor process. Pitocin infusion may be added if the amniotomy alone does not promote labor progress.

The nurse needs to use therapeutic communication with the patient to help the woman identify her anxieties and beliefs about the labor process. Many women become very tired and anxious during this time when they become aware that their labor is not progressing as it should. The nurse will also take measures to support treatment (prevent infection, assess for prolapsed cord, regulate IV therapy, monitor pitocin infusion, etc).

Hypertonic contractions are less common and often affect first-time mothers in early labor. These contractions are uncoordinated, erratic, and painful. They are ineffectual in the progression of labor. Management depends on the cause, and relief of pain is often the primary treatment. A warm shower or soak in a Jacuzzi tub can be relaxing, and for some women this is enough to promote labor. Some women may be given low doses of systemic analgesics to promote relaxation and rest.

Ineffective maternal pushing can be due to many causes, including maternal exhaustion, fear of injury, a decreased or absent urge to push, or a psychological "unreadiness" to the birth of the baby. Management focuses on the causes contributing to ineffective pushing. Nursing care is aimed at helping the mother push more effectively. Changing positions, encouraging the woman to rest between pushes, and coaching her when it is time to push may help with pushing efforts. Talking with the woman about sensations felt during delivery may help alleviate her concerns about injury. Providing a supportive environment during the critical time can help prevent unnecessary surgical interventions.

Problems with the passenger, or fetus, associated with dysfunctional labor include fetal size, fetal presentation or position, multifetal pregnancy, and fetal anomalies.

The macrosomic infant (> 4000 g or 8 lb, 13 oz) may not be able to adapt to the pelvis, although that is relative. Small women may not be able to deliver even a small fetus, whereas others may be able to pass a much larger fetus. With a large infant, the shoulders of the infant may become impacted above the maternal symphysis pubis; this is referred to as ***shoulder dystocia.***

Shoulder dystocia is an urgent situation because the umbilical cord can be compressed between the fetal body and maternal pelvis. Also, although the head is out of the birth canal, the chest is inside and prevents respirations. Preparation for surgical delivery should be initiated while attempts to deliver the baby vaginally are taking place.

Several methods can be used to promote a vaginal delivery. The nurse can help the patient by initiating the McRobert's maneuver, which can be done by bringing the woman's flexed knees up toward her ears, which straightens the pelvic curve, allowing more room for the baby to pass. A supported squat, if appropriate, has a similar effect and adds gravity to the woman's pushing efforts. Another effective method for relieving shoulder dystocia is suprapubic pressure, which pushes the anterior shoulder downward to displace it from above the woman's symphysis pubis.

Fundal pressure should never be used because it will push the anterior shoulder even more firmly against the woman's symphysis pubis and could cause a placental tear or a ruptured uterus.

An ***abnormal fetal presentation,*** or position, may interfere with cervical dilation or fetal descent. An occiput posterior (OP) or occiput transverse (OT) position can interfere with the cardinal movements of labor.

"Back labor" is the result of an OP fetal position. This makes labor more uncomfortable for the woman as she feels more pressure on her back, coccyx bone, or legs and is often poorly relieved with analgesics. The nurse can apply pressure to the woman's coccyx or have the woman's partner roll a tennis ball in circles over the coccyx. This counterpressure often relieves the pain associated with back labor. Frequent position changes may also help to relieve some of the discomfort.

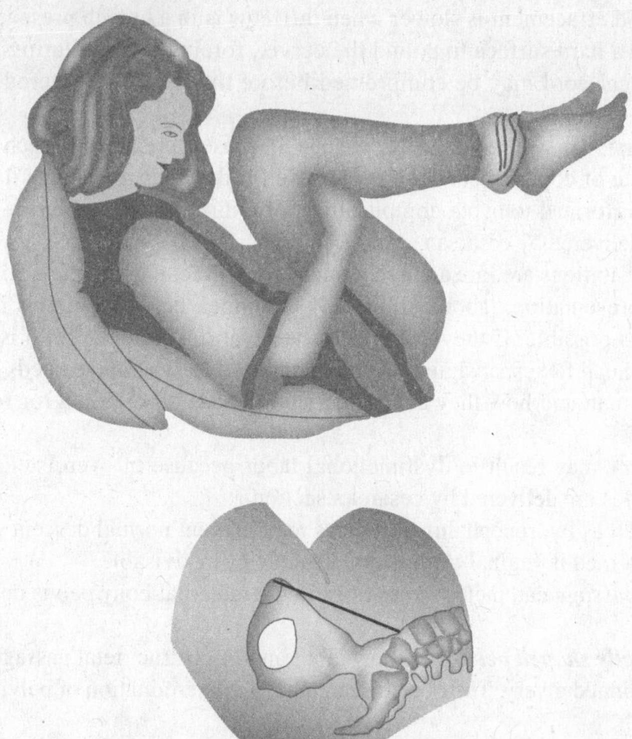

Figure 14.1 Methods that may be used to relieve shoulder dystocia. McRobert's maneuver. The woman flexes her thighs sharply against her abdomen, which straightens the pelvic curve somewhat. A supported squat has a similar effect and adds gravity to her pushing efforts.

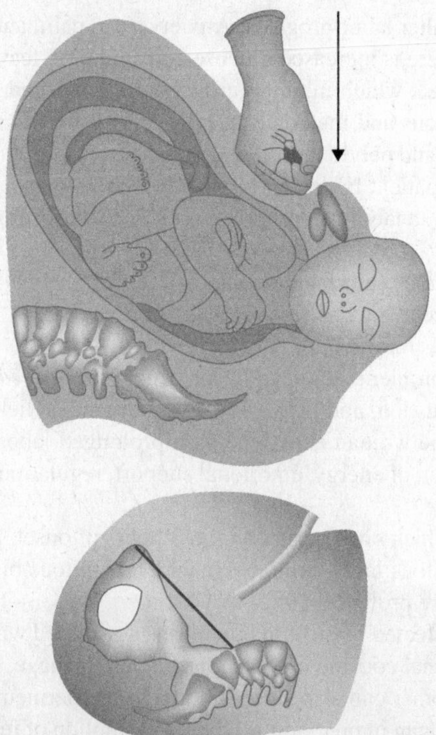

Figure 14.2 Methods that may be used to relieve shoulder dystocia. Suprapubic pressure by an assistant pushes the fetal anterior shoulder downward to displace it from above the mother's symphysis pubis. Fundal pressure should not be used because it will push the anterior shoulder even more firmly against the mother's symphysis.

Cervical dilation and effacement is slower when the fetus is in a breech presentation. The soft, rounded buttocks do not provide a hard surface to pound the cervix, forcing it open during labor. Also, with breech presentation the umbilical cord may be compressed before the head is delivered, making it a dangerous situation.

External cephalic version may be attempted to change the presentation from breech to cephalic several weeks prior to the estimated date of confinement (EDC). However, if the fetus remains in the abnormal presentation, cesarean birth may be performed to avoid complications of a difficult vaginal birth. The fetus remaining in a transverse lie is always delivered by cesarean section.

Face and brow presentations are rare and are associated with fetal anomalies. Diagnosis is made by vaginal exam. With a face presentation, labor will usually be longer, but if the pelvis is adequate and the head rotates, a vaginal birth is possible. If the head rotates backward, a cesarean birth is necessary. With a brow presentation, unless the head flexes, a vaginal birth is not possible. The nurse needs to explain fetal malpositions to the laboring woman and how they can affect labor. Close observation for fetal hypoxia is also very important.

Multifetal pregnancy may result in dysfunctional labor because of overdistention of the uterus. Many pregnancies with multiples are delivered by cesarean section.

Fetal anomalies such as hydrocephalus or tumors may prevent normal descent of the fetus during labor. A cesarean birth is performed if vaginal birth is not possible or inadvisable.

Problems with the passage can include variations in the maternal bony pelvis or soft tissue problems that inhibit fetal descent.

A ***small or abnormally shaped pelvis*** can slow labor and/or obstruct fetal passage. The gynecoid pelvis is the most suitable for vaginal delivery. The obstetrician makes a determination of pelvic size at the first prenatal visit by vaginal exam.

A ***full bladder*** is the most common soft tissue obstruction in the laboring woman. The full bladder reduces the space available for the fetus to pass through the pelvis. The nurse needs to encourage the patient to empty her bladder every 2 hours to prevent soft tissue obstruction. Women who have had epidural placement may not be able to void; in those cases, a straight catheter should be placed by the nurse to empty the bladder.

Problems of the psyche can alter labor progress. Anxiety, fear, pain, and other stressful feelings can interfere with labor in many ways. There is increased glucose consumption, leaving less energy for the contracting uterus; catecholamines are released, which inhibit uterine contractions and heighten the perception of pain by the woman; and uterine contractions and maternal pushing efforts are less effective because those efforts are working against tense abdominal and pelvic muscles.

The nurse needs to help the patient by trying to allay her anxiety and fear, provide pain relief measures, help the woman to relax her body so labor can progress, and be a comforting support to the woman during this stressful time.

An ***unusually long or short labor*** can result in maternal, fetal, or neonatal problems. Prolonged labor is one in which normal progress is not occurring once a woman is in active labor (1.2 cm dilation of the cervix per hour for the nullipara and 2 cm per hour for the multipara).

Possible maternal and fetal problems that can occur from a ***prolonged labor*** include maternal infection, neonatal infection, maternal exhaustion, and higher levels of fear and anxiety during a subsequent labor.

Nursing care measures for the woman experiencing a prolonged labor include assessment for infection, promotion of comfort, conservation of energy, emotional support, regular position changes, and assessment for compromised fetal oxygenation.

Precipitous labor is one in which birth occurs within 3 hours of onset. Although not the same as a precipitous birth, a woman with precipitous labor may also have a precipitous birth. A precipitous birth is one that occurs unattended (by a health care professional).

The mother or fetus can be affected by several conditions associated with precipitous labor. These include abruption, fetal meconium, maternal cocaine use, postpartum hemorrhage, low Apgar scores, and intracranial hemorrhage in the infant. The mother can also suffer trauma to her perineum (lacerations and hematomas).

Priority nursing care for a woman in precipitous labor is promotion of fetal oxygenation and maternal comfort. If the physician or midwife does not arrive in time to deliver the infant, the nurse should put on gloves and support the baby's body as it emerges while also supporting the perineum.

Objective C: To Understand Intrauterine Infection

14.3 Intrauterine Infection

Infection can occur in both normal and dysfunctional labors. The labor and delivery nurse needs to constantly be aware of measures to prevent infection when taking care of the laboring patient. Strict hand washing before and after contact with the patient is imperative to reduce the transmission of organisms.

Limiting the number of vaginal exams reduces the amount of organisms entering the uterine cavity. Keeping the pads under the laboring patient as dry as possible eliminates a moist environment where bacteria can grow. The nurse should periodically clean the woman's perineum from excess secretions to limit contamination and promote the patient's comfort.

Signs that a woman has become infected include fetal tachycardia, maternal tachypnea or tachycardia, increased maternal temperature, and cloudy amniotic fluid with a strong odor. Maternal vital signs should be taken as per hospital policy, typically every 4 hours if membranes are intact, every 2 hours if membranes are ruptured. Fetal heart rate (FHR) is typically taken every hour if the patient is not on an external fetal monitor.

If signs of infection are noted, the nurse needs to contact the physician or midwife. Aerobic and anaerobic cultures are usually collected from the uterine cavity. Antibiotic therapy can then be initiated. The newborn nursery staff, as well as the neonatologist, should be alerted that signs of infection are noted and antibiotics begun. The nurse should take a swab and obtain cultures of the baby once it is born (under the arm and groin). The infant may be taken to the neonatal intensive care unit (NICU) if he or she exhibits any sign of infection for treatment to prevent neonatal sepsis or may be taken there for observation. If the results of the maternal or neonatal cultures indicate that no infection is present, antibiotics are usually discontinued.

Objective D: To Understand Premature Rupture of the Membranes

14.4 Premature Rupture of the Membranes

Rupture of the amniotic sac before the onset of true labor is called premature rupture of the membranes (PROM). Preterm premature rupture of the membranes (PPROM) refers to the rupture of the membranes before 37 weeks' gestation. PPROM is associated with preterm labor and birth. The greatest risk is to newborns before 34 weeks' gestation, when the fetal lungs are mature.

The exact cause of PROM is unclear. Several conditions are associated with it, including maternal infections (bacterial, group B streptococcus, chlamydia, gonorrhea, and *Gardnerella*), chorioamnionitis, fetal abnormalities or abnormal presentations, previous preterm birth, over distention of the uterus, maternal nutritional deficiencies, maternal stress, and low socioeconomic status.

Management of PROM depends on the gestational age and whether evidence of infection or other fetal compromise exists. The first step is to identify if membranes have truly ruptured, as increased vaginal secretions and urinary incontinence are common and may make a woman think her membranes have ruptured when they have not. A nitrazine or ferning test may be done to verify that the fluid is indeed amniotic. A transvaginal ultrasound may be performed to measure cervical length, and tests for fetal lung maturity may also be done.

If the woman is near term and her cervix is soft, labor may be induced if it does not begin spontaneously. If the gestation is preterm, the physician weighs the risk of maternal-fetal infection against the newborn's risks for complications of prematurity. With very early gestations, management is complex.

Antibiotics are usually prescribed for the woman with PROM because of the increased risk of infection for herself and the fetus. Drugs to correct infection will depend on culture and sensitivity test results.

Membranes that rupture before term may form a seal, stopping the leaking fluid and allowing the amniotic fluid cushion to become reestablished. In cases where the fluid continues to leak, there can be umbilical cord compression or reduced lung volume, or deformities resulting from compression may occur.

If preterm birth occurs, the infant is more likely to develop respiratory distress syndrome (RDS). The greatest danger is to the fetus before 34 weeks' gestation, especially if the woman did not receive steroids to accelerate fetal lung maturity.

The nurse will need to monitor the woman with PROM very carefully. The woman may be hospitalized until birth and depending on the gestation, may be in store for a long hospital stay. The nurse must be vigilant for signs of infection along with signs of impending labor. Vital signs should be taken every 4 hours, including FHR. Abdominal pain, cramping, pelvic pressure, change in vaginal secretions, constant lower back pain, and a sense of "not feeling well" or "coming down with something" are all signs that labor may be impending. These should be reported to the physician, and the patient should be evaluated immediately.

To help prevent preterm labor, nothing should be inserted into the vagina, and vaginal exams should be limited. Activity restrictions should be maintained. The woman should be taught to avoid breast stimulation, as the oxytocin that would be released would stimulate contractions. The woman should be instructed to observe the vaginal discharge for a strong odor or for a cloudy or yellow appearance.

Objective E: To Understand Preterm Labor

14.5 Preterm Labor

Preterm labor is defined as labor that begins after the 20th week of gestation and before the 37th week of pregnancy. It can result in the birth of an infant who is ill equipped for adjusting to extrauterine life. Preterm birth ranks second as the leading cause of neonatal mortality in the United States.

Just as the cause of labor is unknown, so is the cause of preterm labor. Over half of the women with preterm labor do not show risk. However, certain associated factors have been identified in cases of preterm labor, including conceptions assisted with reproductive technology; present and past obstetric complications; fetal conditions such as growth retardation, inadequate amniotic fluid volume, and chromosomal abnormalities; social and environmental factors, such as inadequate or absent prenatal care, maternal smoking, and homelessness; chronic hypertension; preexisting diabetes; connective tissue disorders; and drug abuse.

Signs and symptoms of preterm labor are usually subtle, and the woman may not detect them or may be only vaguely aware that something is different. Women who are more aware of the consequences of a preterm birth may be more likely to take action to prevent it. Signs and symptoms of preterm labor include uterine contractions that may or may not be painful; cramping; pelvic pressure; constant low backache; pain, discomfort, or pressure in the vagina or thighs; change or increase in vaginal discharge; and a sense that the patient is "coming down with something" or "just not feeling well."

Management includes identifying those that may be at risk for preterm birth, identifying preterm labor early, delaying birth, and accelerating fetal lung maturity. Once the diagnosis of preterm labor is made, management focuses on stopping uterine activity and resulting dilation > 3 cm. Initial determination of whether any maternal or fetal conditions contraindicate continuing the pregnancy, such as preeclampsia, serious infection, or signs of the inability to correct a nonreassuring FHR tracing, are made.

Initial measures to stop preterm labor include activity restriction, identifying and treating infections, stopping contractions, and promoting fetal lung maturity. The woman will be admitted to the hospital, admission bloods drawn (including a type and cross-match in case of emergency cesarean section surgery), cultures taken, and an IV started. The woman will be hydrated and will need to start on IV tocolytic therapy with medication in an attempt to stop contractions. She will have a baseline internal vaginal exam done.

It is important for the nurse to explain everything that is happening to the patient. The patient will be anxious and afraid. Knowing what is happening may help relieve some of the patient's anxiety.

IV hydration to stop preterm labor contractions has not been demonstrated to be beneficial for all women; however, dehydration can make the uterus irritable, often in those that may have an infection or some other condition (eg, diarrhea). IV fluid is given according to the expected benefit. The nurse should administer IV fluid by infusion pump so fluid and medication can be monitored. High-volume IV infusions may cause fluid overload and/or may cause maternal respiratory distress if a drug such as magnesium sulfate is being administered because the drug may also reduce the respiratory rate.

Tocolytic therapy will be initiated if preterm labor occurs before the 34th week of gestation because the infant's risk for respiratory and other complications for prematurity is high if the infant is born during this time. Delay of preterm birth allows time to give maternal corticosteroids to reduce respiratory distress in the newborn. Four drugs are used for tocolysis: magnesium sulfate, calcium antagonists, prostaglandin synthesis inhibitors, and beta-adrenergics. The lowest possible dose that inhibits contractions is administered.

Magnesium sulfate therapy has a well-established record of safety during pregnancy. It is given intravenously in a loading dose of 4 to 6 g over 20 minutes; the maintenance dose is 1 to 4 g/h for 24 hours. It is continued until contractions are no more than four to six per hour. Continuing magnesium sulfate therapy for 48 hours may be done to allow the woman to receive the whole course of corticosteroids to hasten fetal lung maturity. Side effects include respiratory or cardiac depression, depression of deep tendon reflexes, lethargy, headache, nausea, blurry vision, sensation of heat or flushing, reduced FHR variability, and hypotonia in the infant.

The nurse needs to assess the patient closely with hourly vital signs, deep tendon reflexes, and heart and lung sounds, and assess for urine output of at least 30 mL/h. Serum magnesium levels guide maintenance of therapeutic levels. Calcium gluconate (10%) must be readily available to reverse magnesium toxicity and prevent respiratory arrest if serum levels become high. Calcium is needed for muscular contractions, so by giving calcium channel blockers, such as nifedipine, contractions can be reduced in the preterm labor patient. Side effects include flushing of the skin, headache, a transient increase in maternal and FHR, and hypotension and may make the woman in preterm labor who is probably already very anxious very uncomfortable. Nurses need to give extra support to these patients.

Because prostaglandins stimulate uterine contractions, prostaglandin synthesis inhibitors can be used to inhibit them. Indomethacin is the drug of choice in this class used for tocolysis therapy. Side effects include nausea, vomiting, heartburn, and prolonged bleeding time. Fetal adverse effects are more serious and include constriction of the ductus arteriosus, pulmonary hypertension, and oligohydramnios.

The only beta-adrenergic drug currently approved in the United States for tocolysis is ritodrine (Yutopar). It is not used often because of its significant side effects and minimal increase in the length of pregnancy. Terbutaline (Brethine), although considered an investigational drug, is more widely used due to its low cost and longer duration of action between doses. It can be given intravenously, subcutaneously, or orally.

Tolerance may develop, and magnesium may need to be substituted. The main side effects of beta-adrenergic drugs are cardiorespiratory in nature. Maternal and fetal tachycardia is common. The nurse needs to reassure the woman that the feeling she may experience related to the tachycardia is normal. Some women may be discharged home on oral Brethine if they are able to tolerate the tachycardia and the contractions have stopped.

Objective F: To Understand the Process of Accelerating Fetal Lung Maturity

14.6 Accelerating Fetal Lung Maturity

Corticosteroids are usually ordered to hasten fetal lung maturity if birth before 34 weeks' gestation appears to be inevitable. Betamethasone (Celestone) or dexamethasone (Decadron) may be used for this purpose.

Recommendations for corticosteroids for threatened preterm birth are as follows: betamethasone 12 mg 2 doses intramuscularly (IM), 24 hours apart; or dexamethasone 6 mg., 4 doses IM, 12 hours apart. Side effects include an increase in leukocytes, glucose intolerance, nervousness, insomnia, fever, elevated pulse rate, shortness of breath, and pulmonary edema.

The nurse needs to observe the patient for signs and symptoms of side effects that may be subtle. Women who are diabetic may need to increase their insulin.

Objective G: To Understand Postterm Labor and Birth

14.7 Postterm Labor and Birth

A ***postterm pregnancy*** is one that continues past the 42nd week of gestation. Postterm pregnancies may adversely affect both the mother and fetus. Maternal risk includes large size of the infant at birth, which can cause trauma and increase the chance that the mother will have a cesarean birth. Other risks are shoulder dystocia, postpartum hemorrhage, and infection.

Fetal risks associated with a postterm pregnancy include macrosomia, shoulder dystocia, brachial plexus injuries, cephalopelvic disproportion, uteroplacental insufficiency, meconium aspiration, and intrauterine infection. The biggest risk associated with postterm pregnancies is decreased amniotic fluid, which reduces the cushioning effect and increases the possibility of cord compression.

Nursing interventions for the patient with a postterm pregnancy during the intrapartum period include assessing and monitoring the FHR in order to identify potential fetal distress, maintaining the patient in the left lateral position as much as possible to maximize placental blood flow, inserting an IV to keep the patient well hydrated to maximize placental perfusion and to have quick access in case an emergency cesarean delivery becomes necessary, and assessing the characteristics of the amniotic fluid (color, amount, and odor) to identify previous fetal hypoxia and preparation for prevention of meconium aspiration. Because patients with a postterm pregnancy may have dysfunctional labor patterns, labor may be induced.

The nurse needs to educate the patient and family about the complications that can occur during labor and offer encouragement and support.

Objective H: To Understand Induction and Augmentation of Labor

14.8 Induction and Augmentation of Labor

Many women need help to initiate or sustain the labor process. Labor induction involves the stimulation of the uterus to promote contractions before the onset of spontaneous labor or to enhance ineffective contractions after labor has begun. There are many indications for inducing labor, the most common being postterm gestation. Other indications for induction include prolonged PROM, gestational hypertension, renal disease, chorioamnionitis, dystocia, intrauterine fetal demise, isoimmunization, diabetes, and convenience.

Evidence suggests that elective induction of labor significantly increases the woman's risk of instrument-assisted delivery, use of epidural anesthesia, cesarean birth, and NICU admission for infants.

Contraindications to labor induction include complete placenta previa, abruptio placentae, transverse lie, prolapsed umbilical cord, a prior classic uterine incision that entered the uterine cavity, pelvic structure abnormalities, previous myomectomy, vaginal bleeding with unknown cause, invasive cervical cancer, active genital herpes infection, and abnormal FHR patterns.

Cervical ripeness is an important variable when labor induction is being considered. A favorable or "ripe" cervix is one that is shortened, anterior, softened, and partially open. The ***Bishop score*** helps to identify successful candidates for induction. The score is based on these cervical characteristics and fetal station, with each given a score of up to 2 points. A score ≥ 8 indicates a favorable cervix; a score < 8 indicates that a cervical ripening method should be given prior to induction.

Three prostaglandins are used for cervical ripening: dinoprostone inserts (Cervidil), misoprostol (Cytotec), and dinoprostone gel (Prepidil). Some prostaglandins can be taken orally, and others can be inserted intravaginally. The side effect of prostaglandins is their ability to produce excessive uterine contractions. Frequently, a woman is brought into the hospital the night before a scheduled induction to ripen her cervix with one of the prostaglandin agents.

Nonpharmacologic methods of labor induction are not widely used in the United States. They include herbal agents, castor oil, hot baths, enemas, sexual intercourse, and nipple stimulation.

The nurse needs to ask the patient who comes to the labor and delivery unit if she has used any of these methods prior to coming to the hospital. In some cultures, these measures may be employed before the patient comes to the hospital for delivery.

Mechanical methods are used to open the cervix and move labor along. An indwelling catheter may be used for this purpose and is inserted into the endocervical canal. The mechanism of action is to apply pressure, which stimulates the release of prostaglandins to ripen the cervix.

Surgical methods used to ripen the cervix and induce labor include stripping the membranes and amniotomy. Stripping of the membranes is accomplished by inserting a finger through the internal cervical os and moving it around in a circular motion, which causes the membranes to detach. An amniotomy involves inserting a cervical hook (amnihook) to rupture the membranes.

Risks associated with these procedures include umbilical cord prolapse or compression, maternal or neonatal infection, FHR deceleration, and bleeding. The nurse needs to document the color of the amniotic fluid, carefully monitor the FHR, and assess for cord prolapse.

Pitocin is one of the most widely used drugs for labor induction in the United States. Synthetic pitocin mimics the actions of naturally occurring oxytocin. Responses to pitocin vary widely, and some women are sensitive to even small amounts. Pitocin is administered via an IV infusion, on a pump, and is piggybacked into the main IV line. Usually 10 units of pitocin are added to 1000 mL of isotonic solution. The mixture is titrated by pump to administer 1 mU/min initially and may be increased by 1 to 2 mU/min every 30 to 60 minutes until contractions are every 2 to 3 minutes, or as by hospital protocol.

The nurse needs to explain to the patient and her partner the induction or augmentation procedure, including that the process also includes bed rest, continuous electronic FHR monitoring, significant discomfort from stimulating uterine contractions, epidural anesthesia, and a prolonged stay on the labor and delivery unit.

The nurse needs to monitor the maternal and fetal status very carefully. Maternal vital signs should be taken every 1 to 2 hours and FHR every 15 minutes during the active phase of labor and every 5 minutes during the second stage. The nurse needs to monitor uterine contractions for frequency, duration, intensity, and resting tone and make adjustments to the pitocin infusion accordingly. Pitocin infusion should be discontinued if there is hyperstimulation of the uterus or if a nonreassuring FHR pattern develops; if this occurs, the physician or midwife should be called.

Pain should be assessed regularly and analgesics given as ordered. Because continuous fetal monitoring is necessary for a woman during an induction, many nonpharmacologic pain relief methods would not be available to her, such as ambulating. However, other methods can be employed before drug administration, such as diversionary methods (eg, deep breathing exercises and imagery).

The nurse needs to provide explanations and information regarding the process of labor induction/augmentation and offer support and encouragement as needed.

Objective I: To Understand the Labor and Delivery of a Multiple Gestation Pregnancy

14.9 Labor and Delivery of a Multiple Gestation Pregnancy

On admission to the labor and delivery unit, the woman with a multiple gestation pregnancy is given an IV line for administering fluids and treatment in the event of hemorrhage or the need for emergency delivery and anesthesia. Prophylactic antacids may be given to reduce gastric pH and volume in case surgery is needed.

In many hospitals, cesarean birth is standard practice for multiple gestation pregnancies. A bedside ultrasound scan on admission will be done to assess the presentation and estimated fetal weight for each infant. Continuous, simultaneous external fetal monitoring will be done.

If the patient is to try to deliver vaginally, pitocin augmentation is often given because multiple gestation pregnancies are at high risk for dysfunctional labor. It may also be given to enhance descent of the second twin (or multiple). Twin B is at greater risk for delivery-related complications, such as umbilical cord prolapse, malpresentation, and abruptio placentae.

Double set-ups should be done—a set of equipment for each infant (warmers, ambu bags, oxygen, suction, laryngoscopes, etc)—and the operating room should be made available and ready at the time of delivery. Extra personnel need to be available to attend to the needs of each newborn.

Ultrasound examination is often done after the delivery of the first multiple to reassess the position of other multiples, as well as to guide version if needed to facilitate vaginal delivery. Cesarean delivery may be necessary even after vaginal delivery of the first multiple.

The nurse needs to encourage verbalization and address specific concerns the patient and family may have. The nurse will also need to prepare the patient and family for the intensive care environment in case the infants need to be taken there instead of the well-baby nursery.

Objective J: To Understand Birth-Related Procedures

14.10 Birth-Related Procedures

Amnioinfusion is a technique in which a volume of warmed, sterile, normal saline or Ringer lactate solution is introduced into the uterus through an intrauterine pressure catheter to increase the volume of fluid. This procedure is indicated for cases of oligohydramnios, postmaturity or ruptured membranes, severe variable decelerations, and thick meconium in the amniotic fluid. It helps cushion the umbilical cord and dilutes thick meconium.

There is no standard of practice for the administration of amnioinfusion. Overdistention of the uterus is a risk, so the amount of fluid infused should be monitored closely.

The nurse needs to instruct the patient on the procedure and the goal of treatment, including explaining that the patient must remain in bed for the procedure and that the fetus must be assessed continuously. The nurse needs to monitor the FHR pattern to determine whether or not the amnioinfusion is improving the fetal status, along with the patient's discomfort level.

Intrauterine resuscitation is a term used to describe interventions when a nonreassuring FHR tracing is detected. When intrauterine resuscitation is under way, the priorities are to increase blood flow and volume of the maternal and fetal vasculature and to optimize oxygenation. Interventions include changing position, increasing the rate of IV fluid, and providing oxygen via face mask (8–10 L). Stimulation may be done to elicit an acceleration of the FHR (15 beats per minute lasting at least 15 seconds) that occurs in response to a tactile stimulus. Acceleration will not occur in the presence of fetal distress or acidosis.

Scalp stimulation is conducted by applying pressure with the fingers to the fetal scalp during a vaginal exam. ***Vibroacoustic stimulation (VAS)*** is accomplished by placing a fetal acoustic stimulation device on the maternal abdomen directly over the fetal head for 1 to 2 seconds. Acceleration of the FHR in response to the stimulation is usually indicative of fetal well-being. Lack of acceleration warrants further evaluation.

Fetal scalp blood sampling can be conducted to assess the fetal pH, blood oxygen level (PO_2), and carbon dioxide level (PCO_2). A small sample of capillary blood is taken from the fetal scalp as it presents at the dilated cervix. An internal fetal scalp electrode can be placed to get a more accurate FHR at this time. If the fetus is hypoxic, there is a drop in the pH (acidosis). A scalp blood pH < 7.20 is acidotic and is recognized as an indicator of fetal distress. A scalp blood pH > 7.25 is considered normal for a fetus during labor.

The nurse needs to maintain a calming presence, offer factual, simple explanations for her actions, provide ongoing support for the laboring woman, and keep her informed of her labor progress and fetal status.

Forceps or a ***vacuum extractor*** may be used to apply traction to the fetal head or to provide a method of rotating the fetal head during birth. The indications for use of forceps or a vacuum extractor are similar and include a prolonged second stage of labor, a nonreassuring FHR pattern, failure of the presenting part to fully rotate and descend into the pelvis, limited sensation, and inability to push effectively. The use of forceps or a vacuum extractor poses risks to both mother and newborn. Maternal trauma may include lacerations of the cervix, vagina, or perineum; hematoma; extension of an episiotomy incision into the anus; and hemorrhage. Potential newborn trauma includes facial and scalp lacerations, facial nerve injury, cephalohematoma, and caput succedaneum.

Forceps are stainless steel instruments, shaped like salad tongs, with rounded edges that fit around the fetus's head. They have a locking mechanism that prevents the blades from compressing the fetal skull.

A vacuum extractor is a cup-shaped instrument attached to a pump. The suction cup is applied to the occiput of the fetal head, and the pump is used to create suction. The woman is instructed to push, and the physician or midwife applies traction until the fetal head emerges from the vagina.

Prevention is key to avoiding the use of these devices. The nurse needs to change the patient's position frequently, have the patient empty her bladder frequently (to allow more room for the fetus to descend), and make sure the patient is hydrated well throughout labor. The woman needs to rest frequently between contractions so she is not exhausted and unable to push effectively.

The nursery needs to observe the infant delivered by forceps or a vacuum for any signs of nerve damage. Postpartum nurses need to assess the patient's perineum more carefully, as the woman may have internal injuries and may be at greater risk of infection due to instrumentation.

A ***cesarean birth*** is the delivery of the fetus by an incision in the abdomen and uterus. The low-transverse incision is the most common approach used in the United States. Cesarean birth may be indicated in any situation where safe passage of the fetus through the birth canal or that compromises maternal or fetal well-being is evident. Such cases include active genital herpes, macrosomia, fetopelvic disproportion, prolapsed umbilical cord, placenta previa or abruptio placentae, previous classical cesarean incision, gestational hypertension, diabetes, positive human immunodeficiency virus (HIV) status, and dystocia. Fetal indications include malpresentation, congenital anomalies, hydrocephalus, and fetal distress.

Cesarean birth is a major surgical procedure with increased risks compared to vaginal birth. The patient is at greater risk for infection, hemorrhage, aspiration, pulmonary embolism, urinary tract trauma, thrombophlebitis, paralytic ileus, and atelectasis. Fetal injury and transient tachypnea of the newborn may also occur.

The nurse's role is to help prepare the patient for surgery and to provide postop care. Care should be centered on the family and not on the surgery. Providing explanations for what is going on, listening to the patient's and family's concerns, and providing emotional support are important. The patient and family will be anxious, so eye contact, the use of touch, therapeutic communication, and genuine caring in helping the parents have a positive birth experience are essential at this time.

Vaginal birth after cesarean (VBAC) describes a woman who delivers vaginally after having at least one previous cesarean birth. Most women can attempt a trial of labor if they have a low-transverse uterine scar and are in an environment capable of handling the acute emergency of uterine rupture. Contraindications to VBAC include a prior classical incision, prior transfundal uterine scar, contracted pelvis, and inadequate staffing or facility if a cesarean birth is required.

Nurses need to monitor FHR tracings carefully to identify nonreassuring FHR patterns and to assess for the need for emergency delivery.

Objective K: To Understand Obstetric Emergencies

14.11 Obstetric Emergencies

Women with placental abnormalities may experience hemorrhage during the intrapartum period. Critical nursing actions are required when the intrapartum period is complicated by placenta previa or abruptio placentae because it puts the woman at risk for hemorrhage and shock and puts the fetus at risk for hypoxia.

If the laboring woman with a ***low-lying placenta*** has stable vital signs, stable FHR sounds, and is not bleeding, the woman is managed with expectant watching. If the woman is greater than 37 weeks and is bleeding, immediate birth by cesarean section is always indicated. Women diagnosed with ***partial placenta previa*** who have no bleeding will be allowed to attempt a vaginal birth.

When a cesarean birth is planned, nursing responsibilities include continuous maternal and fetal assessment and preparing the woman for surgery. Vital signs are assessed for signs of hemorrhage (decreasing blood pressure, tachycardia, changes in the level of consciousness, and oliguria). Continuous external fetal monitoring is used to assess for fetal hypoxia. The nurse needs to provide emotional support to the woman and her family while assisting with medical management.

Abruptio placentae (placental abruption) may occur as late as the first or second stage of labor. The primary cause of premature placental separation is unknown, but predisposing factors include maternal hypertension, cocaine use (vasoconstriction), direct trauma, and a history of previous placental abruption.

Treatment for abruptio placentae depends on the severity of maternal blood loss and the fetal maturity and status. If the abruption is mild and the fetus is less than 36 weeks and not in distress, expectant management may be implemented.

When the fetus is at gestation or the bleeding is moderate to severe and the woman or fetus is in jeopardy, delivery is facilitated. The physician may elect to artificially rupture the membranes or augment the labor with IV pitocin to hasten the birth. Artificial rupture of the membranes allows a slow, steady release of amniotic fluid, preventing sudden change in intrauterine pressure, which can cause further placental separation.

Vaginal birth is desirable, especially in the case of fetal death. If birth does not appear imminent, a cesarean birth is the delivery method of choice. Cesarean birth should be reserved, though, for cases of fetal distress or other obstetric complications and should not be attempted if the woman has severe and uncorrected coagulopathy (disseminated intravascular coagulation [DIC]).

Nursing care includes continuous maternal-fetal monitoring, keeping the patient in the left lateral position to prevent pressure on the vena cava and facilitate blood flow, preventing vaginal exams to avoid further damage to the injured placenta, blood and fluid replacement to maintain urine output of at least 30 cc/h, insertion of a Foley catheter, and emotional support. If DIC has developed, surgery poses a major threat. Fibrinogen or cryoprecipitate (which contains fibrinogen) may be given to raise the maternal fibrinogen level.

The patient with uncontrolled bleeding is vulnerable to complications of a ***Couvelaire uterus*** (also called uteroplacental apoplexy) and DIC. A Couvelaire uterus is a rare condition in which the uterus takes on a bluish tinge as blood extravasates into the myometrium. Contractility is lost and may result in a hysterectomy.

The maternal prognosis depends on how quickly interventions are initiated and how effective they are in controlling the bleeding. Death can occur from massive hemorrhage that leads to shock or renal failure from circulatory collapse. Fetal prognosis depends on the severity of hypoxia caused by the hemorrhage.

14.12 Disseminated Intravascular Coagulation

Disseminated intravascular coagulation (DIC) is a disorder of blood clotting. In DIC, anticoagulation and procoagulation are activated simultaneously, resulting in an inability of the blood to clot. Signs the patient may be going into DIC include bleeding from multiple sites (IV site, puncture site, site of urinary catheter insertion, spontaneous nosebleed, bleeding gums, etc), petechiae, and bruising. Lab values reveal low platelets, low hemoglobin and hematocrit, fibrinogen, and elevated fibrin split.

Priority of treatment for DIC includes correcting the underlying cause and replacing fluids and essential clotting factors.

Nursing care includes continuous maternal-fetal monitoring; administration of the prescribed fluids, heparin, and blood products; and assessment for complications from the administration of the replacement products. The nurse positions the woman on her left side to maximize placental perfusion, and oxygen may be administered at 8 to10 L/min. A Foley catheter needs to be inserted to monitor urinary output, as renal failure can occur. The patient and family will need ongoing explanations and emotional support during this time.

14.13 Umbilical Cord Prolapse

An umbilical cord prolapse occurs when a loop of the umbilical cord slips alongside (occult) or below the presenting part of the fetus (covert). Cord prolapse is rare and occurs in 0.14 to 0.62 percent of all births in most studies. It is more common in pregnancies involving malpresentations, growth restriction, prematurity, ruptured membranes with a fetus at a high station, hydramnios, multiparity, and multifetal gestation.

The danger with cord prolapse is that it usually leads to total or partial occlusion of the cord, resulting in rapid deterioration of fetal perfusion. Occlusion of blood flow to and from the fetus for more than 5 minutes can result in central nervous system damage or fetal death.

Prompt recognition of a prolapsed cord is essential to reducing the risk of fetal hypoxia. Prolapse is suspected with changes in FHR, such as variable decelerations or bradycardia.

When cord prolapse occurs, it is the priority to relieve pressure on the cord until delivery. To relieve pressure on the cord, the examiner places gloved fingers into the vagina and manually lifts the presenting part off the umbilical cord. The nurse should assist the patient into a position that lifts her hips higher than her head, shifting the presenting part toward her diaphragm. These include extreme Trendelenburg, the knee-to-chest position, or maintaining the left side-lying position with her hips elevated on pillows. The nurse needs to administer oxygen at 8 to 10 L/min via face mask to improve oxygenation to the fetus. Often a tocolytic agent is ordered to reduce uterine activity, which the nurse will administer.

If the cord is protruding from the vagina, no attempts to place the cord back into the vagina should be made; instead, the nurse should cover the exposed segment of umbilical cord with warm, sterile saline compresses to prevent drying.

The prognosis is good for the woman and for the fetus, the biggest risks being those associated with cesarean section.

14.14 Uterine Rupture

Uterine rupture is a catastrophic tearing of the uterus at the site of a previous scar into the abdominal cavity. Conditions associated with uterine rupture are uterine scars, prior cesarean births, prior rupture, trauma, prior invasive molar pregnancy, history of placenta percreta or increta, malpresentation, labor induction with excessive uterine stimulation, and crack cocaine use.

Uterine rupture is rare. Sudden fetal distress is the most common sign and often happens prior to the onset of abdominal pain or vaginal bleeding. Other signs are acute and continuous abdominal pain with or without epidural, vaginal bleeding, hematuria, irregular abdominal wall contour, and hypovolemic shock.

Because the signs may be nonspecific, the management will be the same as that for any acute fetal distress delivery by cesarean birth. Maternal death is a real possibility, and newborn outcome after rupture depends largely on the speed with which the surgical rescue is executed.

The nurse needs to monitor maternal vital signs for tachycardia, which might indicate hypovolemic shock. The nurse needs to assist in preparing for an emergency cesarean section by alerting the operating room staff, anesthesia provider, and neonatal team. Two IVs with large-bore needles should be inserted, as well as a Foley catheter. A tocolytic may be ordered to reduce excessive contractions. A woman with a large uterine rupture requires a hysterectomy. Blood is replaced as needed. The nurse needs to inform the woman and her family of the seriousness of this event and remind them that the health care team will be working quickly to ensure her health as well as the baby's. The nurse needs to provide emotional support and try to keep the woman calm.

14.15 Anaphylactoid Syndrome/Amniotic Fluid Embolism

Pregnancy-related ***anaphylactoid syndrome,*** or ***amniotic fluid embolism,*** occurs when amniotic fluid enters into the maternal circulation and is carried to the lungs. It is a rare complication of the intra- and postpartum periods that is associated with a high incidence of maternal and fetal death. For women, the mortality rate is as high as 80%; for neonates, it is as high as 50%. Neonates who survive this event very often have neurologic impairment.

The cause of anaphylactoid syndrome is unknown, but it is thought that amniotic fluid containing particles of fetal debris (meconium, hair, vernix, or skin cells) escapes into the maternal circulation and causes the release of endogenous mediators, such as histamine, prostaglandins, and thromboxane. Obstruction of the pulmonary vessels leads to respiratory distress and circulatory collapse. Hemorrhage, DIC, and pulmonary edema are present to some degree in women who experience anaphylactoid syndrome.

Although anaphylactoid syndrome is not preventable, certain maternal and fetal factors have been associated with the condition, including multiparity, abruptio placentae, tumultuous labor, macrosomia, meconium passage, and fetal death. The first symptom is frequently acute dyspnea, followed by severe hypotension. Other symptoms are restlessness, cyanosis, tachycardia, respiratory arrest, shock, and cardiac arrest.

The nurse needs to recognize the early signs of anaphylactoid syndrome and the rapidly deteriorating maternal condition and seek immediate help. The maternal prognosis depends on the size of the embolism and the speed of intervention by the health care team. If the woman survives the initial insult, she will be taken to the intensive care unit for hemodynamic monitoring.

Once the signs and symptoms are recognized, supportive care should be implemented: oxygenation (resuscitation and 100% oxygen), circulation (IV fluids, inotropic medications to maintain cardiac output and blood pressure), control of hemorrhage and coagulopathy (oxytocic agents that control uterine atony and bleeding), and administration of steroids (Solu-Cortef) to control the inflammatory response. The family needs to be supported and allowed to express their feelings.

Although rapid delivery is paramount to save the fetus, a delay in delivery usually occurs to stabilize the mother. In the event of maternal cardiopulmonary arrest, a cesarean section delivery should occur within 5 minutes.

Objective L: To Understand Intrauterine Fetal Demise

14.16 Intrauterine Fetal Demise

Perinatal death, whether it occurs before delivery, during delivery, or as a neonatal death, presents a unique set of physical and psychosocial problems. The developmental task of attachment and preparing for parenthood is abruptly interrupted, and parents suddenly find themselves faced with issues of grief and mourning. The physical process of labor and delivery, as well as the handling of the infant after delivery, requires extreme sensitivity on the part of the nurse and the perinatal team.

Bereavement care must be given to the patient and her family. The nurse and perinatal team must remember that in a cultural context, there are many views of death and different ways of grieving. Tears and emotional outbursts are common to some cultures, whereas in others, grief is quiet and introspective. All patients should be treated with sensitivity, respect, and caring.

The care for patients experiencing a perinatal loss is covered more extensively in Chapter 13.

Review Questions

Completion

1. Dysfunctional labor is characterized by ineffective changes in ____________, ____________, and ____________.
2. The powers of labor include ____________ and ____________.
3. The powers of labor are important in ____________ and ____________.
4. A treatment for hypotonic contractions may include ____________.
5. Hypertonic contractions are characterized by ____________ and ____________ contractions.
6. Fetal anomalies such as ____________ and ____________ can prevent vaginal delivery.
7. "Back labor" can be relieved by ____________ on the lower back or over the coccyx bone.
8. Soft tissue obstruction can be relieved by ____________.
9. A precipitous labor is one in which birth occurs within ____________ hours of onset.
10. Amniotic fluid that is cloudy or has a strong odor is indicative of ____________.
11. Preterm premature rupture of the membranes (PPROM) is associated with ____________ and ____________.
12. Conditions associated with premature rupture of the membranes (PROM) include ____________, ____________, and ____________.
13. A ____________ or ____________ test is used to make a definitive diagnosis of rupture of the membranes.
14. The cause of preterm labor is ____________.
15. Delay of preterm birth allows time to give maternal ____________ to reduce respiratory distress in the newborn.
16. The drug of choice for tocolysis in preterm labor is ____________.

17. The antidote for magnesium sulfate toxicity is ________________.

18. ________________ are used to hasten fetal lung maturity if birth before 34 weeks' gestation appears inevitable.

19. The biggest risk associated with postterm pregnancies is ________________.

20. ________________ involves the stimulation of the uterus to promote contractions before the onset of spontaneous labor.

21. There are many indications for inducing labor, the most common being ________________.

22. Contraindications to labor induction include ________________, ________________, and ________________.

23. Surgical methods to ripen the cervix to induce labor include ________________ and ________________.

24. Risks associated with artificial rupture of the membranes include ________________, ________________, and ________________.

25. The ________________ assesses cervical characteristics in order to determine successful candidates for induction.

26. ________________ is one of the most widely used drugs for labor induction in the United States.

27. Pitocin mimics the actions of naturally occurring ________________.

28. If there is hyperstimulation of the uterus or a nonreassuring fetal heart rate (FHR) pattern develops during labor induction, the nurse's best action would be to ________________ ________________.

29. A woman who is admitted to the labor and delivery unit with a multiple gestation pregnancy will need an intravenous (IV) line for administering fluids and treatment in the event of ________________ or the need for ________________.

30. ________________ is a technique in which a volume of warmed, sterile saline or Ringer lactate solution is introduced into the uterus through an intrauterine pressure catheter to increase the volume of fluid.

31. ________________ of the uterus is a risk when administering amnioinfusion.

32. ________________ is a term used to describe interventions used when a nonreassuring fetal heart pattern is observed on a tracing.

33. In determining fetal hypoxia, a scalp blood pH > ________________ is considered normal.

34. The use of forceps or vacuum extractor poses risks to ____________________.

35. A ________________ birth is the delivery of the fetus by an incision in the abdomen and uterus.

36. ____ describes a woman who delivers vaginally after having at least one previous cesarean birth.

37. Disseminated intravascular coagulation (DIC) is a disorder of ________________________.

38. When cord prolapse occurs, the priority intervention is to ________________________ until delivery.

39. If the cord is prolapsed, the nurse should help the patient into a position where ______________.

40. The most common sign of uterine rupture is ________________.

41. ________________________ occurs when amniotic fluid enters into maternal circulation and is carried to the lungs.

42. ________________ can be done to elicit an acceleration of the FHR.

43. ________________________ is a method of relieving shoulder dystocia.

44. Multifetal pregnancy may result in dysfunctional labor because of ______________.

45. Signs and symptoms of preterm labor include ______________, ______________, and ______________.

46. ________________________ ranks second as the leading cause of neonatal mortality in the United States.

47. Corticosteroids such as ______________ and ______________ may be used for fetal lung maturity in a woman with preterm labor.

48. The side effect of prostaglandins used for cervical ripening is their ability to produce ____________.

49. Side effects of magnesium sulfate therapy for preterm labor include ____________, ____________, and ____________.

Answers

Completion

1. Effacement, dilation

2. Contractions, maternal pushing efforts

3. Pushing the fetal head down, putting pressure on the cervix, helping the cervix dilate, helping to expel the fetus at delivery

4. IV, activity, position changes, amniotomy, pitocin infusion

5. Uncoordinated, erratic

6. Hydrocephalus, tumors

7. Counterpressure

8. Emptying the bladder

9. Three

10. Infection

11. Preterm labor, preterm birth

12. Maternal infections, chorioamnionitis, fetal abnormalities or abnormal presentations, previous preterm birth, overdistention of the uterus, maternal nutritional deficiencies, maternal stress, low socioeconomic status

13. Nitrazine, ferning

14. Unknown

15. Corticosteroids

16. Magnesium sulfate

17. Calcium gluconate

18. Corticosteroids

19. Decreased amniotic fluid

20. Labor induction

21. Postterm gestation

22. Placenta previa, abruptio placentae, transverse lie, prior classical uterine incision, pelvic structure abnormalities, previous myomectomy, vaginal bleeding with unknown cause, invasive cervical cancer, active genital herpes, abnormal FHR pattern

23. Stripping the membranes, amniotomy

24. Prolapsed cord, umbilical cord prolapse, umbilical cord compression, maternal or fetal infection, FHR decelerations, bleeding

25. Bishop score

26. Pitocin

27. Oxytocin

28. Stop pitocin administration

29. Hemorrhage, cesarean section

30. Amnioinfusion

31. Overdistention

32. Intrauterine resuscitation

33. 7.25

34. Both mother and baby

35. Cesarean

36. Vaginal birth after cesarean (VBAC)

37. Blood clotting

38. Keep pressure off the cord

39. Hips are higher than the head

40. Sudden fetal distress

41. Anaphylactoid syndrome

42. Stimulation

43. Suprapubic pressure, McRobert's maneuver, or supported squat

44. Overdistention of the uterus

45. Constant backache; pain, discomfort, or pressure in the vagina or thighs; change or increase in amount of vaginal secretions

46. Preterm birth

47. Celestone, dexamethasone

48. Hyperstimulation of the uterus

49. Depresses respiratory or cardiac status; depressed deep tendon reflexes; lethargy; blurry vision; nausea; headache; sensation of heat or "flushing"; reduced FHR variability; hypotonia in the infant

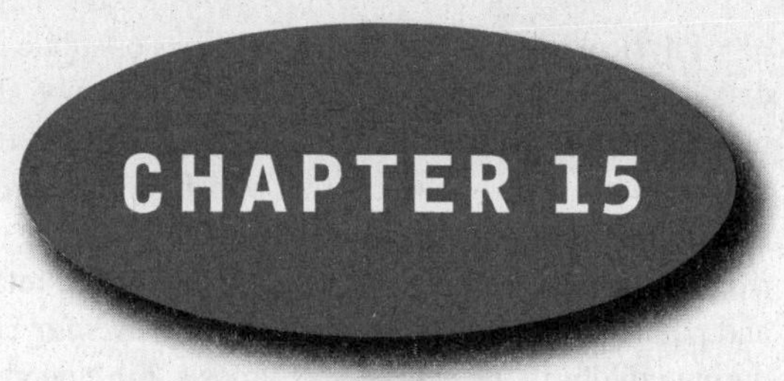

High-Risk Postpartum

Objective A: To Understand the Role of the Nurse in the High-Risk Postpartum Period

15.1 Postpartum and the Role of the Nurse

Childbirth is a natural occurrence from which most women recover fairly quickly. Complications, however, can occur in the immediate postpartum period and some after discharge, or even up to 1 year postpartum. The nurse needs to be aware of problems that may occur and understand that they can affect the whole family. This includes being cognizant of the subtle changes that may occur postpartum so early treatment can be given. The nurse needs to teach the patient and her family about the signs and symptoms of potential complications and encourage them to seek medical assistance as needed.

Objective B: To Understand Postpartum Bleeding Complications

15.2 Postpartum Bleeding Complications

Postpartum hemorrhage is one of the leading causes of death in women who deliver after 20 weeks' gestation. It occurs in ~5% of all deliveries worldwide. Approximately one third of maternal deaths are related to postpartum hemorrhage.

Postpartum hemorrhage is defined as blood loss > 500 mL for a vaginal birth and 1000 mL after a cesarean birth. Another definition of hemorrhage is a decrease in hematocrit of 10% or more since admission to the birth facility. Immediate (early) postpartum hemorrhage occurs in the first 24 hours after delivery, and late postpartum hemorrhage occurs after the first 24 hours following delivery, usually at 7 to 14 days of the postpartum period. The major causes of postpartum hemorrhage are uterine atony, lacerations of the genital tract, hematomas, retained placental fragments, uterine inversion, and blood coagulation disorders.

A review of the labor and delivery history may help with recognition of a cause and help aid in the course of treatment. Postpartum hemorrhage is associated with a precipitous or prolonged first or second stage of labor; overdistention of the uterus; drugs administered; toxins; trauma from the use of forceps or other intravaginal manipulations; past placenta previa or acreta; pregnancy-induced hypertension; uterine malformation; maternal exhaustion, malnutrition, or anemia; defects in the decidua; manipulation of the placenta that occurs when the placenta is not delivered intact and manual extraction is necessary; rapid fetal descent; coagulation disorders; grand multiparity; and uterine infection.

Physical findings that may be obvious or subtle include ***uterine atony,*** which presents as a large, boggy uterus, expelled clots, and bright red bleeding that may be slow and steady or sudden and massive; ***lacerations,*** which are usually present with a firm uterus and bright red bleeding in the form of a steady stream or trickle of unclotted blood; a ***hematoma,*** which may cause a bluish bulging area just under the skin surface of the perineum, a firm uterus, extreme perineal or pelvic pain, difficulty in voiding, unexplained tachycardia, and hypotension; ***retained placental fragments*** in the case of a placenta not delivered intact, a uterus that remains large, and bleeding that is bright red and painless; signs of ***disseminated intravascular coagulation (DIC),*** which may include uncontrolled bleeding during childbirth, petechiae, ecchymosis, prolonged bleeding from the gums and venipuncture sites, tachycardia, oliguria, signs of acute renal failure, convulsions, and coma; decreased systolic blood pressure; cold, clammy skin; profound hypotension; signs of metabolic acidosis; and anxiety and restlessness.

The nurse assesses the patient in the hours after delivery and is responsible for initial management of uterine atony. If the uterus is not firmly contracted, the first nursing intervention is to massage the fundus until it is firm and to express clots that may have accumulated in the uterus. The nurse should encourage the mother to place the baby on the breast if the woman is breastfeeding, as this will release oxytocin and help the uterus contract. To massage the uterus, one hand is placed just above the symphysis pubis to support the lower uterine segment, while the other hand firmly massages the fundus in a circular motion.

If the uterus does not remain contracted as a result of uterine massage or is displaced, the problem may be a distended bladder. A full bladder lifts the uterus and prevents contraction. The nurse should help the patient to void or catheterize if she is unable to urinate.

Pharmacologic measures may be used to maintain contraction of the uterus. A rapid intravenous (IV) infusion of dilute pitocin often increases uterine tone and controls bleeding. Methergine may be given intramuscularly (IM), but it elevates blood pressure and should not be given to a woman who is hypertensive. Analogues of prostaglandins (Hemabate, Prostin) are very effective when given IM if pitocin is ineffective at controlling uterine bleeding. Prostin E2 (dinoprostone) or Cytotec (misoprostol) given rectally may also be used to control bleeding.

If uterine massage and pharmacologic measures are not effective in stopping uterine bleeding, the physician or midwife may use bimanual compression of the uterus to stop the bleeding. In this procedure, one hand is inserted into the vagina, while the other compresses the uterus through the abdominal wall. A balloon may be inserted into the uterus to apply pressure to the uterine wall, or packing may be used and left inside the uterus for 24 hours.

The patient may be taken back to the operating room for exploration of the uterine cavity and removal of placental fragments (dilatation and curettage [D&C]) that interfere with uterine contraction.

Ligation of the uterine or hypogastric artery or occlusion of pelvic arteries may be necessary if other measures are ineffective. Hysterectomy is the last resort measure to save the life of a woman with uncontrolled postpartum hemorrhage. The nurse is often responsible for obtaining properly typed and cross-matched blood and inserting large-bore IV lines that are capable of carrying whole blood. Hemorrhage requires prompt replacement of intravascular fluid volume, lactated Ringer solution, whole blood, packed red blood cells, normal saline, or other plasma extenders.

Along with frequent, careful monitoring of vital signs, the nurse should be assessing the fundus for firmness, height, and midline position of the uterus often, as per institution policy. Pads should be checked frequently, and pad counts may be initiated (or weighed; 1 g = 1 mL). Lochia should be monitored for color, odor, amount, consistency, and clots. The patient should be maintained in a flat position to promote the supply of blood to the heart and brain. She should be turned when assessing postpartal bleeding so blood does not pool and go unnoticed underneath her.

Accurate records of intake and output need to be kept. Insertion of a Foley catheter can help keep the bladder from getting full and displacing the uterus, and it allows for an accurate measure of urine output. Enough fluid should be given to maintain a urine flow of at least 30 mL/h, preferably 60 mL/h. Wide-spectrum antibiotics are usually given to prevent infection.

The nurse needs to explain everything to the patient and her family as it is taking place to help alleviate anxiety. Information should be given in the form of clearly understood, brief statements. The nurse should stay with the patient as much as possible to offer reassurance and support and to keep the family informed of the patient's status.

After the hemorrhage has been controlled, the patient needs to be assessed frequently for resumption of bleeding. She will be fatigued and may be anemic. Allow for frequent rest periods and encourage her to eat foods high in iron. Because she may experience orthostatic hypotension when first getting out of bed, encourage the patient to rise slowly to a seated position, dangle her legs over the edge of the bed, then stand up carefully with assistance.

Late postpartum hemorrhage can be dangerous for the unsuspecting patient. The nurse should teach the patient about the normal duration and characteristics of lochia. She should be instructed to call her health care provider if bleeding persists, becomes unusually heavy, or returns to a bright red color.

15.3 Trauma

Trauma to the birth canal is the second most common cause of early postpartum hemorrhage. Trauma can include vaginal, cervical, or perineal lacerations, as well as hematomas. Small cervical lacerations occur frequently and generally do not need repair. Lacerations of the birth canal should be suspected if the uterine fundus is firm and is at the expected location. Hematomas occur when rapid bleeding into the loose connective tissue occurs while overlying tissue remains intact. Small hematomas usually reabsorb naturally, whereas large hematomas often require incision and evacuation. Often a bleeding vessel needs ligation.

15.4 Hypovolemic Shock

When blood loss is excessive, hypovolemic shock can ensue. During and after giving birth, a woman can tolerate a blood loss equal to the volume of blood added during pregnancy (~1500–2000 mL).

Recognition of hypovolemic shock may be delayed because the body tries to compensate and masks the severity of the problem. Early signs of tachycardia or hypotension may not appear until up to 25% of a woman's blood volume is lost. Skin changes also provide early clues, making the skin cool to the touch and pale, progressing to cold and clammy. As shock progresses, the patient becomes very anxious, then confused, and finally lethargic.

Therapeutic management is focused on controlling bleeding and preventing hypovolemic shock from becoming irreversible.

15.5 Subinvolution

Subinvolution of the uterus refers to a slower than expected return of the uterus to its nonpregnant size after childbirth. The most common cause of subinvolution is retained placental fragments and infection.

Signs of subinvolution include prolonged discharge of lochia, excessive uterine bleeding, pelvic pain, feelings of pelvic heaviness, fatigue, and persistent malaise. On exam, the uterus feels bigger than normal for the time of the postpartum course.

Management is to correct the cause of subinvolution. Methergine is given orally to maintain contraction of the uterus. Antibiotics are given for infection. Because subinvolution may be subtle, it is important when doing discharge teaching to instruct the patient in the normal course of uterine discharge during the postpartum period. Patients should be instructed to call their health care provider when there is a deviation in the amount, appearance, odor of the lochia, or other signs such as pelvic pain, pressure or fullness, and back pain.

Objective C: To Understand Thromboembolic Disorders in the Postpartum Period

15.6 Thromboembolic Disorders

The most common thromboembolic disorders seen postpartum are ***superficial venous thrombophlebitis (SVT), deep vein thrombosis (DVT),*** and, occasionally, ***pulmonary embolism (PE).***

SVT generally involves the saphenous venous system and is confined to the lower leg. DVT can involve veins from the foot to the iliofemoral region. The incidence of thromboembolic disease in pregnancy and postpartum is

1 per 1000 to 2000 pregnancies, and it remains a major cause of maternal death in the United States. A thrombus is a collection of blood factors, primarily fibrin and platelets, on a vessel wall. Thrombi can form wherever the flow of blood is impeded. The three major causes of thrombosis are

1. Venous stasis
2. Hypercoagulable blood
3. Injury to the endothelial surface of the blood vessel

SVT is usually associated with varicose veins and limited to the calf area. It may also result from IV therapy in the arms. Signs and symptoms of SVT include swelling of the involved extremity, redness, tenderness, and warmth.

Nursing interventions include rest, elastic support, and analgesics. Elevation of the lower extremity helps with venous return. Warm packs may be applied to the affected area. After a period of rest with the extremity elevated, the woman can ambulate gradually if symptoms have disappeared. She should be encouraged to avoid standing or sitting for long periods and should continue to wear support hose. If the thrombosis remains in the superficial veins of the leg, there is little chance of PE.

Signs and symptoms of a DVT are absent 75% of the time in those patients affected. DVT is caused by an inflammatory process and obstruction of venous return. Swelling of the leg, erythema, heat, and tenderness over the affected area are the most common signs seen in those with a DVT. A positive Homan sign is not a positive indicator of a DVT.

Factors that increase the risk of thrombosis include inactivity, prolonged bed rest, obesity, cesarean birth, sepsis, smoking, history of previous thrombosis, varicose veins, diabetes, trauma, prolonged labor, prolonged time in stirrups during the second stage of labor, maternal age over 35 years, increased parity, dehydration, use of forceps, air travel, antiphospholipid antibody syndrome, inherited thrombophilias, and first-degree relative with thrombosis.

Diagnosis is made with a venous ultrasonography with vein compression and Doppler flow analysis of the deep veins of the upper legs.

Treatment for DVT includes anticoagulants, analgesics, and bed rest with the affected leg elevated. Therapy may begin with an IV infusion of standard unfractionated heparin (UH) and is later changed to subcutaneous UH. The drug will not dissolve clots but will prevent enlargement of any that are present. During the postpartum period, warfarin is started before heparin is stopped to provide continuous anticoagulation. Warfarin therapy is typically continued from 6 weeks to 6 months. Warfarin is safe for lactating mothers.

Discharge teaching should include lifestyle changes that improve circulation. The patient should be encouraged to avoid wearing tight clothing or girdles for a full 6 weeks until the uterus heals. Wearing restrictive clothing prevents the uterus from getting proper blood flow needed for healing and can cause blood clot formation. The postpartum woman should not sit for long periods with legs dependent in order to prevent stasis. If sitting is required for long periods, walking for a short time hourly or moving the feet and legs frequently will help prevent circulatory stasis. The patient should stay well hydrated, as dehydration can be a causative factor in clot formation.

Objective D: To Understand Infections During the Postpartum Period

15.7 Infections During the Postpartum Period

Puerperal infection is a term used to describe a bacterial infection after childbirth. Postpartum infection occurs in ~6% of births in the United States and is still a leading cause of death in under-developed countries. The definition of a puerperal infection is a temperature of 100.4°F (38°C) or higher after the first 24 hours that occurs on at least 2 of the first 10 days following childbirth.

The most common type of postpartum infection is endometritis. Other infections seen in the postpartum period are wound infections, urinary tract infections, mastitis, and septic pelvic thrombophlebitis. The most common causative agents of postpartum infections are anaerobic streptococcus, *Clostridium,* group A or B hemolytic streptococcus, *Escherichia coli, Klebsiella, Gardnerella vaginalis, Chlamydia trachomatis,* and *Staphylococcus aureus.*

Risk factors for postpartum infections include a history of previous infections, colonization of the lower genital tract by pathogenic organisms, cesarean birth, trauma, prolonged rupture of the membranes, prolonged labor, frequent vaginal exams, internal fetal monitoring, catheterization, retained placental fragments, hemorrhage, poor general health, poor hygiene, medical conditions (diabetes, preeclampsia, anemia, etc), low socioeconomic status, droplet infection from personnel, and a break in aseptic technique.

Genital tract infections involving the muscle of the uterus (metritis), at the placental site (endometritis), pelvic connective tissue (parametritis), tubes (salpingitis), or ovaries (oophoritis) usually exhibit the following signs and symptoms: temperature of 38.5° to 39.5°C (101–103°F); large, tender uterus; lower abdominal pain; malaise; anorexia; chills; extreme lethargy; backache; increased pulse rate (100–140 bpm); foul-smelling lochia; and diaphoresis.

Genital tract infections involving the perineum, vulva, vagina, or cervix may produce the following signs and symptoms: a low-grade fever of 38° to 38.5° (100.4–101°F), site of infection red and warm to the touch, dysuria, localized pain, edema, and white blood cell count (WBC) count > 30,000/mm^3 after the first day. Drainage may or may not be present.

Urinary tract infections and cystitis may produce the following signs and symptoms: a low-grade fever of 38.5°C (101°F), small voiding volume or inability to void, pain on urination, hematuria, overdistended bladder, increased vaginal bleeding, boggy fundus, backache, and restlessness.

Wound infections from cesarean delivery or dehiscence may produce the following signs and symptoms: elevated temperature on the third or fourth postpartum day; drainage of pus or blood from the wound; red, inflamed appearance of repaired edges; presence of cellulitis; and wound opened and abdominal contents exposed to air.

Breast infection, or mastitis, is usually unilateral and may produce the following signs and symptoms: acute pain, tenderness or inflammation, temperature elevation to 40°C (104.1°F), chills, malaise, engorgement, cracked nipples, and lack of proper breast support.

Nursing interventions include obtaining specimens for culture and sensitivity; administering antipyretics and antibiotics; assessing vital signs frequently; using aseptic technique; using proper and frequent hand washing; using the semi-Fowler's position to facilitate drainage; assessing the fundus for involution; monitoring and recording input and output; encouraging frequent rest periods; maintaining an intact wound; facilitating complete bladder emptying; facilitating keeping the breasts empty; assisting with breast and perineal care; changing linens frequently; explaining care measures to the patient; allowing the patient time to verbalize her feelings and concerns; keeping the patient's family informed at all times; promoting bonding with the infant; and allowing the patient's family and friends to visit or telephone if the patient has sufficient energy.

Many of these infections appear after discharge, so it is important to teach the patient about their signs and symptoms and to urge her to contact her physician immediately so that treatment can be initiated early. The nurse should stress that infections must be treated with antibiotics. Although alternate methods of treatment (eg, cabbage leaves and tea bags placed on the breasts) may provide short-term relief of pain, they will not clear up an infection.

Objective E: To Understand Postpartum Mood Disorders

15.8 Mood Disorders

Mood disorders are disturbances in function, affect, or thought processes. For the postpartum mother, they include postpartum depression (PPD), postpartum psychosis, and postpartum anxiety disorders. ***Postpartum "blues"*** is a transient, self-limiting mood disorder seen in the postpartum mother in the first week after childbirth. It commonly coincides with discharge from the birth facility and the realization that the family must take home and care for a new family member. The new father may also experience "the blues."

PPD differs from the "blues" in that it can affect a family as seriously as a physiologic problem and is a more serious disorder that requires intervention to resolve. It is defined as a period of depression that begins after childbirth and lasts for at least 2 weeks. PPD can occur at any time during the first postpartum year and is considered a major mood disorder. The greatest risk occurs at approximately the fourth postpartum week.

PPD is one of the most common complications of childbirth. According to the U.S. Department of Health and Human Services, ~20% of postpartum women suffer from PPD. PPD can last up to 3 years. The cause of PPD is unknown; however, the biggest predictor of PPD is prenatal depression, followed by problems with child care and life stressors.

The woman with PPD shows a depressed mood that tends to become worse over time. She exhibits a loss of interest in her usual activities, as well as a loss of her usual emotional response toward her family. The woman may have intense feelings of anxiety, unworthiness, guilt, agitation, and shame and feel that she is not worthy to be a mother and that she cannot do a good job caring for her infant. The woman may complain of generalized fatigue, irritability, and nonspecific health problems and have difficulty making decisions. She often has little interest in food and experiences sleep disturbances (insomnia or excessive sleeping).

Partners of depressed women report the loss of the woman and the relationship they had known previously, along with feelings of loss of control, anger, and frustration. Depressed women interact differently with their infants than those who are not depressed. They are more tense, are more irritable, and feel less competent as mothers. They may not be able to pick up their infants' cues and may therefore fail to meet their infants' needs. Depressed women are more likely not to provide healthy feeding and sleep practices or positive enrichment activities for their infants. Major depression interferes with normal mother–infant bonding and puts the infant at risk for later cognitive, emotional, and behavioral problems.

Most experts agree that a combination of therapies is best in treating PPD. Counseling and medication are encouraged, as well as family therapy in some instances. It is important to identify family and cultural issues when treating depression. In some cultures, it is shameful for new mothers to admit that they are feeling depressed and may not ask for assistance. It is important for families to be educated about PPD and encouraged to seek assistance, as PPD affects the whole family.

A very small percentage of women (1 or 2 in 1,000) suffer a rare and severe form of perinatal depression called ***postpartum psychosis.*** Women who have bipolar disorder or other psychiatric problem may have a higher risk for developing it. Symptoms of postpartum psychosis include extreme confusion, hopelessness, insomnia even when exhausted, anorexia, distrust of others, seeing or hearing voices that are not there, and thoughts of hurting themselves or their infants. This form of depression is considered a medical emergency, and families need to know they must seek immediate care should a new mother exhibit these signs and symptoms.

Postpartum anxiety disorders include obsessive-compulsive disorder (OCD), panic disorder, and posttraumatic stress disorder (PTSD).

In ***OCD,*** anxiety and depression are the chief cause. The postpartum mother has consuming thoughts that she might harm the baby and may be afraid to be left alone with the baby. The woman may perform compulsive behaviors, such as checking on the baby constantly. In some cases, the mother may totally avoid her infant in order not to act on her thoughts. Treatment includes antianxiety and antidepressant medications and therapy.

Panic disorder manifests itself as episodes of palpitations, shortness of breath, fear of dying, or feelings of "going crazy" and interferes with the woman's daily life. Treatment includes antianxiety and antidepressant medication and counseling.

In ***PTSD,*** women view childbirth as a traumatic event. They may have nightmares or "flashbacks" of the birth, avoid talking about it, and become depressed. Women often report a "lack of caring" on the part of their health care providers, a lack of communication, and having a birth different from what they expected. These women need to talk about their experiences in counseling, and medication may be necessary.

Early identification and treatment of postpartum mood disorders is a significant factor in the duration of the condition. Women should be assessed for depression during pregnancy, at the birth facility, and during follow-up visits postpartum.

Assessment tools, such as the Postpartum Depression Predictors Inventory–Revised (2002), may be used to identify factors that can predict the likelihood that a woman will develop PPD. Other screening tools are the Edinburgh Postnatal Depression Scale (1987) and the Postpartum Depression Screening Scale (2000).

The woman should be assessed for objective signs and symptoms, such as poor personal hygiene, crying, sleeplessness, and inability to follow directions or to concentrate. It should be determined whether or not the woman has family support. Single mothers may not have a significant other who is involved and may feel increasingly isolated, which causes stress above the normal level experienced postpartum.

Conveying a caring attitude is an important nursing strategy to help patients decrease their emotional distress and to guide them in regaining their well-being during the postpartum period. The nurse needs to help the new mother verbalize her feelings, model behavior to show the mother how to respond to the infant's cues, provide anticipatory guidance, and help family members adjust to their new roles and identify ways they can help the new parent(s).

Review Questions

True/False

1. _______ Postpartum hemorrhage is one of the leading causes of death in women who deliver after 20 weeks' gestation.

2. _______ Postpartum hemorrhage occurs in approximately 5% of all deliveries.

3. _______ There is only one cause for postpartum hemorrhage.

4. _______ Hematomas may be a subtle cause of a postpartum hemorrhage.

5. _______ The first intervention for a boggy uterus is to increase intravenous (IV) fluids.

6. _______ Methergine can be given to anyone experiencing a postpartum hemorrhage.

7. _______ Postpartum infections need to be treated with antibiotics.

8. _______ Mastitis usually occurs in both breasts.

9. _______ Thrombophlebitis is an infection of the lining of a vessel that attaches to the vessel wall.

10. _______ Depression during pregnancy or previous postpartum depression is a strong predictor of postpartum depression.

11. _______ Postpartum depression can occur any time during the first year postpartum.

12. _______ Postpartum depression is a major mood disorder.

13. _______ Superficial thrombophlebitis is usually associated with varicose veins and limited to the calf area.

14. _______ During pregnancy, compression of the large vessels of the legs and pelvis by the enlarging uterus causes venous stasis.

15. _______ Thrombus formation is nine times more likely to occur if birth is by cesarean section.

Completion

1. The greatest risk of postpartum depression occurs approximately ________________ after childbirth.

2. ________________ refers to a slower than expected return of the uterus to its prepregnant state.

3. The most common thromboembolic disorders seen postpartum are ________________, ________________, and ________________.

4. Postpartum ________________ is a self-limiting mood disorder.

5. The woman with endometritis should be placed in the ________________ position to facilitate drainage.

Multiple Choice

1. Supportive measures for a mother with mastitis include

   A. Maintaining her normal routine

   B. Applying moist heat or ice packs

   C. Avoiding breastfeeding

   D. Separating the infant from the infected mother

2. Risk factors for postpartum depression include (choose all that apply)

   A. Depression in pregnancy

   B. Poor coping skills

   C. Single-parent status

   D. Strong family support

3. The first nursing intervention for a patient with a boggy uterus is

   A. Catheterization

   B. Increasing intravenous (IV) fluids

   C. Massaging the fundus

   D. Calling the health care provider

4. The most common causative agents of postpartum infection are (choose all that apply)

   A. *Escherichia coli*

   B. *Staphylococcus aureus*

C. Anaerobic streptococcus

D. *Klebsiella*

5. Urinary tract infections in postpartum women may have all of the following physical findings except

A. High fever

B. Pain with urination

C. Small voiding volume

D. Backache

Answers

True/False

1. True
2. True
3. False. There are many causes of postpartum hemorrhage.
4. True
5. False. The first nursing intervention for a boggy uterus is to massage the fundus.
6. False. Methergine should not be given to someone with an increased blood pressure, as it raises blood pressure.
7. True
8. False. Mastitis is usually unilateral.
9. True
10. True
11. True
12. True
13. True
14. True
15. True

Completion

1. Four weeks
2. Subinvolution
3. Superficial venous thrombosis (SVT), deep vein thrombosis (DVT), and pulmonary embolism (PE)
4. "Blues"
5. Semi-Fowler's

Multiple Choice

1. B
2. A, B, C
3. C
4. A, B, C, D
5. A

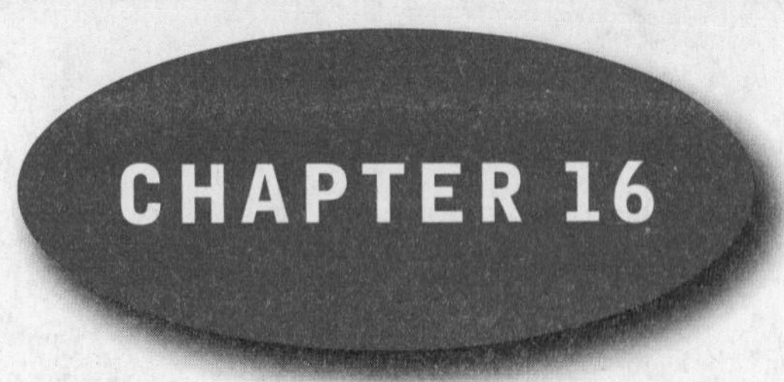

The High-Risk Newborn

Objective A: To Understand the Role of the Nurse in Caring for the High-Risk Newborn

16.1 The Nurse and the High-Risk Newborn

Maternity nurses identify and care for the high-risk newborn until the neonatal intensive care unit (NICU) team can assume responsibility. If a complication is expected, often the neonatologist and intensive care nurses will be at the delivery.

Care for infants with problems at birth often involves collaboration with many different professionals. Nurses are often the coordinator for this care and explain and clarify it to the parents. Because care in the NICU is costly, case managers are assigned to follow these infants from admission to discharge to identify or prevent situations that may interfere with progression toward discharge. Clinical pathways for expected outcomes of care are delineated and followed so as to ensure that discharge can occur as soon as possible.

Approximately 9% of all newborns are sick enough at birth to require intensive care. Problems seen in newborns at birth can be associated with gestational age and development or can be acquired or congenital conditions.

Objective B: To Understand Complications Associated with Gestational Age and Size

16.2 Complications Associated with Gestational Age and Size

Preterm infants are those born before the end of the 37th week of gestation. Particularly those born before 34 weeks are at high risk because of immaturity of all organ systems, numerous physiologic handicaps, and significant morbidity and mortality. Disorders related to short gestation and low birth weight are the second leading cause of infant mortality, congenital anomalies being the leading cause. In 2010, 12.3% of all births were preterm in the United States.

The exact cause of preterm birth is unknown, but all risk factors during pregnancy are potential causes. Measures to prevent preterm births include reducing barriers to prenatal care for all women, assessing for risk factors to promote changes such as smoking cessation, teaching women and their partners about subtle signs and symptoms of preterm labor, and empowering women to take an active approach to seeking medical care if they have signs or symptoms of preterm labor.

Characteristics of preterm infants vary by gestational age. Some characteristics that are common to all preterm infants are the appearance of being frail and weak; under-developed flexor muscles and resulting poor muscle tone (lie in an extended position; poor suck and gag reflex); head that is large in comparison with the rest of the body; the lack of subcutaneous fat, making the skin appear translucent, with blood vessels clearly visible; abundant vernix and lanugo; nipples and areolae that are barely visible and often flat, red, and shiny; and pinnae of the ear that are flat, red, and shiny with little cartilage. In females, the clitoris and labia minora appear large and are not covered by the labia majora; in males, the scrotum may be small, red, shiny, and smooth, with undescended testes. These infants tire easily from environmental stress.

Additional findings of the premature infant include the inability to maintain body temperature; limited ability to excrete solutes in the urine; increased susceptibility to infection, hyperbilirubinemia, and hypoglycemia; and periodic breathing, hypoventilation, and periods of apnea.

Among organ systems, the respiratory system is one of the last to mature, so the preterm infant is at risk for numerous respiratory problems. The presence of surfactant in adequate amounts is of primary importance because it reduces surface tension in the alveoli and prevents the lungs from collapsing. It allows the lungs to inflate with lower negative pressure, decreasing the work of breathing. Infants born before 34 weeks' gestation, when adequate surfactant production is completed, may develop ***respiratory distress syndrome (RDS).***

Nursing interventions for the premature infant in terms of respiratory care include assessing the respiratory status frequently and auscultating for adventitious sounds or absent breath sounds. Periodic breathing needs to be differentiated from apneic spells, in which there is a lack of breathing lasting more than 20 seconds accompanied by cyanosis, a drop in heart rate, and a decrease in oxygen saturation.

The nurse should provide frequent position changes for the infant, as it helps drain air passages and prevents stasis of secretions. Infants should be repositioned every 2 to 3 hours to the side-lying or prone position, which facilitates drainage of respiratory secretions and regurgitated feedings. The infant is suctioned only when necessary; the suctioning should be gentle to avoid traumatizing mucous membranes. The mouth is suctioned before the nose because stimulation of the nares causes reflex inspiration that can cause aspiration of fluids in the infant's mouth. Adequate hydration is essential to keep secretions thin so they can be removed easily.

RDS is a developmental respiratory disorder affecting preterm newborns with a lack of lung surfactant. In RDS, there is diffuse atelectasis with congestion and edema in the lung spaces. On deflation, the alveoli collapse, and there is decreased lung compliance. Clinical signs of RDS begin shortly after birth. Breathing is rapid (tachypnic) and labored and is often accompanied by respiratory grunting. Arterial blood gas values show oxygenation deficits and metabolic acidosis if left untreated.

Mechanical ventilation is used for preterm newborns who have little capacity to ventilate the alveoli on their own. An endotracheal tube (ET) is placed orally or nasally to create an open secure airway in which to ventilate the newborn. The administration of synthetic surfactant within 15 to 30 minutes of birth is required. It is administered through a catheter in the ET. Continued mechanical ventilation after administration helps the medication to be spread throughout the lung tissue. Newborns are weaned from mechanical ventilation as soon as possible to avoid complications from oxygen, such as ***bronchopulmonary dysplasia (BPD)*** and ***retinopathy of prematurity (ROP).*** They are often placed on continuous positive airway pressure (CPAP), an alternative oxygen source.

BPD, or chronic lung disease, is a condition in which the newborn becomes oxygen dependent past 36 weeks' gestation and is a complication of prolonged oxygen use. Although oxygen is needed by the preterm infant, supplemental oxygen can cause damage to lung tissue by suppressing compliancy. It results in the infant's needing oxygen via cannula for an extended period of time, sometimes for a few years. The infant is discharged home on oxygen after the parents have been educated in oxygen administration.

ROP is an alteration in vision leading to partial or total blindness. It typically results from prolonged exposure to high concentrations of oxygen or fluctuations in oxygen administration levels. Such fluctuations lead to rapid vasodilation and vasoconstriction of immature, fragile retinal blood vessels. Nurses taking care of preterm infants receiving supplemental oxygen must prevent fluctuations in arterial concentrations of oxygen. They must wean the preterm infant off supplemental oxygen as soon as possible. In treating ROP, bright lighting should be avoided in the preterm infant's environment. A blanket can be placed over the infant's incubator during the day. Nap time and night time can be designed so that lights are lowered, and other environmental stimuli are greatly decreased. The nurse needs to explain the condition and its treatment to the infant's parents and instruct them on the need for follow-up eye examinations.

The cardiovascular system undergoes transition at birth from the fetal to the neonatal circulatory pattern, and preterm delivery can adversely affect this transition. If oxygen levels remain low, the fetal pattern of circulation may persist, causing blood flow to bypass the lungs. Preterm infants have a higher incidence of patent ductus arteriosus. The foramen ovale may remain open if pulmonary vascular resistance is high. Preterm infants have impaired regulation of blood pressure, and fluctuations in cerebral blood flow are common, predisposing to the rupture of fragile blood vessels in the brain and causing intracranial hemorrhage, as well as predisposing to the development of ROP.

Nursing care of the preterm infant includes closely assessing all body systems; anticipating the need for endotracheal intubation and mechanical ventilation; administering oxygen and monitoring transcutaneous oxygen levels; instituting measures to maintain a neutral thermal environment (keeping extremities close to the body, using an incubator); administering medications to support respiratory and cardiac function; monitoring fluid and electrolyte balance; administering intravenous (IV) fluid as ordered; using firm but gentle touch when handling the infant and avoiding rubbing and stroking; doing cluster care (doing all nursing care at one time to allow infant to rest); administering nutritional therapy as ordered; providing nonnutritive sucking via a pacifier as appropriate; providing education, support, and guidance to the parents and family; and assisting with referrals for supportive services.

Necrotizing enterocolitis (NEC) is a serious inflammatory condition of the intestinal tract that may lead to cellular death of areas of intestinal mucosa. The ileum and proximal colon are the areas most affected. It occurs in 1% to 5% of infants admitted to NICUs. The mortality rate is 25% to 30%, and 25% of survivors have long-term gastrointestinal (GI) problems.

Although the exact cause of NEC is unknown, immaturity of the intestines is a major factor in preterm infants. The condition is less common in infants whose mothers received prenatal steroids. The incidence is higher in infants who have received feedings, especially those given too early or where the amount of feedings has been increased too quickly. Breast milk, which contains immunoglobulins, leukocytes, and antibacterial agents, may have a preventive effect on the development of NEC.

Signs of NEC include increased abdominal girth, respiratory difficulty, apnea, bradycardia, increased gastric residuals, decreased or absent bowel sounds, loops of bowel seen through the abdominal wall, vomiting, bile-stained residuals or emesis, abdominal tenderness, signs of infection, occult blood in the stools, temperature instability, lethargy, hypotension, and shock. On x-ray, there may be loops of bowel dilated with air, which is characteristic of the condition.

Treatment of NEC includes antibiotics, discontinuation of oral feedings, continuous or intermittent gastric suction, and use of parenteral nutrition to rest the intestines. Surgery may be necessary if lack of improvement or perforation occurs. The necrotic area is removed, and an ostomy may be performed. Infants who have had large portions of bowel removed may develop short bowel syndrome, which may result in malabsorption and malnutrition.

Nursing care includes encouraging mothers to pump their breasts so breast milk can be given to their infants, as breastfed infants are less likely to develop NEC. The nurse needs to monitor constantly for changes in status and to withhold a feeding if changes are noted while notifying the neonatologist. Abdominal girth should be monitored regularly and frequently (as per facility protocol), and IV fluids and parenteral nutrition need to be managed. The infant should be positioned on his or her side to minimize the effects of the pressure on the diaphragm from the distended intestines. During recovery, the nurse needs to monitor for signs of feeding intolerance.

16.3 Postterm or Postmature Infants

The term ***postterm*** or ***postmature infants*** refers to neonates born after 41 completed weeks of gestation. The greatest risk to the fetus is the aging placenta, which after term begins to collect calcium deposits, making the placenta unable to function and reducing the oxygen, fluids, and nutrients that reach the fetus. Some postterm fetuses grow to more than 4000 g (8 lb, 13 oz), also placing them at great risk for birth injuries or cesarean birth.

Because of the incidence of placental degeneration, postterm neonates are susceptible to perinatal asphyxia and meconium passage and possibly meconium aspiration. Intrauterine hypoxia can trigger increased red blood cell (RBC) production, leading to polycythemia, which causes sluggish perfusion in organ systems and hyperbilirubinemia resulting from the breakdown of excessive numbers of RBCs.

The postmature neonate is susceptible to hypoglycemia because of the rapid depletion of glycogen stores. Because of the depleted subcutaneous fat, the neonate is also susceptible to cold stress.

Physical assessment findings of the postmature neonate include an alert, wide-eyed look; absence of vernix caseosa; dry, peeling, parchmentlike skin; long fingernails; profuse scalp hair; long, thin body; decreased or absent subcutaneous fat; and meconium staining.

Nursing care for the postterm neonate is primarily prevention of complications and monitoring for changes in status. Signs of postmaturity syndrome are usually noted during the initial assessment. Respiratory problems may be seen and necessitate continuing respiratory care. The neonate should be assessed for hypoglycemia soon after birth and as per hospital policy. Early and frequent feedings need to be initiated. Temperature must be monitored frequently, and parents need to be taught about prevention of cold stress. Because polycythemia increases the risk of hyperbilirubinemia, the infant should be monitored for increasing levels of jaundice.

16.4 Small for Gestational Age

Small for gestational age (SGA), also known as ***intrauterine growth restriction (IUGR),*** infants are those who fall below the 10th percentile in size on growth charts. They have failed to grow in utero as expected. Infants who are SGA may be preterm, full term, or postterm.

There are many risk factors associated with SGA. Chromosomal abnormalities, congenital malformations, multiple gestations, poor placental function, fetal infections, such as rubella and cytomegalovirus (CMV), and illness in the mother, such as preeclampsia and severe diabetes, can impair fetal growth. Smoking, drug or alcohol abuse, and malnutrition can also impair fetal growth.

Because the causes of growth restriction are so varied, nursing care must be tailored to meet the individual infant's needs. Parents must be educated and given emotional support.

16.5 Large for Gestational Age

Large for gestational age (LGA), also known as ***macrosomic,*** infants, are those who are above the 90th percentile on growth charts. They tend to weigh more than 4000 g (8 lb, 13 oz) and are usually born at term, although they can be postterm or even preterm.

LGA infants are born to large parents, multiparas, members of certain ethnic groups known to have large infants, and diabetic mothers. They may have birth injuries such as fractures, nerve damage, and bruising as a result of their size. LGA infants are more likely to be delivered by cesarean section. Additionally, they may have hypoglycemia and polycythemia.

The nurse must carefully assess the LGA infant for injuries and other complications, such as hypoglycemia and polycythemia. Nursing care is directed toward problems presented. Parents need to be educated and given emotional support.

Objective C: To Understand Acquired Conditions Associated with the High-Risk Newborn

16.6 Asphyxia

Asphyxia is a lack of oxygen and an increase in carbon dioxide in the blood. It can occur in utero, during delivery, or after birth and can result in ischemia to major organs. The lack of oxygen in cells leads to the production of lactic acid. Respiratory acidosis occurs as carbon dioxide accumulates. Vasoconstriction caused by low oxygen levels decreases blood flow to all organs except the brain, myocardium, and adrenal glands. The ductus arteriosus and foramen ovale may remain open because of the low oxygen level in the blood, high resistance to blood flow through constricted pulmonary vessels, and elevated pressure on the right side of the heart.

When asphyxia occurs after birth, rapid respirations are followed by cessation of respirations (primary apnea) and a rapid fall in heart rate. Stimulation alone or with oxygen may restart respirations. If asphyxia continues without intervention, the infant may enter into a period of secondary apnea in which oxygen levels continue to decrease, the infant loses consciousness, and stimulation is ineffective. Resuscitative measures must be initiated immediately to prevent permanent brain damage or death.

An infant may be at risk for asphyxia any time there are problems during pregnancy, labor, or birth. If the mother receives narcotics less than 4 hours prior to delivery, the infant's central nervous system (CNS) may be too depressed for spontaneous breathing. Trauma during delivery (forceps, vacuum extraction, cord around the neck, shoulder dystocia, etc) may leave the infant asphyxiated.

The nurse must be prepared for situations in which asphyxia may occur and be ready to begin resuscitative measures. Maintenance of thermoregulation is important during resuscitative care. The nurse may assist with intubation, insertion of an umbilical catheter, and administration of medications. Additionally, the infant must be closely monitored for changes in status. Infants with asphyxia often have other problems, such as hypoglycemia, feeding problems, temperature instability, seizures, hypotension, pulmonary hypertension, metabolic acidosis, renal problems, and fluid and electrolyte imbalances. The nurse needs to offer explanations to the parents and provide emotional support. These infants are usually taken to the NICU immediately after birth.

16.7 Transient Tachypnea of the Newborn

Transient tachypnea of the newborn (TTN), also known as ***type II respiratory distress syndrome*** or ***"wet lung,"*** is a mild respiratory condition in neonates developing within hours after birth and lasting approximately 72 hours. Although the exact cause of TTN is unknown, it is thought to result from a delay in absorption of fetal lung fluid by the pulmonary capillaries and lymph vessels. This leads to decreased lung compliance and air trapping and produces signs and symptoms similar to RDS.

Neonates at greater risk for TTN include those born by cesarean section, neonates whose mothers have asthma or smoked during the pregnancy, neonates of diabetic mothers, SGA neonates, premature neonates, and those born precipitously vaginally.

Assessment findings include increased respiratory rate (> 60 breaths/min), expiratory grunting, nasal flaring, slight cyanosis, retractions, tachypnea, increased carbon dioxide levels, and an x-ray that reveals streaking.

Nursing care for the neonate with TTN includes monitoring the neonate's respiratory rate, heart rate, and oxygenation status; providing respiratory support, including mechanical ventilation, if necessary; instituting measures to maintain a neutral thermal environment; providing nutritional support via gavage feedings or parenteral nutrition; minimizing stimulation by dimming lights and reducing noise levels; educating the parents about the condition; and providing emotional support to the parents and family. Antibiotics may be given until sepsis is ruled out.

16.8 Meconium Aspiration Syndrome

Meconium aspiration syndrome (MAS) involves aspiration of meconium into the lungs and typically occurs with the first breath or while the neonate is in utero. Neonates with MAS increase respiratory efforts to create greater intrathoracic pressures and improve air flow to the lungs.

Hyperinflation, hypoxemia, and acidemia cause increased peripheral vascular resistance, and right-to-left shunting commonly follows. Chemical pneumonitis results, causing the alveolar walls and interstitial tissues to thicken and preventing adequate gas exchange. Cardiac efficiency can be compromised from pulmonary hypertension.

Assessment findings may include green staining of the amniotic fluid upon rupture; fetal hypoxia, as indicated by fetal heart rate tracings; green staining of the neonate's skin at delivery; signs of distress at delivery, including the neonate appearing limp, cyanotic, and pale; Apgar scores < 6; respiratory distress; and coarse crackles when auscultating the neonate's lungs. A chest x-ray may show patches or streaks of meconium in the lungs, air trappings, or hyperinflation.

Nursing interventions include assisting with immediate endotracheal suctioning during delivery; monitoring lung status closely; assessing vital signs frequently; administering treatment modalities, such as oxygen, respiratory support, surfactant therapy, and antibiotics; instituting measures to maintain a neutral thermal environment; teaching the parents about the condition, the treatment, and procedures, as well as what to expect; and providing emotional support to the parents and family members.

16.9 Persistent Pulmonary Hypertension of the Newborn

Persistent pulmonary hypertension of the newborn (PPHN), also known as ***persistent fetal circulation,*** is a condition in which the vascular resistance of the lungs does not decrease after the birth, and normal changes to neonatal circulation are impaired.

The cause of PPHN may be abnormal lung development, hypoxia, or maternal use of nonsteroidal antiinflammatory drugs (NSAIDs). The condition is often associated with hypoxemia and acidosis from conditions such as asphyxia, meconium aspiration, RDS, sepsis, polycythemia, diabetes, and diaphragmatic hernia. It is also associated with preterm or postterm births, LGA infants, Asian and African American infants, and in maternal conditions such as obesity and asthma.

Infants with PPHN usually develop signs within the first 12 hours after birth. Assessment findings include tachypnea, respiratory distress, and progressive cyanosis that become worse with handling. Oxygen saturation is decreased, carbon dioxide level is increased, and acidosis is present. Other signs may be present resulting from associated conditions. An echocardiogram reveals shunting.

Treatment includes high-frequency ventilation, surfactant therapy, inhaled nitric oxide, or extracorporeal membrane oxygenation (ECMO) therapy if conventional therapies are unsuccessful.

Nursing care is similar to that for infants with severe respiratory disease. Because neonates with PPHN become hypoxic with handling, the nurse must be sure to keep activity, as well as noise and other stimuli, to a minimum. The nurse needs to pay particular attention to preventing cold stress, as this can increase the metabolic rate and need for oxygen, which causes additional pulmonary vasoconstriction. Additionally, the nurse must monitor for hypoglycemia, hypocalcemia, and anemia as per hospital policy.

16.10 Sepsis

Sepsis occurs when pathogenic microorganisms or their toxins are present in the blood or tissues. The nurse must constantly be alert for signs and symptoms of infection in the newborn. Infection is a major cause of death during the neonatal period. Bacterial infection affects 1 to 4 infants in every 1,000 live births in developed countries. The incidence in preterm infants is 3 to 10 times that of full-term infants.

Newborns can acquire infections before, during, or after birth. During pregnancy, organisms causing rubella, CMV, syphilis, human immunodeficiency virus (HIV), and toxoplasmosis may pass across the placenta and infect the fetus through vertical transmission from the mother. During labor and birth, organisms in the vagina such as group B streptococcus, herpes, and hepatitis may enter the uterus after rupture of the membranes or infect the infant during passage through the birth canal. Infections that occur after birth are acquired from hospital staff, contaminated equipment, family members, or visitors. Such infections can result in sepsis neonatorum, a systemic infection from bacteria in the bloodstream. Common causative agents of neonatal sepsis are group B streptococcus, *Staphylococcus aureus,* methicillin-resistant *S. aureus, Escherichia coli, Aerobacter,* and *Klebsiella.*

Assessment findings include subtle, nonspecific behavioral changes, such as lethargy and hypotonia; temperature instability; feeding pattern changes, such as poor sucking and decreased intake; apnea; hyperbilirubinemia; skin color changes, including mottling, pallor, and cyanosis; and positive blood cultures.

Treatment includes urine, skin, blood, and nasopharyngeal cultures; lumbar puncture to rule out meningitis; gastric aspiration; and wide-spectrum antibiotics given intravenously until the causative agent is identified; specific antibiotics can then be given depending on the causative organism.

Of particular importance in nursing care is meticulous hand washing when interacting with the ill infant, as well as between interactions with other infants, to prevent the spread of infection. All family members and visitors need to be instructed on the importance of good hand washing before and after touching the infant. The nurse is responsible for obtaining or assisting in obtaining specimens and for administering antibiotics as prescribed. The nurse is also responsible for assessing vital signs frequently, providing a neutral thermal environment, administering IV fluids, and keeping intake and output records. Other care may include administering oxygen or other respiratory care as needed. Gavage feedings may be necessary if the infant is unable to take oral feedings. Keeping parents informed about the infant's treatments and changes in condition, along with involving them in the care of the infant, is important. Providing emotional support and guidance to parents and other family members is also important in the care of an ill neonate.

16.11 Infant of a Diabetic Mother

The ***infant of a diabetic mother (IDM)*** faces many risks that depend on the type of diabetes and how well it was controlled. The neonatal mortality rate is five times higher than that of infants born to nondiabetic mothers. Congenital anomalies are three times greater in IDMs. Cardiac, urinary tract, GI, and neural tube anomalies are frequently seen. IDMs are large (> 4000 g) and at risk for birth injuries.

IDMs have a higher risk of asphyxia and RDS. They are at risk for hypoglycemia and hypocalcemia, and their magnesium levels may be low. Polycythemia may occur as a response to chronic hypoxia in utero and may lead to hyperbilirubinemia.

The IDM demonstrates a characteristic appearance. The face is round, the skin is often very pink or red (ruddy; plethoric), and the body is obese. The infant often has poor muscle tone at rest but becomes irritable and may have tremors when disturbed.

Nursing care includes assessment for signs of complications, trauma, and congenital anomalies at delivery and in the early hours after birth. Respiratory problems may develop. Infants should be fed early and frequently (as per hospital policy) to prevent hypoglycemia. Cold stress needs to be prevented. Infants with polycythemia need adequate hydration to prevent sluggish blood flow. IDMs are usually poor feeders, and the parents may not understand why. The nurse needs to educate the parents on the characteristics of the IDM and what to expect. The mother may feel guilty and needs emotional support. Allowing the parents to discuss their feelings and ask questions may help alleviate some of their anxiety, and the nursing staff needs to allow them to do so.

16.12 Polycythemic Infants

Polycythemic infants have excessive red blood cells and a hematocrit > 65%. Polycythemia is a more common finding in infants who are LGA, in those with IUGR, and in those who are postterm. It also occurs more frequently in infants whose mothers were diabetic, hypertensive, or smoked.

There is increased viscosity of the blood in infants with polycythemia. The increased viscosity can cause decreased blood flow and resistance in the blood vessels, which can result in decreased blood flow to organs and result in organ damage. Most infants are asymptomatic. Those with symptoms exhibit ruddy (dark red) skin, respiratory distress, lethargy, poor suck, vomiting, cyanosis, exaggerated startle reflex, hypoglycemia, hypocalcemia, or jaundice (yellowing of skin).

Treatment is supportive but in some cases may include an exchange transfusion.

Nursing care includes maintaining good hydration to prevent dehydration, which could slow blood flow even further, monitoring bilirubin levels, and, if a transfusion is given, monitoring for signs of complications.

16.13 Hyperbilirubinemia (Pathologic Jaundice)

Hyperbilirubinemia, or ***pathologic jaundice***, is seen in infants in the first 24 hours of life. It is of greater concern than physiologic jaundice, which occurs on the second or third day of life in 60% of newborns, in that it may lead to acute bilirubin encephalopathy, or bilirubin toxicity (***kernicterus***). Bilirubin encephalopathy is the most serious complication of hyperbilirubinemia.

Jaundice appears when the infant's bilirubin levels exceed 4 to 6 mg/dL before it is visible in the skin. Almost all newborns have elevated serum bilirubin levels > 2 mg/dL (the normal level in adults is ≤1.3 mg/dL).

In kernicterus, yellow staining of the brain tissue occurs and creates morphologic changes in brain cells, which results in irreversible damage. Although kernicterus is rare today because of advanced treatment measures, the mortality rate among affected infants is ~50%. Those infants who survive may suffer from cerebral palsy, sensorineural hearing loss, mental retardation, gaze paresis, dental dysplasia, and other neurologic deficits. The condition is generally thought to occur at bilirubin levels in excess of 20 mg/dL in full-term neonates.

The most common cause of pathologic jaundice is hemolytic disease of the newborn resulting from incompatibility between the mother's and infant's blood types. The mother with Rh-negative blood forms antibodies when blood from an Rh-positive fetus enters her circulation. Antibodies can develop from a previous pregnancy and after an injury, abortion, amniocentesis, or transfusion. The antibodies cross the placenta and attach to the fetal RBCs and destroy them. Excessive hemolysis causes erythroblastosis fetalis.

Infants with erythroblastosis fetalis are anemic. Severely affected newborns may develop hydrops fetalis, a severe anemia that results in heart failure and generalized edema.

ABO incompatibility also causes pathologic jaundice. Mothers with type O blood have natural antibodies to type A and B blood. The antibodies cross the placenta and cause hemolysis of fetal RBCs, although less severe than that seen in Rh incompatibility.

Other causes of nonphysiologic jaundice are infection, hypothyroidism, polycythemia, structural and enzyme defects of RBCs, drug toxicity (chemical hemolysis), hypothermia, hypoglycemia, deficient glucuronyl transferase activity, decreased albumin binding sites, and biliary atresia. It is also more likely to occur in infants who suffered hypoxia or respiratory acidosis during labor and/or delivery.

Therapeutic management is prevention of bilirubin encephalopathy and kernicterus. During pregnancy, an Rh-negative mother is given Rho (D) immune globulin, such as RhoGAM, to prevent her from forming antibodies against Rh-positive blood. Once an infant is born, if he or she is jaundiced, the infant's blood type and a direct Coombs test are performed on the cord blood. A positive test indicates that antibodies from the mother have attached to the infant's RBCs. The health care provider will draw bilirubin levels and take other factors, such as gestational age, into consideration to assess risk and determine if therapy needs to be initiated.

The most common treatment of jaundice is phototherapy, which involves placing the newborn under fluorescent lights. During phototherapy, bilirubin in the skin (yellowing) absorbs the light and changes into water-soluble products that are then excreted in bile and urine.

Phototherapy can be delivered in several ways. The most common is to place a bank of fluorescent lights within 45 to 50 cm (18–20 in) of an infant placed in an incubator. The infant wears only a diaper, to ensure maximal exposure of skin to the lights and to protect the reproductive organs. Patches are placed over the infant's eyes to protect them from constant light. More than one set of lights may be used if the bilirubin level is very high. A phototherapy blanket may be placed under the infant in the incubator, or the infant can be swaddled in the blanket so the mother can hold the child.

Side effects of phototherapy include frequent, loose green stools that result from increased bile and peristalsis. Although this promotes more rapid excretion of bilirubin, it can also cause fluid loss and skin irritation (erythematous macular skin rash).

Nursing care for the newborn includes maintaining a neutral thermal environment, providing adequate nutrition, protecting the eyes and reproductive organs, enhancing response to therapy, detecting complications, and teaching parents. Warding off cold stress, which can cause acidosis and decrease the number of binding sites available for bilirubin, and maintaining an appropriate distance between the neonate and the lights are priorities. Although it is standard practice to place a probe on the infant to ensure temperature regulation, the nurse should also monitor the infant's axillary temperature every 2 to 3 hours.

Infants under phototherapy should receive feedings every 2 to 3 hours, by breast or bottle. Breastfeeding does not need to be stopped because an infant is under phototherapy. Frequent feedings help promote GI motility and prompt emptying of bilirubin from the intestines. The infant should be monitored for signs of dehydration. The infant's eyes should be closed and patches placed over the eyes to prevent retinal damage from the lights. The nurse should check the position and fit of the eye patches, as they may become displaced and cause skin irritation or respiratory difficulty. The eye patches should be removed when the infant is taken for feedings or other care.

To enhance response to phototherapy, the nurse needs to expose as much skin as possible to the light. The infant should be turned every 2 hours to expose all areas of the skin and to prevent irritation. The infant's skin should be kept as dry as possible, as the use of creams or lotions can cause burning. Drawing regular bilirubin levels, as per hospital protocol, provides data for determining the effectiveness of treatment and the appropriate time to discontinue phototherapy. The nurse needs to monitor for signs and symptoms of bilirubin encephalopathy, which include lethargy, decreased muscle tone, decreased or absent Moro reflex, poor feeding, high-pitched cry, and seizures.

Parents should be taught about jaundice and phototherapy and be allowed to hold the infant during feedings to allow for attachment. They may be frightened, but encouraging them to see the infant and participate in the infant's care may decrease their worry.

Exchange transfusions are rarely needed but are performed when phototherapy has not reduced dangerously high bilirubin levels quickly. This treatment removes maternal antibodies, unconjugated bilirubin, and sensitized (antibody-coated) RBCs. The transfusion provides fresh albumin with binding sites for bilirubin and corrects severe anemia. Small amounts of blood are removed from the infant and replaced with an equal amount of donor blood. Complications that may occur from exchange transfusions include fluid and electrolyte imbalances, infection, hypoglycemia, hyperglycemia, cardiac dysrhythmias, bleeding, thrombocytopenia, and NEC.

The nurse must carefully assess the infant during an exchange transfusion and observe for adverse reactions. Explaining the procedure to parents is important in helping to reduce their anxiety.

16.14 Neonatal Abstinence Syndrome

Neonatal abstinence syndrome (NAS) is a disorder in which drug-exposed neonates demonstrate signs of drug withdrawal. Substance abuse affects the fetus at any time during pregnancy. Most drugs readily cross the placenta and can cause a variety of problems. Maternal substance abuse may be identified before an infant is born or suspected from the woman's behavior during delivery or if she has not had prenatal care. If drug abuse is suspected, it is often facility protocol to obtain a urine sample and have it tested for toxicology. The infant should be tested soon after delivery because some drugs are excreted quickly, whereas others are not. Meconium may also be tested.

Signs of drug exposure usually occur in the first 24 to 72 hours after birth. Symptoms vary and depend on the specific drug, the dose, and the time of the mother's last use. The nurse should keep in mind that polydrug use is common and that the infant may not show abnormal signs until after the first week of life.

Infants with NAS may be irritable and have hyperactive muscle tone, poor coordination of suck and swallow, frequent regurgitation or vomiting, diarrhea, tremors, and failure to gain weight. Congenital anomalies or other effects of prenatal drug exposure may be present at birth, such as IUGR, prematurity, respiratory distress, and jaundice.

Therapeutic management includes treating the complications. Drug therapy may be indicated for 50% to 60% of infants. Drugs commonly used include morphine, tincture of opium, methadone, and phenobarbital. Medication is gradually tapered until the infant no longer needs it. IV or gavage feedings may be necessary due to the infant's uncoordinated suck and swallow. Some infants need more calories because of their hyperactivity, and formula (24 kcal/oz) may be given.

The drug-exposed neonate's respiratory status and suck and swallow coordination must be assessed. If he or she is too agitated, has rapid respirations, or cannot suck and swallow adequately, the infant will need gavage feedings. When the infant is able to take feedings orally, he or she may need cheek and chin support similar to that used for preterm infants. The neonate should be swaddled to prevent excessive movement, and other types of stimulation should be avoided (bright lights, loud noise, rocking, etc). Excessive activity and poor sleep pattern interfere with drug-exposed neonates' need to rest. The nurse must take a calm approach when caring for these infants. The nurse should follow a cluster care routine, in which all of the care is done at one time, to avoid overtiring the infant. Keeping lights dimmed and reducing noise helps soothe the infant. Swaddling and a pacifier for nonnutritive sucking may also prove soothing.

Because child abuse, neglect, and failure to respond appropriately to an infant are associated with alcohol and drug abuse, child protective services will become involved. The infant will not be released to the mother until her ability to care for the infant safely is assessed by social services.

Because the mother may eventually become the infant's primary caregiver, it is important for the nurse to constantly assess her willingness and ability to care for the infant. The number of times the mother visits the child, as well as her bonding behaviors, such as calling the infant by name, smiling, and kissing the infant, should be noted. The nurse should encourage the mother to participate actively in infant care during visits. The mother needs the same instructions given to all new parents, as well as special techniques necessary to meet the needs of the drug-exposed infant. Because some withdrawal symptoms may continue for up to 6 months, the mother needs to know how to handle them. Family and friends who may be assisting in the care of the infant also should be taught techniques necessary to meet the needs of the drug-exposed infant.

Objective D: To Understand the Care of the Infant with Congenital Conditions

16.15 Congenital Heart Defects

Congenital heart defects (CHDs) are some of the most frequently seen congenital defects in infants and children, with the incidence reported in ~1% of pregnancies and 5 to 8 per 1000 live births. The heart and the great vessels develop during the first 3 to 8 weeks of gestation. The fetus is most vulnerable to cardiac malformations during this period. CHDs are the leading cause of death from congenital anomalies.

Genetic disorders that cause heart defects are categorized into three major groups:

1. Chromosomal disorders (trisomy 21, Down syndrome)
2. Single-gene disorders, which can be either autosomal dominant or autosomal recessive
3. Polygenic disorders resulting from multiple genetic or environmental influences

Cardiac defects or lesions are categorized as acyanotic (oxygenated blood is shunted to the body, but the infant remains "pink") or cyanotic (unoxygenated blood is shunted to the body, causing the infant to be "blue").

Children with certain genetic defects, including those with chromosomal aberrations, have an extremely high incidence of cardiac disorders; in Down syndrome, the incidence of congenital heart disease is ~50%. Children with fetal alcohol syndrome are at a 25% to 30% incidence, and IDMs are at an increased risk for CHDs. A family history of CHD, especially if the family member is a parent or a sibling, increases the risk for giving birth to a child with CHD. Acyanotic defects include patent ductus arteriosus (PDA), atrial septal defects, ventricular septal defects, and coarctation of the aorta.

Patent ductus arteriosus (PDA) is an anatomical and functionally open shunt between the pulmonary artery and the aorta. PDA occurs in 5% to 10% of all cases of CHD in full-term neonates. PDA becomes functionally closed within the first 12 hours of life in the full-term infant. The closure is complete by 2 to 3 weeks of life.

Physical findings include a harsh systolic murmur, which becomes continuous, that is heard at the left upper sternal border and posteriorly. Also, bounding peripheral pulses and a widened pulse pressure with a low diastolic pressure are found.

Management depends on whether the shunt is hemodynamically significant. Conservative measures are generally used initially. Fluid restriction, diuretics, and positive end-expiratory pressure (PEEP) may be instituted, and NSAIDs may be used. In surgical management, surgical ligation via thoracotomy is done.

An ***atrial septal defect (ASD)*** is an opening in the septum between the atria that occurs as a result of improper septal formation in early fetal cardiac development. ASDs account for 5% to 10% of all congenital heart disease.

Physical findings depend on the severity of the defect. A low-pitched diastolic murmur is heard at the left lower sternal border. If the defect is small, clinical follow-up is indicated because the defect may close spontaneously. If the defect is large or associated with intractable congestive heart failure (CHF), surgical repair is done with the patient on cardiopulmonary bypass.

A ***ventricular septal defect (VSD)*** is an opening in the septum between the right and left ventricles that results from imperfect ventricular formation during early fetal development. VSD is the most commonly occurring form of CHD, with an incidence of 20% to 25% among neonates with cardiac defects. VSD frequently occurs in association with other cardiac defects.

Neonates with a small VSD usually show no signs other than a holosystolic murmur in the area of the lower left sternal border. The infant may have normal growth and development patterns. In a neonate with a large VSD, a holosystolic murmur is heard accompanied by a thrill. Fifty percent to 75% of small VSDs close spontaneously. With mild CHF, treatment consists of diuretics and digoxin. Surgery is indicated if the infant has failure to thrive or intractable CHF.

Coarctation of the aorta is a narrowing of the upper thoracic aorta that produces an obstruction to the flow of blood through the aorta. It accounts for 8% of all cases of congenital heart disease. The coarctation can be opposite, proximal to, or distal to the ductus arteriosus switch procedure.

Physical findings depend on the location of the coarctation. Findings include diminished or absent femoral pulses, higher blood pressure in the upper extremities, respiratory distress, pallor, blowing systolic murmur at the left upper sternal border, and poor weight gain in the first 2 to 6 weeks of life.

Interventions include aggressive management of CHF, prostaglandin E1 to dilate the ductus arteriosus, palliative balloon angioplasty in a critically ill neonate, and/or surgical correction.

Cyanotic CHDs include tetralogy of Fallot (TOF), transposition of the great arteries, and hypoplastic left heart syndrome or single ventricle.

Tetralogy of Fallot (TOF) is the most common type of cyanotic heart disease, accounting for 10% of all cases. It is characterized by a combination of four defects:

1. VSD
2. An overriding aorta
3. Right ventricular outflow obstruction
4. Hypertrophy of the right ventricle

Physical findings include respiratory distress (tachypnea) and cyanosis, with the degree directly related to the extent of the right ventricular outflow obstruction. Crying and feeding increase cyanosis and respiratory distress due to increased shunting of unoxygenated blood from the right side of the heart to the left as a result of pulmonary artery obstruction. A harsh systolic murmur may be heard at the left upper and lower sternal borders. Signs of CHF may be apparent if the VSD is large.

Current trends in interventions are complete repair of the TOF, which includes repair of pulmonary stenosis and closure of the VSD. Palliative surgical intervention such as placements of shunts can be used to control cyanosis. Shunts temporarily increase blood flow to the pulmonary artery from the aorta.

Transposition of the great arteries (TGA) accounts for 5% of congenital heart disease. In TGA, the aorta originates from the right ventricle, and the pulmonary artery originates from the left ventricle. On physical assessment, tachycardia, tachypnea, and pansystolic murmur are present. Other symptoms include progressive cyanosis that worsens with crying and feeding.

Survival is dependent on early diagnosis and aggressive treatment. If left untreated, the infant will become critically ill.

Interventions include correction of acidosis, inotropic therapy, prostaglandin E1 (PGE1) via continuous IV infusion, no supplemental oxygen to prevent the PDA from closing, immediate transfer to a tertiary care facility with cardiac expertise, and surgical correction with a physiologic correction of the vessels, called an atrial switch procedure.

Hypoplastic left heart syndrome occurs when parts of the left side of the heart (mitral valve, left ventricle, aortic valve, and aorta) do not develop completely. This includes valvular or vascular obstructive lesions on the left side of the heart that impede left-sided filling or emptying. It accounts for 7% to 9% of all CHDs.

These neonates are commonly asymptomatic at birth but become symptomatic within 1 to 2 days of life. Symptoms include a soft, systolic, ejection murmur; respiratory distress, especially tachypnea and dyspnea; pallor; diminished pulses; cyanosis; and mottling leading to vascular collapse and acidosis as the PDA begins to close.

Interventions may include inotropic therapy, PGE1 IV infusion to maintain a PDA, hypoventilation, maintenance of acid–base balance, and cardiac transplantation.

Nursing care for the neonate with CHDs is focused on reducing the infant's need for oxygen and assessing for changes in condition. The infant's response to activity is evaluated, and the nurse must promote frequent rest periods with small amounts of cluster care. Infants with rapid respirations may need to be fed by gavage to prevent aspiration. Oxygen at the lowest maintenance level required may need to be given during feedings or other activity. Support should be offered to the mother who desires to express breast milk for the infant. Often, formula with added calories is given to the infant, as weight gain is slow due to the child's tiring easily. Maintaining a neutral thermal environment is important to avoid the need for increased oxygen consumption. Accurate intake and output records are necessary for infants with heart defects.

The nurse needs to educate the parents and family members about the infant's condition, treatment, care, prognosis, and outcome. They need to be encouraged to support each other in their feelings of loss and grief, which is an appropriate response to the loss of the fantasized newborn. The nurse needs to promote attachment by encouraging parents to hold and care for the infant. Teaching parents to bathe, clothe, position, feed, and monitor the newborn according to individual needs is a priority. Parents need to be taught techniques for accurate administration of medication, as the range between therapeutic and toxic dosage of the drugs is often narrow. Teaching parents and other family members infant cardiopulmonary resuscitation (CPR) is also encouraged. Discharge planning should be done from admission and assistance given in planning care to be provided in the home. Nursing home care visits should be set up to provide assistance to parents in the home setting. Parents should be referred to support groups for families of children with heart anomalies.

16.16 Central Nervous System Congenital Anomalies

Congenital anomalies of the central nervous system (CNS) include neural tube defects and hydrocephalus.

Spina bifida is a general term used to describe defects in closure of the neural tube associated with malformations of the spinal cord and vertebrae. It is the most common congenital malformation of the CNS. (Spina bifida has three main types: meningocele, myelomeningocele, and myeloschisis.)

In ***meningocele spina bifida,*** there is a sac containing meninges and cerebrospinal fluid (CSF); however, the spinal cord and nerve roots are normal in their structure and position within the spinal canal. Typically, these infants do not demonstrate neurologic deficits.

Myelomeningocele is the most common form of spina bifida. The occurrence rate is 1 to 1.5 per 1000 live births. It is a protrusion of a membrane-covered sac through the spina bifida. The sac contains meninges, nerve roots, spinal cord, and spinal fluid. The degree of paralysis depends on the location of the defect. Typically, the infant will show neurologic deficit below the level of the lesion.

In ***myeloschisis,*** there is no cystic covering; the spinal cord is open and exposed. Therapeutic management includes surgery as soon as possible to prevent infection. A shunt is placed to divert CSF if hydrocephalus develops. Antibiotics are given to prevent infection. Long-term follow-up care is necessary, with physical therapy and other care as needed.

Nursing care of the infant includes placing the torso in a sterile plastic bag or covering the defect with a sterile saline dressing and plastic to prevent drying. The infant needs to be handled carefully and positioned prone or to the side to prevent trauma to the sac. The nurse needs to monitor for signs and symptoms of infection. Particular care should be given to prevent contamination from urine and feces. Every shift, or as per policy, the infant's head should be checked for increasing head circumference, bulging fontanelles, separation of sutures, intermittent apnea, and other signs of increased intracranial pressure to identify early hydrocephalus. The nurse should promote attachment behavior in the parents by encouraging them to hold the infant and participate in the infant's care.

Women should be encouraged to increase folic acid intake before and during future pregnancies to reduce the risk of recurrence.

In congenital ***hydrocephalus,*** there is a problem with absorption of or obstruction to the flow of CSF in the ventricles of the brain, causing compression of the brain and enlargement of the head. On physical assessment, the fontanelles may be full or bulging, and sutures may be separated. The head may be enlarged, especially the frontal area. The infant is usually irritable and feeds poorly. The "setting sun" sign is usually apparent (sclera visible above the pupils of the eyes).

Therapeutic management consists of surgery. A ventriculoperitoneal shunt to drain the fluid into the peritoneal cavity is most often done. The shunt will need revision as the child grows.

Nursing care of the infant with hydrocephalus includes monitoring head circumference daily, preventing pressure areas, and observing for signs of infection and intracranial pressure. The nurse should teach the parents how to care for the shunt and observe for signs of increased intracranial pressure.

16.17 Gastrointestinal Congenital Anomalies

Gastrointestinal (GI) congenital anomalies include cleft lip and palate, esophageal atresia, tracheoesophageal fistula, abdominal wall defects, diaphragmatic hernia, and imperforate anus. Cleft lip and palate are the most common congenital anomalies. They can occur together or separately. The defects are a result of failure of fusion during the fourth and eighth week of gestation.

Cleft lip affects about 1 of every 600 live births. ***Cleft palate*** alone occurs in 1 out of every 1000 newborns and occurs more frequently in females. Cleft deformities are more prevalent among people of Asian descent. Both genetic and environmental factors are included in the causes. Risk factors for this anomaly include maternal use of phenytoin (Dilantin), alcohol, retinoic acid (Accutane), and cigarette smoking. There is a 40% chance of clefting in siblings of a child with a cleft lip or palate.

Physical findings include a unilateral or bilateral visible defect, flattening or depression of the midfacial contour in cleft lip, a fissure connecting the oral and nasal cavities in cleft palate, difficulty in sucking, expulsion of formula or breast milk through the nares, dehydration, and poor weight gain or loss.

Repairing a facial anomaly as soon as possible is important to facilitate bonding between the parents and the newborn and to improve nutritional status. Lip surgery is performed between 6 and 12 weeks of age. Palate repair surgery is done by 1 year to minimize speech problems. Long-term follow-up is necessary for speech therapy and dental work and to assess for possible hearing problems. Infants with these anomalies are susceptible to respiratory and ear infections.

Nursing care of the infant with cleft lip and/or palate includes determining a feeding approach. This will depend on the severity of the defect.

If the infant has a cleft lip only, the mother should be encouraged to breastfeed if she so desires (soft tissue fills in the cleft lip). The infant should be fed in an upright position to prevent aspiration and infection. A special nipple and bottle should be used with bottle-fed infants, and a higher-calorie formula may be needed. Feedings should be limited to 30 to 45 minutes to avoid fatigue, and the infant should be burped frequently. Milk curds should be washed away with water after feedings.

The nurse should encourage the parents to verbalize feelings about the defect and feeding frustrations. They need to be supported in their loss of the idealized baby. The nurse can provide role modeling while interacting with the infant so that the parents can internalize positive interaction. They should be referred to community agencies and support groups.

Esophageal atresia and ***tracheoesophageal fistula (TEF)*** are congenital malformations in which the esophagus terminates before it reaches the stomach and/or a fistula is present that forms an unnatural connection with the trachea.

The cause is unknown; there is failure of normal development during the fourth week of pregnancy. Esophageal atresia with or without TEF occurs in 1.2 to 4.67 in 10,000 live births, with no difference by gender. Nearly half of infants born with esophageal atresia have other associated anomalies of the cardiac, GI, and central nervous systems.

Physical findings include excessive oral secretions, coughing, choking, vomiting, abdominal distention, and failure to pass a suction catheter or nasogastric (NG) tube at birth.

Esophageal atresia and TEF are considered a critical surgical emergency. Therapeutic treatment is surgical repair.

Nursing care differs preoperatively and postoperatively. Preoperatively, prevention of aspiration is a priority. The infant is elevated at a 30-degree angle while supine to decrease reflux. As part of preparation for surgery, he or she is kept NPO (nothing by mouth) and hydrated with IV fluids. Continuous suction should be used.

In the immediate postoperative period, monitoring respiratory status, providing nutrition and fluid balance, maintaining thermoregulation, providing pain relief, monitoring for infection, and promoting bonding with parents are priority nursing care interventions. Long-term follow-up is needed for esophageal reflux and dilation of strictures that form at the surgical site (staged surgery).

Abdominal wall defects include omphalocele and gastroschisis.

An omphalocele, a defect of the umbilical ring, occurs when the intestines protrude into the base of the umbilical cord. Other anomalies are often seen with omphalocele. The incidence is 1.5 to 3 per 10,000 live births.

Gastroschisis is a defect of the umbilical ring that allows evisceration of the bowel through a defect in the abdominal wall with no membrane covering.

Therapeutic management includes placing an NG tube to decrease air in the stomach. Gastric suction, parenteral nutrition, and antibiotics are necessary. Surgery is performed as soon as the infant is stable. A Silastic pouch may be used to replace the intestines gradually over a period of days. The abdomen is closed when the contents have been replaced into the abdominal cavity.

Nursing care includes covering the intestines with a warm sterile dressing wrapped with plastic or lacing the infant's torso in a plastic bag immediately after birth to prevent heat and water loss. The infant should be positioned to avoid pressure or trauma to the intestines. Prevention of infection is also a priority measure. Administration of IV fluids and monitoring of glucose and electrolytes are imperative, as well as maintaining a neutral thermal environment.

Congenital diaphragmatic hernia (CDH) is a malformation that consists of herniation of the abdominal contents into the thorax cavity via a defect in the diaphragm. The incidence is ~2.5 to 3.8 per 10,000 live births, with a mortality rate of 45% in live-born infants. CDH and neonatal lung lesions often occur together. Abdominal contents in the thorax can cause a mediastinal shift that can result in impairment of cardiovascular function.

Physical findings include mild to severe respiratory distress at birth (difficulty initiating respiration, gasping respirations, retractions and nasal flaring, and decreased or absent breath sounds on the side of the hernia), cyanosis, large or barrel chest, scaphoid abdomen (concave), bowel sounds heard in the chest, and asymmetric chest expansion.

The neonate should be immediately intubated with suction; bag and mask ventilation must be avoided because air can be forced into the intestine, which will further compromise lung space in the chest. Mechanical ventilation (extracorporeal membrane oxygenation [ECMO]) pressures should be kept at a minimal level to avoid pneumothorax. An orogastric tube is also placed for decompression of the stomach. Pulmonary hypertension needs to be managed with bicarbonate.

Surgery to reposition the intestines and repair the defect is performed when the infant is stable, usually 6 to 18 hours after birth.

Monitoring respiratory status is a priority. Nursing care includes positioning the infant on the affected side to allow the unaffected lung to expand. The head should be elevated to decrease pressure on the heart and lungs. Postoperatively, the nurse gives routine care and monitors for infection, respiratory distress, and feeding difficulties. The nurse needs to support the parents mourning the loss of a perfect child, provide accurate information, and encourage them to see and touch the infant. When providing discharge teaching, referral to support groups may be helpful.

An ***imperforate anus*** is any congenital malformation of the anorectal area. The rectum may end in a pouch that does not connect to the colon, or there may be fistulas between the rectum and the perineum.

Imperforate anus occurs in 1 out of every 5000 live births. The malformations occur in early fetal development and are associated with anomalies in other body systems. Surgical intervention is needed. Surgery often involves a colostomy in the newborn period, with corrective surgery performed in stages to allow for growth.

Nursing care preoperatively includes maintaining NPO status, monitoring gastric decompression, administering IV therapy and antibiotics, and parent teaching. Postoperatively, the nurse needs to provide pain relief, maintain NPO status and gastric decompression until normal bowel function is restored, and provide colostomy care if needed.

16.18 Genitourinary Structural Anomalies

Genitourinary (GU) structural anomalies are usually not life-threatening, but they can pose problems.

Hypospadias involves the abnormal positioning of the meatus on the underside of the penis. It is often accompanied by a downward bowing of the penis (chordee), which can lead to urination and erection problems in adulthood.

Hypospadias is a relatively common birth defect that occurs in ~1 in every 300 males in the United States each year. The abnormality is the result of incomplete fusion of the urethral folds and occurs between 9 and 12 weeks' gestation. The cause is unknown but thought to be of multifactorial inheritance, as it frequently occurs in more than one male in the same family. Hypospadias can be corrected surgically within the first year of life to prevent any body image problems in the child.

Epispadias is a rare congenital genitourinary defect occurring in 1 of 117,000 male births and 1 of 484,000 female births. In boys, the urinary meatus is on the top or on the side of the penis. In girls, the meatus is between the clitoris and the labia. Surgical correction is necessary, and male newborns should not be circumcised. Nursing care for newborns is to provide accurate information and support to parents.

In ***bladder exstrophy,*** the bladder protrudes onto the abdominal wall because the abdominal wall failed to close during embryonic development. Virtually all affected males have associated hypospadias. The upper urinary tract is usually normal. The incidence is ~1 in 24,000 to 40,000 live births.

Treatment is surgical repair in several stages. Initial bladder closure is completed within 48 hours of birth, with epispadias repair taking place at the same time if possible. Surgery to reconstruct the bladder neck and reimplant ureters is performed between 2 and 3 years of age.

Nursing care for the newborn with bladder exstrophy includes covering the bladder with a sterile, clear, nonadherent dressing to prevent hypothermia and infection; irrigating the bladder surface with sterile saline after each diaper change to prevent infection; assisting in inserting and monitoring a suprapubic catheter to drain the bladder; administering antibiotic therapy as prescribed; assessing the newborn frequently for signs of infection; maintaining a modified Bryant traction for immobilization after surgery; administering antispasmodics, analgesics, and sedatives as prescribed to prevent bladder spasm and provide comfort; educating the parents on care of the catheter; promoting bonding by encouraging the parents to visit and care for the newborn; and referring the parents to a support group.

16.19 Musculoskeletal Anomalies

Clubfoot and congenital dysplasia of the hip are two common congenital anomalies of the musculoskeletal system. These anomalies can be identified at birth or soon after and need early intervention, as they can impede mobility as the child grows.

Clubfoot, or ***talipes equinovarus,*** is a congenital malformation of the lower extremity that affects the lower leg, ankle, and foot. The incidence is 1 in 1000 live births. Boys are affected more than girls, with a ratio of 2:1 in the United States. It is bilateral in more than half of cases.

On examination, the heel is internally rotated, making the soles of the feet face each other when the deformity occurs bilaterally.

Treatment starts with serial casting, which is needed due to the rapid growth of the newborn. Casts are changed weekly and are applied until the deformity responds and is fully corrected. If serial casting is not successful, surgical intervention is necessary between 4 and 9 months of age.

Nursing care focuses on pain management, education, and anticipatory guidance. The parents need to be educated about their newborn's condition and the treatment protocol to reduce anxiety. Challenges associated with activities of daily living need to be addressed with parents so they know what to expect and learn how to handle the infant. Encouraging a calm, quiet environment to promote relaxation and sleep for the newborn should be discussed with the parents.

Developmental dysplasia of the hip (DDH) involves abnormal growth or development of the hip that results in instability. This instability allows the femoral head to become easily displaced from the acetabulum. Normally, the infant is otherwise healthy.

The etiology of DDH is unclear, but associated factors include racial background (highest in Native Americans), genetic transmission (runs in families), gender (female), oligohydramnios, birth order (first born), and postnatal carrying positions (tight swaddling). The incidence is ~10 in 1000 live births.

DDH is not always identified during the newborn exam. Two methods used to detect hip instability in the newborn are Ortolani's maneuver and Barlow's maneuver. Ortolani's maneuver elicits the sensation of the dislocated hip reducing; Barlow's maneuver detects the unstable hip dislocating from the acetabulum. Additional physical signs of DDH are an asymmetric number of skinfolds on the thigh, an apparent short leg, and limited hip abduction.

Treatment is started as soon as DDH is identified. The newborn will be referred to an orthopedist. The goal of treatment is to relocate the femoral head in the acetabulum to facilitate normal growth and development. The Pavlik harness is the most widely used device; it prevents adduction while allowing flexion and abduction to accomplish the treatment goal. The harness is worn continuously until the hip is stable, which takes several months. If harnessing is not successful, surgery is necessary.

Nursing care of the newborn with DDH starts with identification and early reporting. The nurse needs to educate the parents on how to care for their infant in a harness. The nurse needs to stress compliance with treatment and emphasize that frequent clinical visits for monitoring progress are essential. Limb defects are common in children and are of great concern to parents. Most alterations of arms/hands and legs/feet are mild variations of normal posturing, but some are severe anomalies or abnormalities.

Limb deformities result from birth anomalies and sometimes from trauma. These defects can take many forms, including webbing (syndactyly) or extra digits (polydactyly), absence of all or part of an extremity, genu valgum ("knock knees"), genu varum (bowleg), and clubfoot.

Mild limb defects frequently occur as a result of positioning—either in utero or from the sitting and sleeping positions of young children. Mild limb deformities resolve without treatment. Splints, exercises, special shoes, or casts may be prescribed. Surgical interventions may be required for more severe cases.

Nursing care includes teaching the parents about the principles of therapy, skin care, and treatments at home and encouraging them to follow through with treatment even if the child does not like it. The nurse needs to reinforce that periodic follow-up is necessary.

Objective E: To Understand Inborn Errors of Metabolism

16.20 Inborn Errors of Metabolism

Inborn errors of metabolism are genetic disorders that disrupt normal metabolic function. Newborns undergo screening tests in the United States for conditions that result from inborn errors of metabolism and other genetic conditions. With early identification and treatment, infants with these conditions may avoid severe intellectual disability and other problems. The newborn screening is performed on the morning of discharge, usually at least 24 hours after birth. Many of the tests are not accurate unless the infant is 24 hours old, so early discharge of the newborn is usually discouraged until the screening can be done.

Some of the more common conditions that are tested for are phenylketonuria, galactosemia, and congenital hypothyroidism.

Phenylketonuria (PKU) is an autosomal recessive disorder caused by a deficiency of the hepatic enzyme phenylalanine hydroxylase with a subsequent accumulation of amino acid phenylalanine. Incidence is 1 in 15,000 live births. Clinically, newborns appear normal but by 6 months of age show signs of slow mental development. They may have poor feedings, vomiting, failure to thrive, overactivity, irritability, and musty-smelling urine. If not treated, mental retardation can occur. Treatment is lifelong dietary restriction of phenylalanine.

Galactosemia is an autosomal recessive inherited disorder in which an enzyme is deficient, and the infant cannot metabolize lactose ("milk allergy"). It occurs in 1 in 50,000 live births. Clinically, the infant may be vomiting frequently, have poor weight gain, hypoglycemia, frequent infections, hyperbilirubinemia, liver damage, or cataracts. Treatment is lifelong lactose-restricted diet to prevent mental retardation, liver disease, and cataracts.

Congenital hypothyroidism is an absent or under-developed thyroid gland or biochemical defects in thyroid hormone. It occurs in ~1 in 4,000 live births. Physical signs that an infant may have congenital hypothyroidism include a large, protruding tongue; slow reflexes; distended abdomen; a large, open posterior fontanelle; poor feedings; hoarse cry; dry skin; coarse hair; goiter; and jaundice. Treatment is lifelong thyroid replacement hormone therapy and continued monitoring of thyroid levels and response to treatment. If untreated, irreversible cognitive and motor impairment may become evident.

Parents need to be informed of the fact that the infant will have a newborn screening done as per state law, and abnormal results will be sent to their pediatrician. Most of the time, the parents do not hear of the test again because the results are within normal limits. Parents need to be informed of the seriousness of potential findings and the importance of follow-up and treatment should an abnormal finding occur.

Review Questions

True/False

1. _______ Preterm infants are those born before 37 weeks' gestation.

2. _______ Preterm infants are particularly prone to respiratory complications.

3. _______ Retinopathy of prematurity is related to fluctuations in arterial concentrations of oxygen during oxygen administration to the premature infant.

4. ______ Premature infants develop jaundice at a higher rate than do full-term infants due to the extreme immature liver and polycythemia.

5. ______ Postterm newborns are at high risk for the development of meconium aspiration pneumonia and persistent pulmonary hypertension.

6. ______ Necrotizing enterocolitis is a complication that affects mostly preterm infants and is due to an ischemic episode of the bowel.

7. ______ Sepsis in the newborn may be asymptomatic.

8. ______ Nonnutritive sucking is promoted for the preterm infant and high-risk newborn for both physiologic and psychological reasons.

9. ______ Newborns experiencing neonatal abstinence syndrome are lethargic and usually very quiet.

10. ______ Congenital hypothyroidism can lead to mental retardation if not treated.

11. ______ The newborn screening test is a voluntary option offered to parents upon a newborn's discharge from the birth facility.

12. ______ Newborn screening tests are often not accurate until the infant is 24 hours old.

13. ______ Patent ductus arteriosus functionally closes within 12 hours of life in a full-term infant.

14. ______ Mothers of infants with cleft lip should be discouraged from breastfeeding to prevent aspiration.

15. ______ The newborn with congenital developmental dysplasia of the hip is normally otherwise healthy.

16. ______ Repairing a facial anomaly as soon as possible is important to facilitate bonding between parents and newborns and to improve nutritional status.

17. ______ Infants with neonatal abstinence syndrome have uncoordinated suck and swallow.

18. ______ Breast milk may have a preventive effect on the development of necrotizing enterocolitis.

19. ______ Synthetic surfactant should be given to a preterm within 15 to 30 minutes of birth to prevent respiratory distress syndrome.

20. ______ In neonatal abstinence syndrome, symptoms usually occur in the first 24 to 72 hours after birth.

Multiple Choice

1. The priority focus of nursing care for an infant with cleft palate is

   A. Helping the parents deal with the child's defect

   B. Maintaining adequate nutrition

   C. Ensuring privacy for the infant

   D. Preparing the infant for immediate surgery

2. To prevent retinopathy of prematurity, nursing care includes

   A. Covering the infant's incubator with a blanket during the day and nap times

   B. Restricted visiting time with parents

   C. Keeping the infant's eyes covered with eye patches

   D. Placing pictures inside the infant's incubator

3. An infant with untreated jaundice is at risk for bilirubin crossing the blood–brain barrier, causing

   A. Permanent damage to the infant's brain

   B. Permanent yellowing of the infant's skin

   C. Loose stools

   D. ABO incompatibility

4. When caring for an infant with congenital diaphragmatic hernia, the nurse places the infant on the affected side to

   A. Feed the infant easily

   B. Allow the unaffected lung to expand

   C. Make it easier for the parents to see the infant

   D. Prevent sudden infant death syndrome

5. For what condition would measuring abdominal girth be part of the nursing assessment?

   A. Respiratory distress syndrome

   B. Necrotizing enterocolitis

   C. Jaundice

   D. Neonatal abstinence syndrome

6. When examining a newborn upon admission to the newborn nursery, the nurse finds a tuft of hair over the base of the infant's spine. The nurse would suspect

   A. A postterm infant

   B. Spina bifida

   C. Mongolian spots over the body

   D. Cardiac defects

7. Newborns with asphyxia often have other problems, such as (choose all that apply)

   A. Hypoglycemia

   B. Temperature instability

   C. Hypotension

   D. Metabolic acidosis

8. The nurse knows that the underlying mechanism in transient tachypnea of the newborn is

   A. Meconium passage

   B. Delayed absorption of fetal lung fluid

   C. Genetic malformations

   D. Cardiac defects

9. Characteristics of a preterm infant include (choose all that apply)

   A. Abundant vernix and lanugo

   B. Lack of subcutaneous fat

   C. Small scrotum in males

   D. Pinnae that are red, flat, and shiny

10. Periodic breathing in preterm infants differs from apneic spells in that (choose all that apply)

    A. Lack of breathing lasts more than 20 seconds.

    B. It is accompanied by a decrease of oxygen saturation.

    C. Cyanosis occurs.

    D. There is a drop in heart rate.

11. Subtle assessment findings that would lead the nurse to suspect that a newborn has an infection include (choose all that apply)

    A. Lethargy and hypotonia

    B. Increased feeding patterns

    C. Ruddiness

    D. Increased urinary output

12. Chordee in an infant can cause problems later in life, including (choose all that apply)

    A. Mobility difficulties

    B. Urination and erection difficulties

    C. Restricted growth of the penis

    D. Altered body image

13. The nurse teaching the parents of an infant with phenylketonuria would stress compliance with treatment consisting of

    A. Increased feedings

    B. Phototherapy

    C. Following a lifelong dietary restriction of phenylalanine

    D. Following a lifelong lactose-restricted diet

14. The postmature infant is susceptible to hypoglycemia due to

    A. Meconium aspiration

    B. Decreased passage of meconium

    C. Rapid depletion of glycogen stores

    D. Inability to breastfeed

15. The nurse caring for a newborn with excessive secretions, coughing, choking, and abdominal distention would suspect what illness in the newborn?

    A. Infection

    B. Cardiac defects

    C. Macrosomia

    D. Esophageal atresia

16. On the morning of discharge, Baby C, who is 3 days old, requires phototherapy. While Baby C is under phototherapy lights, it is imperative for the nurse to (choose all that apply)

    A. Keep Baby C's eyes and gonads covered.

    B. Change Baby C's position every 2 hours.

    C. Discourage breastfeeding.

    D. Limit feedings.

17. Baby C's mother is crying, expresses fear over her baby's health, and states she does not want to leave the infant in the hospital. Which intervention by the nurse would be the most therapeutic at this time?

    A. Encourage the mother to come in and feed and visit her infant as often as she would like.

    B. Encourage the mother to go home to rest.

    C. Explain to the mother that phototherapy is a routine procedure and that she does not have to worry.

    D. Ask her not to cry in the nursery and to come back when she "feels better."

18. A baby is born with suspected coarctation of the aorta. Which of the following assessments should be done by the nurse?

    A. Assess hemoglobin and hematocrit levels.

    B. Take blood pressures in all four extremities.

    C. Limit feeding times to 30 minutes each.

    D. Palpate fontanelles for bulging.

19. A newborn has been diagnosed with a small ventricular septal defect. What would the nurse expect to find upon examination?

    A. Cyanosis with crying

    B. Respiratory distress

    C. Systolic murmur with no other obvious symptoms

    D. Pallor

20. The goal of treatment for an infant with developmental dysplasia of the hip is to

    A. Relocate the femoral head in the acetabulum to facilitate normal growth and development

    B. Cast the affected hip and leg until dislocated hip stays in socket

    C. Intervene surgically as soon as diagnosed to prevent worsening of the condition

    D. Assess the infant for other musculoskeletal disorders

Answers

True/False

1. True
2. True
3. True
4. True
5. True
6. True
7. True
8. True
9. False. The infant would be hyperactive and crying.
10. True
11. False. Newborn screening tests are mandatory by state law.
12. True
13. True
14. False. The breast will mold and fill in the cleft in the lip, preventing aspiration.

15. True

16. True

17. True

18. True

19. True

20. True

Multiple Choice

1. B

2. A

3. A

4. B

5. B

6. B

7. A, B, C, D

8. B

9. A, B, C, D

10. A, B, C, D

11. A

12. B

13. C

14. C

15. D

16. A

17. A

18. B

19. C

20. A

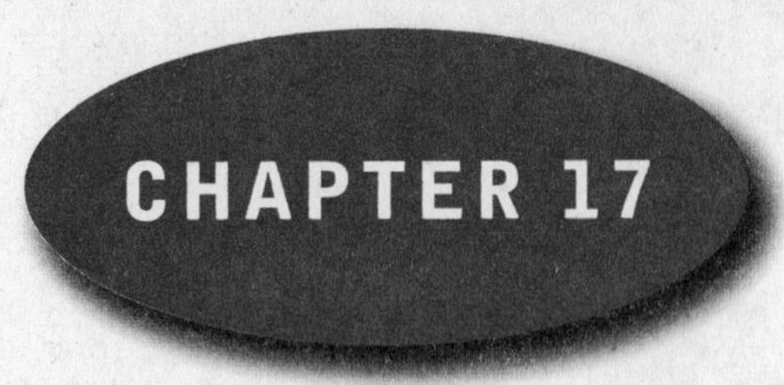

CHAPTER 17

Community-Based Care

Objective A: To Understand Concepts of Community

17.1 Community

Community is often defined as a collection of people sharing common characteristics, interests, needs, resources, and environments that interact with one another. The goals of Healthy People 2020 are to increase quality and years of healthy life and to eliminate health disparities are attainable through community-based health care activities and interventions.

Recent changes in health care financing have reduced hospital stays significantly for women after giving birth. Community-based nursing is part of an effort that extends beyond the birth facility setting. Many women do not feel well when they are discharged and may be uncertain about feeding and caring for their infants. New mothers need to be made aware of available community resources after discharge from the birth facility.

Contemporary nursing parallels today's trend for new families to obtain health care in diverse, familiar settings in which they live, grow, play, work, or go to school. These resources and settings may include telephone consultations with nurses, neighborhood outpatient clinics, home visits, shopping malls, mobile health care units, schools, and faith communities. In community-based settings, the providers of care are concerned not only with the clients who present themselves for service, but also with the larger population of potential or at-risk clients.

Objective B: To Understand Community-Based Nursing

17.2 Community-Based Nursing

Nursing in the United States began as community-based nursing. Self-trained midwives assisted women in laboring and birthing and offered health education. Most of the care nurses provide today for the childbearing family is also given in community settings.

Community-based nursing is the application of the nursing process in caring for individuals and families in community settings. It emphasizes all levels of prevention (primary, secondary, and tertiary). Nurses interested in working in community-based settings must be able to apply the nursing process in a less structured or controlled environment compared to the hospital setting.

Nurses who work in community settings must be aware of the many health issues commonly encountered within their unique communities. Nursing practice in the community setting is similar to that in the acute care setting in that the nurse will be assessing, performing procedures, administering medications, coordinating care services and equipment, and counseling and educating patients and their families. As nurses build their experiences in community-based settings, they will also develop their roles in patient education, case management, collaborative practice, counseling, research, and advocacy.

Objective C: To Understand Community-Based Care for Women and Newborns

17.3 Community-Based Care for Women and Newborns

There are several public policies and programs in the United States that make an attempt to provide equitable care for women, children, and families' health in the community at large. ***Medicaid,*** legislated through Title XIX of the Social Security Act, is a major publicly funded program that helps boost the health status of women, children, and families. Funding is shared between states and the federal government. Medicaid is the largest source of funding for medical and health-related services for people with limited income in the United States.

Another program is the ***Women, Infants, and Children (WIC) program***. WIC assists pregnant women, infants, and children up to 5 years of age who are nutritionally at risk and provides nutritious foods and nutrition counseling and education. The program serves low-income families and those with high-risk conditions, such as anemia and diabetes. The ***Newborn and Mothers Health Protection Act of 1996*** ensures that mothers and their newborns can remain in the hospital at least 48 hours after a vaginal birth, and 96 hours after a cesarean section. The ***Family and Medical Leave Act (FMLA) of 1993*** permits American workers to take up to 12 weeks of unpaid leave per year from their jobs for recovery from a serious illness or to provide care for a sick family member.

Objective D: To Understand Levels of Prevention in Community-Based Nursing

17.4 Levels of Prevention

The concept of prevention is a key focus of community-based nursing care, but care now also encompasses secondary and tertiary care.

The concept of ***primary prevention*** involves preventing the disease or condition before it occurs through health promotion activities. Nurses do much teaching in a vast variety of areas at this level. ***Secondary prevention*** is the early detection and treatment of adverse health conditions. At this level, many screenings are appropriate, such as pregnancy testing, blood pressure readings, and mammograms. Such screenings do not prevent the start of a health problem but are intended to detect them so early treatment can be instituted to prevent further complications. ***Tertiary prevention*** is designed to reduce or limit the progression of a disease or disability after an injury. The purpose of tertiary prevention is to rehabilitate or restore individuals to their maximal potential.

Objective E: To Understand Cultural Issues in Community-Based Care

17.5 Cultural Issues

It is very important for nurses to research and understand the cultural practices of the population in the community in which they will be delivering care so that false assumptions and stereotyping do not lead to insensitive care.

By becoming culturally competent, nurses can become familiar with the values, beliefs, and characteristics of diverse populations. Time orientation, personal space, family dynamics, and language are all important characteristics the nurse needs to be aware of when caring for cultures other than his or her own. The nurse must understand that becoming culturally competent does not mean losing one's own identity for another or ignoring variability within cultural groups. Instead, a respect for differences and a willingness to accept different views of the world maintain objectivity and promote fairness.

Objective F: To Understand Complementary and Alternative Medicine and Nursing Management

17.6 Complementary and Alternative Medicine

There has been a significant increase in the use of complementary and alternative medicine (CAM) during the past decade. Research indicates that one in three pregnant women use CAM therapies, some of which may be potentially harmful. CAM includes diverse practices, products, and health care systems that are not currently considered to be part of conventional medicine in the United States. Some CAM therapies are tied to specific cultural practices.

The nurse should be sensitive to and knowledgeable about CAM and encourage their pregnant patients to check with their health care provider before taking any supplements or "natural" substances. Additionally, the nurse must be familiar with different types of CAM therapies to be able to answer patients' questions accurately. When assessing patients, it is important for the nurse to ask specific questions about supplements or therapies they are taking that have not been ordered by their health care provider.

Review Questions

1. _______ Nursing care in the United States began as community-based nursing.
2. _______ A community can be defined as a collection of people sharing common needs.
3. _______ Community-based nursing responsibilities can include research and counseling.
4. _______ Secondary prevention in community-based nursing involves preventing the disease or condition before it occurs.
5. _______ Personal space is an important characteristic of a culture to be aware of when providing nursing care.
6. _______ Fifty percent of pregnant women use some form of complementary and alternative medicine (CAM).
7. _______ The Women, Infants, and Children (WIC) program provides nutritional support to low-income women.
8. _______ The Family and Medical Leave Act (FMLA) of 1993 allows American workers to take up to 6 months of unpaid leave.
9. _______ It is important for the community-based nurse to be aware of the unique health needs of the people in the community in which he or she administers care.
10. _______ By becoming culturally competent, the community-based nurse can avoid false assumptions and stereotyping about populations to whom he or she will be administering care.

Answers

True/False

1. True
2. True
3. True
4. False. Secondary prevention is the early detection and treatment of adverse health conditions.
5. True
6. False. One in three pregnant women partake in CAM therapy.
7. True
8. False. FMLA provides for up to 12 weeks of unpaid leave to care for a sick family member or for recovery.
9. True
10. True

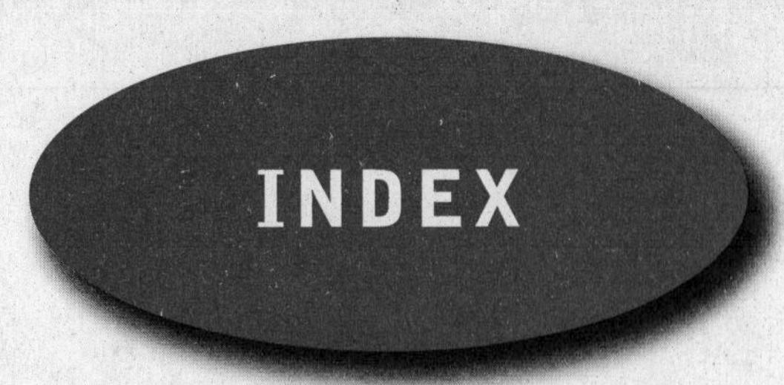

INDEX